OXFORD MEDICAL PUBLICATIONS

Dyspnoea in advanced disease

Dyspnoea in advanced disease

a guide to clinical management

Edited by

Sara Booth

Macmillan Consultant in Palliative Medicine, Lead Clinician in Palliative Care
Cambridge University Hospitals NHS Foundation Trust;

Honorary Senior Lecturer, Department of Palliative Care and Policy
Kings College, London

Deborah Dudgeon

W Ford Connell Professor of Palliative Care Medicine, Queen's University,
Kingston, Ontario, Canada

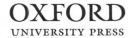

OXFORD
UNIVERSITY PRESS

OXFORD
UNIVERSITY PRESS

Great Clarendon Street, Oxford OX2 6DP

Oxford University Press is a department of the University of Oxford.
It furthers the University's objective of excellence in research, scholarship,
and education by publishing worldwide in

Oxford New York

Auckland Cape Town Dar es Salaam Hong Kong Karachi
Kuala Lumpur Madrid Melbourne Mexico City Nairobi
New Delhi Shanghai Taipei Toronto

With offices in

Argentina Austria Brazil Chile Czech Republic France Greece
Guatemala Hungary Italy Japan Poland Portugal Singapore
South Korea Switzerland Thailand Turkey Ukraine Vietnam

Oxford is a registered trade mark of Oxford University Press
in the UK and in certain other countries

Published in the United States
by Oxford University Press Inc., New York

© Oxford University Press 2006

The moral rights of the author have been asserted

Database right Oxford University Press (maker)

First published 2006

A catalogue record for this title is available from the British Library

Library of Congress Cataloging in Publication Data
Dyspnoea in advanced disease: a guide to clinical
management / edited by Sara Booth and Deborah
Dudgeon.
    p.; cm.
  Includes bibliographical references and index.
  1. Dyspnea. 2. Dyspnea–Palliative treatment.
  [DNLM: 1. Dyspnea–complications. 2. Dyspnea–therapy.
  3. Palliative Care. WF 143 D9983 2005] I. Booth, Sara, Dr. II.
  Dudgeon, Deborah.
  RC776.D9D975 2005
  616.2–dc22
  2005016392

Typeset by SPI Publisher Services, Pondicherry, India
Printed in Great Britain
on acid-free paper by Biddles Ltd, Kings Lynn
ISBN–0–19–853003–X (Pbk)   978–0–19–853003–9 (Pbk)
10 9 8 7 6 5 4 3 2 1

Foreword

The editors (Drs. Booth and Dudgeon), together with their contributors, have produced a major multi-author book on dyspnoea which will have real practical clinical significance, combining the modest pharmacological tools we have at present with other therapeutic strategies. The reader has been brought face to face with both the complexity and severity of the problems. Ameliorating dyspnoea is possible, but at the same time we learn how little we really understand of the genesis of this symptom. The size of the problem of effective therapeutics for dyspnoea is well summarized in the preface. The achievement of increased cooperation between those working in specialist palliative care, oncology, neurology, respiratory and cardiovascular medicine and paediatrics is clearly demonstrated by the contributions of individual authors knowledgeable in their own fields. The result for severely dyspnoeic patients is likely to be "shared care" between the super-specialist and the community practitioner, resulting in improved care.

There remains an astonishing lack of precise information regarding the genesis of dyspnoea. Julius Comroe, a medically qualified physiologist and pharmacologist, wrote the equivalent of a "Foreword": *Dyspnea; Modern Concepts of Cardiovascular Disease* (1956), Vol. 25.9, 347–349. His advice to young investigators was to direct their attention to determining the neuro-biological basis of dyspnoea. There has been some advance along these lines and this is mentioned both in the preface and elsewhere in this book. We need to know where the perception of the symptom is taking place in the brain, so that appropriate medication can be discovered. The modern neuro-psychiatrist is likely to be familiar with this type of question – even if not the answer! The association of Anxiety with Dyspnoea is striking and mentioned in more than one paper in this book. How does this come about? At present we do not understand this phenomenon. Imaging the brain in a functional as well as a structural manner is likely to demonstrate areas activated within the amygdaloid complex in the anterior part of the temporal lobe – an area known to be concerned with anxiety perception in man. Minimising anxiety is likely to reduce the impact of dyspnoea. We need more specific drugs to reduce anxiety.

The editors should be congratulated on what has been achieved. As research is making progress, I suspect that a new edition will be needed within the next five years, to update us on all these matters.

Meanwhile a word of warning is needed! Research in this area is very difficult. Let us neither castigate nor ignore research workers in this area for having only done few studies where the "n" is below an acceptable level of statistical "purity". We need to remember that no two patients are alike in their response to medication for dyspnoea. "Suck it and See" has historically done a great deal for the development of new therapeutics. Rushing to publish such studies is not necessarily a crime.

Professor A. Guz
August 2005

Preface

Dyspnoea is a very common symptom in people with advanced cancer and cardiac, respiratory, and certain neurological diseases. Its prevalence varies according to the stage and the type of the underlying disorder. Breathlessness may be reversible early in the course of the illness but becomes intractable as the disease progresses. Once it is irreversible, in spite of the best medical care dyspnoea can profoundly impair the quality of life not only of the person who suffers with it but also those closest to them. Patients almost universally respond to breathlessness by decreasing their activity to whatever degree will relieve their discomfort. This leads to social isolation, depression, fatigue, generalized dissatisfaction with life and significant emotional distress. Some studies have found that many patients receive little or no medical or nursing assistance with their dyspnoea, leaving them to cope with this debilitating symptom in isolation. Many doctors and nurses, even amongst those who treat the diseases commonly associated with dyspnoea, find it hard to manage chronic intractable breathlessness and this can lead to a sense of nihilism which is often perceived by the patient and family, and possibly further exacerbates any feelings of helplessness and isolation. Unfortunately, even with the interventions of expert teams, dyspnoea is often not as well controlled as pain. Specialists in palliative care are more practiced in managing the dyspnoea associated with advanced cancer (which invariably has a short prognosis when it becomes intractable) than managing patients who live with breathlessness for many months or years. It is heartening that more attention is being paid to improving the quality of life (as well as understanding the medical care) of patients with non-malignant diseases such as heart failure and chronic obstructive airways disease (www.NICE.org.uk). There is also increasing co-operation between those working in specialist palliative care, oncology, neurology, respiratory medicine and cardiology so that patients can receive shared care both in hospital and in the community. There are also exciting advances in imaging of breathlessness with functional MRI and PET scanning beginning to illuminate the way the sensation is processed by the central nervous system.

This synthesis of ideas should lead to a better understanding of the pathophysiology and management of dyspnoea, with an improvement in the quality of life for patients with breathlessness.

This book builds on this shared knowledge to provide clinicians with a practical guide to the management of breathlessness in patients with different common advanced diseases. It provides the latest scientific advances in the understanding of the pathophysiology, assessment and clinical management of this complex symptom. The increasing understanding of the wide-ranging effects on the patient's quality of life is underlined.

The book has been organized to address generalized aspects of breathlessness in advanced illness and more specific underlying aetiologies and managements relevant to particular underlying diseases.

The earlier chapters are concerned with the science and aetiology of breathlessness (as it is presently understood) in specific diseases; others follow which consider assessment and different management strategies and treatments in some depth (scientific and practical aspects); and there is a final summary chapter which gives guidance on integrating scientific and practical clinical care. There is still uncertainty about many aspects of breathlessnes and this is reflected in the discussions.

We hope this book will be of use to those trying to deepen their understanding of this difficult symptom and those who want to improve their clinical care or just check a fact or strategy in clinic. We hope that you will enjoy using this book as much as we have enjoyed editing it. We have learned much from all our contributors and are grateful for the time and energy they devoted to sharing their knowledge with us.

SB
DD
August 2005

Contents

Contributors

Douglas Beach
Division of Pulmonary and Critical
Care Medicine and Department of
Medicine,
Beth Israel Deaconess Medical Center
and Harvard Medical School,
Boston, USA

Sara Booth
Macmillan Consultant in Palliative
Medicine, Lead Clinician in
Palliative Care, Cambridge University
Hospitals NHS Foundation Trust;
Honorary Senior Lecturer,
Department of Palliative Care and
Policy, Kings College, London

Rachel Burman
Consultant in Palliative Medicine,
King's College Hospital Palliative
Care Team,
London, UK

Virginia Carrieri-Kohlman
Professor, Department of
Physiological Nursing,
University of California,
San Francisco, USA

David Currow
Professor, Department of Palliative
and Supportive Services,
Flinders University, South Australia;

Director, Southern Adelaide
Palliative Services,
Daw Park, South Australia

Andrew J. Drain
Specialist Registrar,
Papworth Hospital,
Cambridge, UK

Deborah Dudgeon
W. Ford Connell Professor of
Palliative Care Medicine,
Queen's University, Kingston,
Ontario, Canada

David P. Dutka
Lecturer in Cardiovascular
Medicine and Honorary
Consultant Cardiologist,
Cambridge University Hospitals
NHS Foundation Trust.

Polly Edmonds
Consultant in Palliative Medicine,
King's College Hospital
Palliative Care Team,
London, UK

Miriam J. Johnson
Consultant in Palliative Medicine,
St Catherine's Hospice,
Scarborough, UK

Stephen Liben
Director, Palliative Care Program,
The Montreal Children's Hospital of
the McGill University Health Center;
Associate Professor of Pediatrics,
McGill University, Montreal,
Canada

Fliss Murtagh
Specialist Registrar in
Palliative Medicine, King's College
Hospital Palliative Care Team,
London, UK

Denis O'Donnell
Professor of Medicine and
Physiology; Head,
Division of Respirology and Critical
Care Medicine,
Department of Medicine,
Queen's University,
Kingston, Ontario, Canada

Michelle M. Peters
MSc candidate, Physiology,
Queen's University, Kingston;
Research Associate,
Kingston General Hospital,
Ontario, Canada

Michael Polkey
Consultant Physician and Reader in
Respiratory Medicine,
Royal Brompton Hospital/National
Heart and Lung Institute,
London, UK

Richard M. Schwartzstein
Associate Professor of Medicine,
Harvard Medical School; Clinical
Director,
Division of Pulmonary and Critical
Care Medicine,
Beth Israel Deaconess Medical
Center,
Boston, USA

Anna Spathis
Specialist Registrar in Palliative
Medicine,
Cambridge University Hospitals
NHS Foundation Trust

Nha Voduc
Assistant Professor,
University of Ottawa,
Canada

Rosemary Wade
Consultant in Palliative Medicine,
West Suffolk Hospitals NHS Trust,
Bury St Edmunds, UK

Katherine Webb
Research Associate,
Queen's University,
Kingston, Ontario, Canada

Francis C. Wells
Consultant Cardiothoracic Surgeon,
Papworth and Addenbrooke's
Hospital;
Associate Lecturer in Surgery,
Cambridge University,
Cambridge, UK

1

The genesis of breathlessness
What do we understand?

Douglas Beach and Richard M. Schwartzstein

Understanding the mechanisms of breathlessness: Why should we care?

A 72-year-old former smoker with end stage obstructive lung disease comes to see her physician for a routine visit. She says she feels much worse as of late. Her last spirometry testing revealed her one second forced expiratory volume to be 600 milliliters, a decline in her lung function brought on by her smoking three packs of cigarettes per day for 50 years. She now must wear oxygen even at rest. Even when she feels her best, she is only able to walk up one flight of stairs before she must stop and catch her breath. However, over the past few weeks she can only go up a few steps at a time.

An understanding of the multiple physiologic processes that contribute to the sensation of breathlessness can assist tremendously in the diagnosis and treatment of patients such as the one described above. For example, her underlying disease, emphysema, is primarily characterized by impaired gas exchange, airway obstruction, and hyperinflation of the lungs – all three of these derangements can contribute to dyspnea. As she engages in activity, the damaged lungs may be unable to meet the oxygen demands of metabolically active tissue or to remove the carbon dioxide that is the consequence of aerobic activity. The normal physiologic response to hypoxemia and hypercarbia is to increase both the rate of breathing and the volume of each breath. In patients with obstructive lung disease, this causes a worsening hyperinflation of the lungs (due to airway obstruction) and, more importantly, an increased demand on the muscles of ventilation. Both of these physiological consequences to gas exchange abnormalities may, in their own right, produce breathing discomfort.

The inability to adequately oxygenate the blood and/or to eliminate carbon dioxide, while potentially life-threatening, is not sufficient to explain all breathing discomfort. There are many examples of patients who are limited by breathlessness yet have normal oxygenation and arterial P_{CO2}. Similarly, the work of breathing cannot fully explain breathlessness in all clinical situations since studies have shown that the intensity of breathing discomfort may vary for a given individual maintaining constant ventilation while other variables are modified.[1,2] Thus, the clinician must take a comprehensive view of the physiology of each patient when investigating the cause of breathing discomfort.

The natural course of many cardiopulmonary diseases that lead to breathlessness is a slow steady progression, with superimposed acute episodes of worsening symptoms and physiological changes that are variably reversible. Given the incurable nature of most of these processes, healthcare providers are left with a finite number of therapies to direct at alleviating symptoms (for example: supplemental oxygen to correct gas exchange abnormalities, bronchodilators to lessen airway obstruction). However, if a secondary process is present and can be distinguished from the underlying disease, for example, muscle deconditioning or acute infection, then additional therapies can be targeted. Deconditioning of the skeletal muscles due to the increasingly sedentary lifestyles of patients who experience exertional dyspnea is a progressive and severely debilitating component of almost every cardiopulmonary disease, and can be improved with exercise rehabilitation programs. Furthermore, identification of the physiological derangements that contribute to breathlessness, such as hyperinflation due to rapid breathing patterns, can lead to strategies to ameliorate symptoms even when the underlying disease cannot be corrected. Ultimately, our ability to reduce dyspnea in patients with end-stage cardiopulmonary disease, short of using narcotics, which often have significant side-effects, rests on an understanding of the physiology of the respiratory discomfort, and on our ability to identify the factor that is primarily responsible for the patient's functional limitation.

The multiple origins of breathlessness

The ability to differentiate between the different mechanisms responsible for debilitating breathlessness (for example, airway obstruction, hyperinflation, deconditioning) is crucial for the design of treatment strategies to aid patients. Over the past two decades, our understanding of the physiologic mechanisms responsible for the sensation of breathlessness has increased dramatically. In contrast to sensations such as pain, which are typically the consequence of stimulation of a single receptor, breathlessness arises from the complex integration of information from a multitude of receptors located throughout the respiratory system. Information from these receptors (including mechanoreceptors in the airways, lungs, and chest wall, and chemoreceptors, both central and peripheral) is processed along with sensory signals associated with motor output from the cortex and brainstem. The ultimate product is breathing discomfort that we label as dyspnea. Figure 1.1 is an overview of the multiple interactions involved in the sensation of breathlessness.

Research in the past fifteen years has also revealed that the different physiological mechanisms responsible for dyspnea produce multiple qualitative distinct sensations. For example, receptors in the lung parenchyma may give rise to a sense of chest tightness, chemoreceptors a sense of air hunger, and information from the motor cortex and brainstem a sense of effort. These qualitative descriptors may provide healthcare providers with insight into the underlying problem leading to a patient's functional limitation.

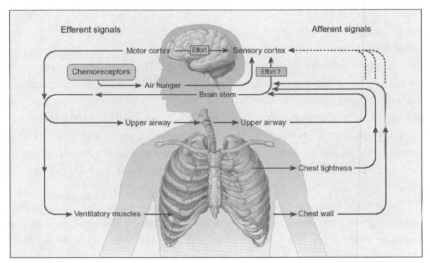

Figure 1.1 Efferent and afferent signals that contribute to the sensation of dyspnea. The sense of respiratory effort is believed to arise from a signal transmitted from the motor cortex to the sensory cortex coincidently with the outgoing motor command to the ventilatory muscles (corollary discharge). The arrow from the brainstem to the sensory cortex indicates that the motor output of the brainstem may also contribute to the sense of effort. The sense of air hunger is believed to arise, in part, from increased respiratory activity within the brainstem, and the sensation of chest tightness probably results from stimulation of pulmonary receptors. Although afferent information from airway, lung and chest wall passes through the brainstem before reaching the sensory cortex, the dashed lines indicate uncertainty about whether some afferents bypass the brainstem and project directly to the sensory cortex. (Used with permission from reference 12).

Language of breathlessness

Patients who present to their physician complaining of chest pain are routinely asked to describe the quality of the pain. Is it a burning sensation, a pressure, or a sharp pain? Clinicians quickly learn to use these qualitative descriptions of pain to gain insight into the pathophysiologic mechanisms underlying the discomfort. For example, burning chest pain may indicate acid reflux into the esophagus, while pressure-like pain is in suggestive of ischemia of the myocardium, and sharp, stabbing pain is characteristic of inflammation of the pleura or pericardium.

The qualitative descriptions of breathlessness offered by patients provide similar insights. Before undertaking a review of the physiologic mechanisms of breathlessness, we will quickly address what is known about the language of breathlessness. For the purposes of this discussion, we will define dyspnea or breathlessness as 'breathing discomfort'. Since there are multiple qualitatively distinct sensations that comprise breathlessness, we believe this definition, which does not imply a particular sensation, is the most generic definition and, therefore, the most appropriate.

Certainly it would be invaluable to know if a certain word or phrase could point to a single cause of breathing discomfort. The approach to this question, however, is complicated by the fact that multiple physiologic abnormalities may be present at a given time in the breathless patient (for example, hypercapnia, bronchoconstriction and hyperinflation in an asthmatic patient). It is conceivable, therefore, that even if a given physiologic derangement is associated with a discrete sensation, more than one phrase may be evident in a patient with cardiopulmonary disease and dyspnea.

The first question is: Do each of the pathophysiologic mechanisms that cause dyspnea produce a unique sensation that can be distinguished by the language used to describe the sensation? An important study by Simon *et al.* attempted to answer this question. Utilizing breathing tasks that were believed to stimulate different receptors in the cardiopulmonary system, investigators induced breathlessness in normal subjects.[3] The tasks included: breath-holding, induced hypercapnia, breathing with a restricted minute ventilation during induced hypercapnia, breathing with a resistive load, breathing with an elastic load, breathing at a voluntarily increased functional residual capacity, breathing with a voluntarily reduced tidal volume, and exercise. Without exception, all subjects volunteered that the varying respiratory tasks could easily be distinguished by the sensations they produced. The data emanating from this study demonstrated three characteristics. First, each task was associated with a unique set of phrases. Second, subjects used the same sensation, in some cases, to describe two or more tasks. Third, each sensation had more

Table 1.1 Descriptors of breathlessness in certain conditions. Adapted from (4)

Descriptors	Asthma	COPD	CHF	ILD	Neuromuscular/ chest wall	Pregnancy	Pulmonary vascular disease
Rapid breathing			×				×
Incomplete exhalation	×						
Shallow breathing					×		
Increased work or effort	×	×		×	×		
Feeling of suffocation			×				
Air hunger		×	×			×	
Chest tightness	×						

than one descriptor associated with it. This was the first clear evidence that there were multiple sensations that contributed to breathlessness, rather than a single sensation that varied only in intensity.

To determine if these results could be translated to the clinical setting, similar questionnaires were used in two studies of breathless patients with a variety of cardiopulmonary diseases (one of these studies also include healthy women who experienced breathing discomfort during pregnancy).[4,5] Again, multiple phrases that clustered in distinct groups were found to be associated with each of the disease states.

The reliability of such questionnaires was demonstrated in a study in which a questionnaire was given on two separate occasions one week apart to patients with chronic obstructive pulmonary disease (COPD). There was a significant correlation between the phrases chosen to describe breathlessness on the two occasions.[6] Data from these and related studies are consistent with the hypothesis that different disease states, characterized by different pathophysiological derangements, are associated with qualitatively distinct sensations. Furthermore, they suggest that attention to the words used by patients to describe their breathing discomfort may provide clues that will be useful in defining the problem producing the sensation.

Physiology of breathlessness

To better understand how the complex interactions of neural pathways and receptors cause breathlessness, we will describe three important concepts that form the elements for a model that clarifies the origins of the intensity and qualities of the sensations of breathlessness. The first concept is that of a 'corollary discharge', a term that describes the hypothesis that a sensory 'copy' of the motor output is sent from the motor cortex to the sensory cortex and imparts a conscious awareness of respiratory effort. The second concept, called 'efferent–reafferent dissociation', describes an hypothesis in which it is postulated that the sensory cortex acts as if it were comparing information received about efferent signals from the motor cortex to ventilatory muscles (via the corollary discharge) with information (afferent signals) arising from receptors stimulated by the mechanical response of the lungs and chest wall to the motor commands. The intensity of breathlessness appears to correlate with the match or mismatch of these signals. The greater the dissociation between the efferent and afferent signals, the greater is the intensity of the breathing discomfort. Finally, the third element in the model postulates that some receptors (mechanoreceptors and chemoreceptors) are responsible for unique sensations, such as 'chest tightness' and 'air hunger'.

Increased work of breathing: the corollary discharge

The sense of breathlessness associated with an increased work of breathing is common among people who have ever tried to breathe through a narrow tube or take a deep breath while someone was pressing on their abdomen. The sense of effort in these situations is similar to the effort you experience when you try to lift a weight. You are trying to move something (in the case of breathing, the lungs and chest wall), but there seems to be an impediment that prevents the ventilatory muscles from shortening to achieve the desired inflation of the respiratory system.

The concept of a 'corollary discharge' is the most widely accepted hypothesis used to explain the origin of the sense of effort. As the motor cortex sends efferent commands to the ventilatory muscles, a neurological 'copy' of these commands is simultaneously sent to the sensory cortex.[7] This exchange between the motor and sensory cortex is called a corollary discharge and is thought to be the mechanism by which conscious awareness of the effort of breathing occurs. Although increased work of breathing is not the sole physiological explanation for dyspnea, increased effort is a common cause of breathing discomfort, since muscle weakness and increased mechanical loads, such as airway obstruction and stiff lungs, are characteristic of many cardiopulmonary conditions.

Descriptors associated with increased ventilatory muscle work

In the language studies by Simon *et al.* on normal subjects, the phrases 'my breathing requires effort' or 'my breathing requires more work' were used by subjects after the addition of an external resistive load (pressure work), as well as during large increases in minute ventilation (volume work) resulting from experimentally induced hypercapnia.[3] Patients with cardiopulmonary disease, when asked to describe which phrases most accurately describe their breathlessness just prior to having to stop an activity, commonly use 'my breathing requires effort' and 'I feel out of breath'. These descriptors appeared to be an element of dyspnea associated with many disease processes.[6] These studies and others have consistently shown that the sense of effort can be reproduced in experimental and clinical settings, and that it may be the most prevalent cause of the sensation of breathing discomfort.

Since the respiratory system is under both voluntary and reflex control, ventilatory muscles may receive neural impulses originating from the cerebral cortex or the respiratory centers in the brainstem. Does the sense of effort vary with the origin of the neural impulse? To answer this question, subjects were asked to breathe at constant, high minute ventilation while end tidal P_{CO2} was varied by modifying the concentration of inspired carbon dioxide.[1] When the P_{CO2} was normal, subjects experienced an intense sense of effort to sustain the elevated levels of ventilation. When the same task was repeated with the patients breathing carbon dioxide, the intensity of the sense of effort was reduced. In the latter condition, ventilation was presumably responding, in part, to output from the chemoreceptors and, as a result, less 'voluntary' work was being done to maintain the target ventilation. The decrease in the intensity of effort with hypercapnia in this experiment is consistent with the hypothesis that brainstem respiratory activity is not associated with the same sensations as cortical or voluntary breathing maneuvers. Specifically, output from the automatic or reflex respiratory centers in the brainstem does not produce the same type of corollary discharge to the sensory cortex as does output from the motor cortex; the sense of effort was reduced despite a constant 'work' of breathing.

The contribution of the sense of effort to breathing discomfort has been identified in patients with several cardiopulmonary diseases. Patients with obstructive airways disease, congestive heart failure, interstitial lung disease, and neuromuscular disease all describe increased work or effort as a factor in their description of breathlessness.[6] The mechanism common to all of these disorders is an increased mechanical load on the ventilatory pump (for example, increased airway resistance or decreased respiratory system compliance), which necessitates a greater neural discharge from the brain to the ventilatory muscles to achieve adequate ventilation for a given metabolic demand.

The sensation of effort can also be affected by the strength of respiratory muscles. Normal subjects who participated in a 6 to 18 week inspiratory muscle training program had a 51 per cent increase in their maximal inspiratory pressure.[8] When asked to rate the intensity of effort associated with breathing with elastic and resistive respiratory loads, the ratings after training were reduced compared to those obtained prior to training. Physiologically, a stronger muscle will generate a greater tension for a given neurological stimulus than a weaker muscle. Thus, to perform a particular task, it requires fewer commands from the motor cortex, hence less corollary discharge to the sensory cortex and less effort, when the muscles are stronger. After a period of detraining, with corresponding loss of muscle strength, the intensity of the sensation of effort returned to the pre-training levels at the same workload.

Efferent–reafferent dissociation

During a voluntary breathing task, the sensory cortex receives information simultaneously from the motor cortex (via the corollary discharge) and afferent information from the peripheral receptors of the respiratory system (reafferent signals). Reafferent signals are neural impulses produced by afferent receptors in response to efferent commands. For example, you take a deep breath. Efferent signals from the motor cortex descend to the ventilatory muscles leading to muscle contraction, a negative intrathoracic pressure and inspiratory flow. The lungs and the chest wall expand. A variety of flow, pressure, and stretch receptors are stimulated by the increasing thoracic volume, and reafferent information is transmitted to the brain.[7] If the mechanical response to efferent stimuli is impaired, such as when smaller tidal volumes result from respiratory muscle weakness, then reafferent signals become dissociated from the efferent output. This concept has been described as efferent–reafferent dissociation.[9]

Using acute hypercapnia to stimulate the automatic or reflex ventilatory control centers of the brain, several studies have examined the dissociation between 'command' and 'response' and its impact on breathlessness.[10,11] Normal subjects were studied during experimentally induced hypercapnia at various levels of ventilation.[10] After a ten minute equilibration period during which ventilation rose in response to the hypercapnia (chemically driven ventilation), the level of ventilation was then voluntarily changed to various levels ranging from 50 per cent below to 50 per cent above the steady state level. All subjects noted that they became increasingly breathless when the level of ventilation was held below or targeted above the chemically determined ventilation level, that is, the ventilation that resulted from hypercapnia with free breathing. A second study demonstrated similar results when hypercapnia was induced in normal subjects who voluntarily limited their tidal volume and respiratory rate to baseline levels.[11] These data are consistent with the hypothesis that efferent–reafferent dissociation can modify the intensity of breathlessness.

The role of respiratory system afferents

While the sense of effort is certainly a prominent component of the sensations of breathlessness, there are clearly other distinct and separable sensations that contribute to breathlessness. 'Chest tightness' associated with bronchoconstriction is the most studied example of this. In investigations of patients with cardiopulmonary disease, the description of chest tightness was significantly associated with asthma,[4] which is thought to arise from the stimulation of receptors in the lung parenchyma.[12] The sensation of chest tightness associated with bronchoconstriction has also been differentiated from the increased work of breathing and sense of effort.[13] The origin of chest tightness may lie with mechanical receptors (rapidly adapting stretch receptors) in the lungs and/or with chemical receptors (C-fibers). Pulmonary receptors may also play a role in the breathlessness associated with pulmonary vascular disease, congestive heart failure, atelectasis (as may occur in association with large pleural effusions) and acute respiratory infections.

Afferent receptors

A well recognized problem with the study of breathlessness is that there is no way to localize and stimulate a single receptor and document the resulting sensory response to the stimulus. However, as researchers have been able to distinguish how different tasks and different physiologic changes in the respiratory system produce different sensations, the function of individual pulmonary receptors have been better defined.

   The following section will review the various receptors that contribute to the sensation of breathlessness. In discussing each type of receptor, we will focus not only on the evidence supporting the existence of each receptor, but on whether the receptor modulates the intensity of breathlessness via efferent–reafferent dissociation or by producing a distinct and separable sensation.

Chemoreceptors

Peripheral chemoreceptors, located in the carotid and aortic bodies, produce the afferent response to changes in P_{CO2}, P_{O2}, and arterial hydrogen ion (i.e., pH).[14,15] The carotid body is more sensitive to increases in P_{CO2} or decreases in P_{O2} or pH, whereas the aortic body is less sensitive to P_{CO2} and P_{O2}, and has the opposite response to pH as the carotid body. In humans, the aortic chemoreceptors appear to have a minimal role in the control of ventilation.

Central chemoreceptors located in the medulla respond to changes in P_{CO2} and arterial pH. In addition, skeletal muscle is also thought to have metaboreceptors, which are not typically described as chemoreceptors, but appear to be capable of detecting changes, at the tissue level, in metabolites produced by anaerobic metabolism.[16]

The contribution of hypercapnia, independent of the ventilatory muscle response to the altered level of carbon dioxide, to the sensation of breathlessness has been studied by inducing hypercapnia in subjects with respiratory muscle paralysis who are mechanically ventilated. In patients with quadriplegia[17] and normal subjects under conditions of total neuromuscular blockade,[18] subjects noted severe 'air hunger' with increasing end tidal P_{CO2} without a change in ventilation. These studies reinforce the concept that the breathing discomfort associated with acute hypercapnia is not a reflection of ventilatory muscle activity, and the stimulation of chemoreceptors by hypercapnia produces a distinct sensation of breathlessness, which is characterized by phrases such as 'air hunger', 'urge to breathe', and 'need to breathe'.[17,18,19]

The degree to which hypercapnia contributes to the sensation of breathlessness in patients with chronic hypercapnia (e.g. neuromuscular disease, COPD) has been questioned.[20] The reduced dyspnea associated with chronic hypercapnia as compared to acute hypercapnia may, in fact, reflect that the discomfort correlates better with hydrogen ion concentrations in the blood and brain, which tend to normalize with time, than with the arterial P_{CO2}.

Compared to acute hypercapnia, acute hypoxemia produces less intense sensations of breathlessness. It is not uncommon to find patients with chronic lung disease to have mild to moderate levels of hypoxemia without breathlessness. Chronos *et al.*, however, demonstrated that during heavy exercise at a constant workload, subjects were more breathless when they inspired hypoxic gas mixtures compared with air, and less breathless when inspiring 100 per cent oxygen.[2] Although subjects did increase their minute ventilation when hypoxemic, the increase in breathlessness occurred before the increase in ventilation was noted. Similar results were produced in patients with COPD,[21] who also experienced increased breathlessness in the setting of hypoxemia.

Although the quality of dyspnea associated with hypoxia has been less well studied than that associated with hypercapnia, hypoxemia appears to be a less potent stimulus for dyspnea than in acute hypercapnia. As with acute hypercapnia, a restriction of ventilation below the level normally associated with a given degree of hypoxemia will intensify the discomfort.

The origin of exercise-induced dyspnea in individuals with normal cardio-pulmonary systems is still debated. Typically, individuals are neither hypoxemic nor hypercapnic during exercise, and metabolic acidosis occurs relatively late in high intensity exercise. Metaboreceptors, located in skeletal muscles, may be a source of afferent neurological signals that lead to a perception of dyspnea. These receptors are believed to respond to local changes in the tissue environment with respect to the byproducts of metabolism. When one reaches the limits of cardiopulmonary fitness, accumulation of these metabolic bypro-ducts may contribute to the sensation of dyspnea, both in normal subjects and patients.[16] As is the case with breathlessness associated with hypoxemia, not enough information is available to determine if metaboreceptors either mod-ify other forms of dyspnea or generate a unique sense of breathlessness.

One's level of fitness, which is a reflection of the ability of the heart to deliver oxygen to the muscles and of the ability of the muscles to extract and utilize oxygen for aerobic metabolism, correlates with an individual's exercise rou-tine. To the extent that patients with chronic cardiopulmonary disease typically become increasingly sedentary, cardiovascular fitness deteriorates (patients become 'deconditioned') and may become the primary cause of the patient's functional limitation. Since fitness is amenable to improvement with a supervised exercise program, the identification of deconditioning as the cause of an individual's breathing discomfort is critical. The sensations 'heavy breathing' and 'huffing and puffing' are typically associated with cardiovas-cular deconditioning.[6]

Mechanoreceptors

There are multiple receptors located in the upper airway, lung parenchyma (including stretch receptors and C-fibers), pulmonary vasculature, and chest wall that contribute to the sensation of breathlessness. We begin by describing upper airway receptors, and continue downward into the lower airways, vasculature, and chest wall.

Upper airway receptors

Upper airway receptors, including facial receptors innervated by the trigem-inal nerve, were thought to be involved in the sensation of breathlessness when it was noticed that patients with cardiopulmonary diseases would obtain relief when sitting near a source of cool air directed onto the face (for example, next to an open window or fan). One study of normal subjects, in whom acute hypercapnia was induced in conjunction with external resistive loads, dem-onstrated a decreased intensity of breathlessness when cold air was directed against the cheek.[22] Stimulation of the receptors in the oral mucosa also appears to decrease the intensity of breathlessness; attenuation of the activity of these receptors may worsen dyspnea. In normal subjects and patients with COPD, the intensity of hypercapnia-induced breathlessness increased when stimulation of oral mucosal receptors was reduced (as occurs when breathing through a mouthpiece, applying topical lidocaine to the mucosa, and breathing warm, humidified air).[23,24] To some degree, the decrease in dyspnea associated with upper airway stimulation may reflect diminution of respiratory drive. The ventilatory response to hypercapnia, for example, is blunted when cool air is used to stimulate nasal airway receptors.[25] The stimulation of upper airway receptors has been shown to clinically reduce breathlessness and increase exercise tolerance in patients with COPD.[24,26] Taken together, these data suggest that upper airway receptors, which monitor the changes of flow in the upper airway by detecting temperature changes, modulate breathlessness. This effect is likely due to changes in efferent–reafferent dissociation; greater stimulation of flow receptors may be perceived by the sensory cortex as evidence of a good mechanical response of the respiratory system to the efferent messages emanating from the motor cortex, thereby reducing the sensation of breathlessness.

Lower airway receptors

The major receptors that reside in the lung parenchyma are characterized as stretch receptors and C-fibers (unmeyelinated nerve endings). These receptors are responsible for detecting a wide variety of pathophysiologic derangements in the lung and transmit information to the CNS via the vagus nerve. Several studies have explored the importance of these receptors in the production of breathlessness.

Stretch receptors are thought to modulate breathlessness by altering efferent–reafferent dissociation. In a study performed on ventilator-dependent, high cervical spinal cord-injured patients, 'air hunger' was induced with acute hypercapnia while tidal volume was varied on the ventilator.[27] At a given end tidal P_{CO2}, and in the absence of chest wall receptor afferent information due to the spinal cord lesions, all patients reported increased air hunger when ventilated with lower tidal volumes. The greater stimulation of stretch receptors associated with the larger tidal volumes was believed to be the mechanism by which the breathing discomfort was relieved.

Further evidence for the role of pulmonary mechanoreceptors has been supplied by studies of patients with COPD, in whom a negative pressure is applied at the mouth leading to dynamic airway compression. This maneuver was associated with increased levels of breathlessness.[28] These data suggest that receptors in the airway are sensitive to changes in transmural pressure across the airway, and that deformation of the airway by a negative transmural pressure leads to a sensation of breathing discomfort. The technique of pursed lip breathing, commonly employed by patients with COPD, and the application of continuous positive airway pressure (CPAP) in patients with emphysema and respiratory distress are examples of how dyspnea may be reduced by diminishing airway compression and stimulation of mechanoreceptors.

The role of lower airway receptors in the modulation of dyspnea was studied in laryngectomized patients with tracheal stomas, in whom dyspnea was induced with acute hypercapnia. When airway receptor information was blocked by administration of aerosolized bupivacaine, the intensity of breathlessness increased.[29] These findings suggest that blocking afferent information from lower airway receptors, possibly flow or stretch receptors, increases the sensation of breathlessness, consistent with the hypothesis that inhibition of afferent information from the airways creates a dissociation between efferent and reafferent neural impulses.

Irritant receptors or C-fibers, located in the airway epithelium, are thought to respond to both mechanical and chemical stimuli, including bronchoconstriction and inhaled irritants. Taguchi *et al.* found that in normal subjects with breathlessness induced by both bronchoconstriction (secondary to inhaled histamine) and external resistive loading, the sensation of breathlessness was reduced following inhalation of aerosolized lidocaine only in the patients with bronchoconstriction.[30] This suggests that airway receptors stimulated by bronchoconstriction modify breathlessness.

Stimulation of pulmonary receptors by bronchoconstriction also appears to produce a qualitatively distinct sensation. The sensation of chest tightness is associated with experimentally induced and naturally occurring bronchoconstriction and is distinct from the sense of effort. Utilizing a 19-item questionnaire to examine the language used by asthmatics during methacholine-induced bronchoconstriction and while breathing on an apparatus that included external resistors, investigators found that the phrases 'chest tightness' or 'constriction' were used almost exclusively when bronchoconstriction was present.[31] In contrast, the descriptors 'work' or 'effort' were employed by subjects during bronchoconstriction and external resistive loading, which is consistent with the increased corollary discharge associated with the mechanical load on the respiratory system that results from airway obstruction. Additional evidence that the sense of effort is separate from the sense of chest tightness was offered by a study in which mechanical ventilation (via a mouthpiece) was used to relieve the work of breathing during methacholine-induced bronchoconstriction in subjects with mild asthma. With mechanical ventilation, as compared to free breathing off the ventilator, the sense of 'chest tightness' was unchanged despite the reduction in the work of breathing. In contrast, the sense of effort was reduced by the implementation of mechanical ventilation.[13] The actual receptors responsible for the sensation of chest tightness, however, remain to be determined.

Other vagally mediated lower airway receptors, such as C-fibers (which include juxtapulmonary or J receptors) and pulmonary vascular receptors likely have an impact on respiratory sensations but little is known about their role in dyspnea. C-fibers are thought to be stimulated by interstitial fluid and probably contribute to the breathing discomfort and rapid, shallow breathing pattern associated with pulmonary edema.[20] There is also evidence that distinct sensations can be attributed to C-fiber stimulation. When lobeline, a substance known to stimulate C-fibers, was given to normal subjects, they reported several types of sensations in the upper airway and throat including 'choking, pressure, or fumes'.[32]

The mechanism by which vascular receptors lead to the sensation of breathlessness is unclear. Although we are not aware of any studies investigating the relationship of vascular receptors to the sensations provoked by acute pulmonary embolism, the observation that breathing discomfort is rapidly relieved by intra-arterial thrombolysis in the absence of hypoxia suggests that stimulation of pulmonary vascular receptors may play a role in breathing discomfort (personal communication J. Markis and R. Schwartzstein). The absence of other significant physiological derangements that might explain the dyspnea associated with pulmonary embolism also argues for the role of pulmonary vascular receptors. Although hypoxemia is frequently seen in patients with pulmonary embolism, relief of the hypoxemia with administration of supplemental oxygen usually has minimal impact on breathlessness. Although bronchoconstriction and airflow obstruction may accompany pulmonary embolism, the vast majority of patients with this disease do not have an acute change in the mechanical properties of the ventilatory pump. Thus, stimulation of vascular receptors may give rise to breathing discomfort in a primary fashion, in a manner analogous to the production of chest tightness by pulmonary receptors during acute bronchoconstriction. For example, a case report of a patient with extreme dyspnea due to acute unilateral pulmonary veno-occlusion, which was relieved by vagotomy on the same side as the occlusion, provides some evidence that dyspnea may be mediated by pulmonary vascular receptors stimulated by the high pulmonary vascular pressures, or by C-fibers stimulated by pulmonary edema, or both.[33]

Chest wall receptors

Receptors located in the joints, tendons, and muscles of the chest wall communicate with the central nervous system and contribute to the sensations of breathlessness. Stimulation of chest wall receptors with a physiotherapeutic vibrator placed over parasternal intercostal muscles has been used to investigate the role of chest wall receptors in respiratory sensation. Normal subjects with experimentally-induced breathlessness, produced with acute hypercapnia or the imposition of external resistive loads, noted decreased intensity of breathlessness with stimulation of chest wall receptors.[34] Application of chest wall vibrators to patients with COPD has also been shown to relieve breathing discomfort.[35] These results suggest that chest wall receptors, like mechanoreceptors in the lungs, decrease breathlessness when stimulated. This effect is likely a consequence of improved matching between the efferent output of the central controller and the afferent information arising from the chest wall.

Dynamic hyperinflation

Dynamic hyperinflation occurs when patients with expiratory flow limitation attempt to increase ventilation during exercise. In order to increase flow, these individuals must breathe at increasingly high lung volumes (lung volumes at which elastic recoil of the lung and the diameter of the airways is increased). The more severe the airflow obstruction, the more likely that hyperinflation will occur. This increase in lung volumes during exercise is termed 'dynamic hyperinflation'. In some cases, patients with flow limitation will be breathing at lung volumes that approximate total lung capacity. Patients with dynamic hyperinflation use descriptors such as 'I can not get enough air in' or their inspiratory effort is 'unsatisfied'.[12,36] Upon further investigation, we find that many of these patients literally cannot get a deep breath at these times because inspiratory capacity is limited by their maximal lung volume. Although the sensation of breathlessness in patients with obstructive airways disease can also be attributed to gas exchange abnormalities or efferent–reafferent dissociation due to weakened muscles, the dynamic hyperinflation due to air trapping may be the primary cause of breathlessness in many of these patients, especially during exercise.[36]

Physiology of breathlessness in advanced disease

Other chapters in this book will address specific types of diseases, such as heart failure, neuromuscular disease, and malignancy. Using the information presented in this chapter, clinicians may approach each disease with a greater understanding not only of the individual pathophysiologic mechanisms responsible for breathing discomfort, but also of the complexity of the physiology of any given patient in whom multiple processes are occurring at once. Patients with lung cancer who develop breathlessness, for example, may have a number of physiologic derangements. Some are irreversible, such as hyperinflation and airflow limitation from underlying COPD, or partially reversible, such as hypoxia and cardiovascular deconditioning. Some, however, may be quite reversible with appropriate treatment. Drainage of a malignant pleural effusion may improve gas exchange, facilitate expansion of the lung, and decrease hyperinflation of the chest wall.

The sensation of breathlessness involves the complex integration of information from throughout the body. Our understanding of how each source of information affects the patient's awareness of breathing discomfort allows a targeted approach to treatment and, in the future, may lead to improved therapeutic options to alleviate breathlessness.

References

1. Demediuk BH, Manning H, Lilly J, *et al.* (1992). Dissociation between dyspnea and respiratory effort. *Am Rev Respir Dis* 146, 1222–5.
2. Chronos N, Adams L, Guz A (1988). Effect of hyperoxia and hypoxia on exercise-induced breathlessness in normal subjects. *Clin Sci* 74, 531–7.
3. Simon PM, Schwartzstein RM, Weiss JW, *et al.* (1989). Distinguishable sensations of breathlessness induced in normal volunteers. *Am Rev Respir Dis* 140, 1021–7.
4. Simon PM, Schwartzstein RM, Weiss JW, Fencl V, Teghtsoonian M, Weinberger SE (1990). Distinguishable types of dyspnea in patients with shortness of breath. *Am Rev Respir Dis* 142, 1009–14.
5. Elliott MW, Adams L, Cockcroft A, MacRae KD, Murphy K, Guz A (1991). The language of breathlessness: use of verbal descriptors by patients with cardiopulmonary disease. *Am Rev Respir Dis* 144, 826–32.
6. Mahler DA, Harver A, Lentine T, Scott JA, Beck K, Schwartzstein RM (1996). Descriptors of breathlessness in cardiorespiratory diseases. *Am J Respir Crit Care Med* 154, 1357–63.
7. McCloskey DI, Gandevia S, Potter EK, Colebatch JG (1983). Muscle sense and effort; Motor commands and judgments about muscular contractions. In: Desmedt JE, ed. *Motor Control Mechanisms in Health and Disease*, 151–67. Raven Press, New York.
8. Redline S, Gottfried SB, Altose MD (1991). Effects of changes in inspiratory muscle strength on the sensation of respiratory force. *J Appl Physiol* 70(1), 240–5.
9. Schwartzstein RM, Manning HL, Weiss JW, Weinberger SE (1990). Dyspnea: A sensory Experience. *Lung* 169, 185–99.
10. Schwartzstein RM, Simon PM, Weiss JW, Fencl V, Weinberger SE (1989). Breathlessness induced by dissociation between ventilation and chemical drive. *Am Rev Respir Dis* 139, 1231–7.
11. Chonan T, Mulholland MB, Cherniack NS, Altose MD (1987). Effects of voluntary constraining of thoracic displacement during hypercapnia. *J Appl Physiol* 63, 1822–8.

12. Manning HL, Schwartzstein RM (1995). Pathophysiology of dyspnea. *N Engl J Med* 333, 1547–53.

13. Binks AP, Moosavi SH, Banzett RB, Schwartzstein RM (2002). 'Tightness' sensation of asthma does not arise from the work of breathing. *Am J Respir Crit Care Med* 165, 78–82.

14. Fidone SJ, Gonzalez C (1986). Initiation and control of chemoreceptor activity in the carotid body. In: Fishman AP, Cherniack NS, Widdicombe JG, Geiger SR, eds *The Handbook of Physiology: The Respiratory System*, pp. 247–312. Section 3, Volume II, Part 2. Bethesda, MD: American Physiological Society.

15. Fitzgerald RS, Lahiri S. Reflex responses to chemoreceptor stimulation. In: Fishman AP, Cherniack NS, Widdicombe JG, Geiger SR, eds *The Handbook of Physiology: The Respiratory System*, pp. 313–63. Section 3, Volume II, Part 2. Bethesda, MD: American Physiological Society.

16. Scott AC, Davies LC, Coats AJ, Piepoli M (2002). Relationship of skeletal muscle metaboreceptors in the upper and lower limbs with the respiratory control in patients with heart failure. *Clin Sci* 102, 23–30.

17. Banzett RB, Lansing RW, Reid MB, Adams L, Brown R (1989). 'Air hunger' arising from increased P_{CO2} in mechanically ventilated quadriplegics. *Respir Physiol* 76, 53–68.

18. Banzett RB, Lansing RW, Brown R, *et al.* (1990). 'Air hunger' from increased P_{CO2} persists after complete neuromuscular block in humans. *Respir Physiol* 81, 1–18.

19. Shea SA, Andres LP, Guz A, Banzett RB (1993). Respiratory sensations in subjects who lack a ventilatory response to CO2. *Respir Physiol* 93(2), 203–19.

20. Manning HL, Schwartzstein RM (1998). Mechanisms of dyspnea. In: Mahler DA, ed. *Dyspnea*, pp. 63–95. Marcel Dekker, New York.

21. Lane R, Cockroft, Adams L, Guz A (1987). Arterial oxygen saturation and breathlessness in patients with chronic obstructive airways disease. *Cli Sci* 72, 693–8.

22. Schwartzstein RM, Lahive K, Pope A, Weinberger SE, Weiss JW (1987). Cold facial stimulation reduces breathlessness induced in normal subjects. *Am Rev Respir Dis* 136, 58–61.

23. Simon PM, Basner RC, Weinberger SE, Fencl V, Weiss JW, Schwartzstein RM (1991). Oral mucosal stimulation modulates intensity of breathlessness induced in normal subjects. *Am Rev Respir Dis* 144, 419–22.

24. Burgess KR, Whitelaw WA (1984). Reducing ventilatory response to carbon dioxide by breathing cold air. *Am Rev Respir Dis* 129, 687–90.

25. Liss HP, Grant BJB (1988). The effect of nasal flow on breathlessness in patients with chronic obstructive pulmonary disease. *Am Rev Respir Dis* 137, 1285–8.

26. Spence DPS, Graham DR, Ahmed J, Rees K, Pearson MG, Calverley PMA (1993). Does cold air affect exercise capacity and dyspnea in stable chronic obstructive pulmonary disease? *Chest* 103, 693–6.

27. Manning HL, Shea SA, Schwartzstein RM, Lansing RW, Brown R, Banzett RB (1992). Reduced tidal volume increases 'air hunger' at fixed P_{CO2} in ventilated quadriplegics. *Respir Physiol* 9019–30.

28. O'Donnell DE, Sanii R, Anthonisen NR, Younes M (1987). Effect of dynamic airway compression on breathing pattern and respiratory sensation in severe chronic obstructive pulmonary disease. *Am Rev Respir Dis* 135, 912–18.

29. Hamilton RD, Winning AJ, Perry A, and Guz A (1987). Aerosol anesthesia increases hypercapnic ventilation and breathlessness in laryngectomized humans. *J Appl Physiol* 63, 2286–92.

30. Taguchi O, Kikuchi Y, Hida W, Iwase N, Satoh M, Chonan T, Takishima T. (1991). Effects of bronchoconstriction and external resistive loading on the sensation of dyspnea. *J Appl Physiol* 71, 2183–90.

31. Moy ML, Weiss JW, Sparrow D, Israel E, Schwartzstein RM (2000). Quality of dyspnea in bronchoconstriction differs from external loads. *Am J Respir Crit Care Med* 162, 451–5.

32. Raj H, Singh VK, Anand A, Paintal AS (1995). Sensory origin of lobeline-induced sensations: a correlative study in man and cat. *J Physiol* 482, 235–46.

33. Davies SF, McQuaid KR, Iber C, *et al.* (1987). Extreme dyspnea from unilateral venous obstruction. *Am Rev Respir Diseases* 136, 184–8.

34. Manning HL, Basner R, Ringler J, *et al.* (1991). Effect of chest wall vibration on breathlessness in normal subjects. *J Appl Physiol* 71, 175–81.

35. Sibuya M, Yamada M, Kanamaru A, *et al.* (1994). Effect of chest wall vibration on dyspnea in patients with chronic respiratory disease. *Am J Respir Crit Care Med* 149, 1235–40.

36. O'Donnell DE, Webb KA (1993). Exertional breathlessness in patients with chronic obstructive airflow limitation. *Am Rev Respir Dis* 148, 1351–7.

Multidimensional assessment of dyspnea

Virginia Carrieri-Kohlman and Deborah Dudgeon

Introduction

Assessment of dyspnea requires an understanding of the multidimensional nature of this distressing symptom and the different pathophysiological mechanisms that can cause it. Like pain, dyspnea is a subjective experience that includes interactions among multiple physiological, psychological, social and environmental factors[1] that modulate both the quality and the intensity of the person's perception of the symptom. These interactions may cause secondary physiological and behavioral responses[1] that should be considered in the assessment process.

The multidimensional assessment of dyspnea involves both a clinical appraisal and measurement of the different factors that impact on the perception of breathlessness and the effects of shortness of breath on the individual. As the American Thoracic Society says, 'Any assessment of dyspnea must take into consideration the question being asked'.[1] Clinical assessments are usually directed at determining the underlying pathophysiology to determine appropriate treatment and evaluate response to therapy. Measurement instruments or tools are used to bring some objectivity and precision to the evaluation of clinical assessments or interventions and to answer research questions. In the setting of advanced disease it is also critical to understand the individual patient's diagnosis and prognosis; the goals of investigations and possible treatments available and their side-effects; the wishes of the patient and family; and the patient's performance status and setting of care. All of these factors will help to determine which clinical assessments and measurements are reasonable to consider.

Clinical assessment

History

Clinical assessment of dyspnea should include a complete history of the symptom. This would take account of: its temporal onset (acute, subacute, or chronic); the persistence or variability of the symptom; the aggravating factors including ambulation, eating, and position; previous exposures; its qualities; any associated symptoms; previous response to medications or other relieving events or activities; and its impact on psychosocial and functional well-being.[2–4] A past history of smoking, underlying lung or cardiac disease or other concurrent medical conditions, allergy history and details of previous medications or treatments should also be elicited.[5,6]

The initial approach to assessment and possible treatment is greatly affected by whether the breathlessness is an acute, subacute, or chronic problem.[4] The differential diagnosis of acute shortness of breath is relatively narrow: pneumonia, pulmonary embolism, congestive heart failure, or myocardial infarction;[4] and this knowledge should guide further questioning, the physical examination and possible investigations. In the setting of advanced disease it is important to determine if the breathlessness is related to the underlying disease and potentially irreversible – i.e. worsening chronic obstructive pulmonary disease (COPD) on maximal bronchodiators – or whether it is completely unrelated and potentially curable (e.g. pneumonia).

It can be helpful in establishing a diagnosis to inquire as to when dyspnea occurs and in which position.[3] Orthopnea, difficulty breathing while lying flat, is very common with symptomatic congestive heart failure, mitral valvular disease and superior vena cava syndrome, but rare in people with emphysema, severe asthma, chronic bronchitis and neurological diseases. Platypnea, difficulty breathing while sitting up and relieved by lying flat, is rare but occurs status post-pneumonectomy, cirrhosis, hypovolemia and with some neurological diseases. Trepopnea, when patients are more comfortable breathing while lying on one side, occurs in people with congestive heart failure or with a large pleural effusion.[3] Studies have shown that patients universally respond to breathlessness by decreasing their activity to whatever degree necessary. It is therefore helpful to ask about shortness of breath in relation to activities such as 'walking at the same speed as someone of your age', 'stopping to catch your breath when walking upstairs', or 'eating'. It is also important to quantify the amount of exercise, or lack of, that is needed for the person to become breathless as this will provide a baseline for comparison to assess progression or improvement.[3]

Physical examination

A careful physical examination focused on possible underlying causes of dyspnea should be performed. Particular attention should be directed to identify signs that are associated with the clinical syndromes identified in the history or common in people with their particular underlying disease. A detailed description of the different syndromes that distinguish these disorders is beyond the scope of this chapter but an example of this would be: on palpation – the decreased fremitus and trachea deviated to the other side; on percussion – the dullness; and on auscultation – the absent breath sounds associated with a pleural effusion in a person with lung cancer. Another example would be the findings of pulmonary edema secondary to congestive heart failure with possible findings of right heart pressures (elevated jugular venous distention, pedal edema, hepatomegaly), an S_3 heart sound, early crackles, and possibly wheezes.[3]

It is important to recognize that dyspnea, like pain, is a subjective experience that may not be evident to an observer. Tachypnea, a rapid respiratory rate, is not dyspnea. Medical personnel must learn to ask and accept the patient's assessments, often without measurable physical correlates. When patients say that they are having discomfort with breathing we must believe they are dyspneic. Gift *et al.*[7] studied the physiological factors related to dyspnea in subjects with COPD with high, medium and low levels of breathlessness. There were no significant differences in respiratory rate, depth of respiration or peak expiratory flow rates at the three levels of dyspnea. There was, however, a significant difference in the use of accessory muscles between patients with high and low levels of dyspnea. This would suggest that the extent of use of accessory muscles is a physical finding that is helpful when assessing breathlessness as it reflects the intensity of dyspnea.

Laboratory evaluation

There are a number of tests that can be done to help determine the etiology of a person's dyspnea but the choice of the appropriate diagnostic tests should be guided by the stage of disease, the prognosis, the risk:benefit ratios of any proposed tests or interventions and the desires of the patient and family.

Oxygen saturation can be measured non-invasively using a pulse oximeter. It should be remembered that pulse oximeters are reasonably accurate (+/– 3%) at high saturations, but less accurate below saturations of about 80 per cent.[8] Oxygen saturation also gives no indication as to whether the person has adequate ventilation, so a person who is retaining carbon dioxide can have normal or near normal oxygen saturations. Arterial blood gas analysis provides information not only of oxygenation (PO_2) and ventilation (PCO_2), but also acid-base balance (pH) and should be considered in appropriate situations.[8]

Possible blood tests include: a complete blood count to diagnose anemia and to help rule out infection and polycythemia (which suggests chronic hypoxemia); and serum calcium, potassium, magnesium and phosphate (all of which can impair the function of the respiratory muscles).[9]

If appropriate, radiological examinations may include: a chest radiograph, ventilation/perfusion scan, CT scan, CT angiogram, MRI or an echocardiogram.

Lung function tests vary from simple spirometry that can be done with hand-held electronic devices, to more complicated tests that require sophisticated equipment in a lung function laboratory. Standardized pulmonary function tests (PFTs) can be helpful to diagnosis the underlying problem and determine its severity and response to treatment. Spirometry can demonstrate two basic patterns of disorder: obstructive and restrictive. Stulbarg has suggested that the relationship of pulmonary dysfunction and the severity of dyspnea is strongest within specific diseases.[4] Mahler and Wells[10] showed that: in patients with COPD measures of maximal expiratory pressure (PEmax) (r = 0.35) and maximal inspiratory pressure (PImax) (r = 0.34) showed the strongest correlations to the intensity of dyspnea as measured by the baseline dyspnea index (BDI); in patients with asthma, FVC (r = 0.78) and FEV_1 (r = 0.77) were highly related to BDI; and in interstitial lung disease (a restrictive disease) PImax (r = 0.51) and FVC (r = 0.44) showed significant correlations with breathlessness. Others have found that maximal voluntary ventilation (MVV) (r = 0.78), the largest volume in liters that can be breathed per minute by voluntary effort, had the greatest correlation with dyspnea in COPD patients, and PImax (r = 0.51) and FVC (r = 0.44) in patients with interstitial lung disease[11] Maximum inspiratory and expiratory measurements can be helpful in assessing respiratory muscle strength but are dependent on patient effort. Unlike others,[12,13] Bruera and colleagues[14] found that in cancer patients with moderate to severe dyspnea, multivariate analysis showed PImax (p = 0.02) was an independent correlate of the intensity of dyspnea.

Cardiopulmonary exercise tests provide additional information to that gathered from lung function tests that are performed at rest. In the appropriate setting, the reason to perform an exercise test is: to identify a cardiac or respiratory cause for exercise limitation, to quantify functional disability, and to assess the response to treatment.[8] Simple measures of exercise capacity include the 6 or 12-minute walking test and the shuttle walking test. For the 6 or 12-minute walk test the person walks as far as they can at their own pace for 6 or 12 minutes on a set course. Walking tests correlate with measures of both dyspnea and exercise capacity.[15] In the shuttle walking test the individual walks around two points at a speed that is controlled by an audiotape and progressively increased. They are to continue until they can't keep up with the tape or have to stop.[8] The shuttle walking test has been validated in comparison with the treadmill exercise test[16] and is a reproducible test of functional capacity in ambulant patients with advanced cancer.[17] Progressive exercise testing has the person exercise on either a cycle ergometer or treadmill with increasing workloads while various parameters are continuously measured. Modern exercise systems can provide varying degrees of sophisticated information to help distinguish the organ system that is limiting exercise capacity.[8] This type of assessment is frequently used to establish a baseline for people entering a pulmonary rehabilitation program, to identify the etiology of exertional dyspnea and to assess interventions.

Qualitative dimensions of dyspnea

In discussing the assessment of dyspnea, it is important to understand that it is not a single sensation. Studies have shown that patients chose different phrases to describe their discomfort with breathing and that there is an association of different descriptors and clusters with different pathophysiological conditions (i.e. 'chest tightness', 'exhalation', and 'deep' with asthma).[18–20] O'Donnell et al., however, found that while descriptor choices were clearly different between health and disease states, there was too much overlap to help distinguish between COPD, restrictive lung disease and congestive heart failure.[21–23] Wilcock and colleagues also did not find that there was sufficient robustness and construct validity to support the use of word descriptors and clusters to help in determining a diagnosis.[20]

Measurement of dyspnea

For many years the assessment of pain has been recognized as an indicator of quality care and most recently has become a mandatory measurement to determine the effect of treatments in many acute care settings.[24] Despite the fact that dyspnea remains the most frequent and distressing symptom for patients suffering from cardiopulmonary disease, it is not yet considered mandatory to assess dyspnea. Dyspnea is increasingly assessed in research studies and in palliative care settings, however, in other clinical settings there remains only sporadic assessment of dyspnea. In addition, this measurement often tends to be qualitative and insensitive with the provider asking only, 'Are you short of breath?,' while neglecting to record the patient response, possible mechanisms, or appropriate treatments.

The assessment of dyspnea must be more frequent if patients with cardio-pulmonary illness or malignant disorders are going to receive quality care. The importance of assessing and monitoring dyspnea is supported by several research studies that found the patient's clinical ratings of dyspnea provides an independent and separate dimension, not measured by pulmonary function tests or dyspnea measured during laboratory exercise.[25–28] Clinical measurement of dyspnea influences and predicts health-related quality of life (HRQL) and survival to a greater extent than do physiological measurements.[29–31] The method used to assess dyspnea depends on the specific purpose (clinical or research), the setting of the assessment, the acuity of the symptom, the phase of illness; and the need to measure not only the symptom itself, but also the impact on quality of life.

Clinically the simplest, yet least sensitive, measure of dyspnea is to ask the patient whether he or she is short of breath. This yes-or-no categorical measurement is a frequently used method of assessing dyspnea, but it gives no information about the severity or quality of the sensation. It should be remembered that patients use different descriptors or words to describe their shortness of breath and these may vary with ethnicity and type of illness.[32,33] More informative and sensitive is a unidimensional quantitative visual ana-logue scale (VAS) or modified Borg scale that can be used to monitor the intensity of dyspnea and the effect of alternative treatments. A quantitative rating of dyspnea can capture the severity of the symptom and associated distress the patient is feeling. These scales can be used in chronic illness as part of a daily diary, in acute episodes of dyspnea, or during the palliative phase of care. Since these scales are not linked to an activity either of them can be used if the patient is bed-bound. During the palliative care phase family or care-givers can be taught how to measure the intensity of shortness of breath by asking the patient to point or say the number corresponding to their shortness of breath. Symptom levels should be monitored and recorded so that patterns of the symptom with titration of medication can be used to predict essential care.

Non-pharmacological treatments may offer relief for the extreme distress but not for the actual intensity of dyspnea. Therefore, if possible the 'anxiety' or 'distress' associated with dyspnea should be measured. The changes in intensity and distress associated with dyspnea can be measured over time to evaluate treatment modalities and fluctuations that will predict changes in the patient's activities and care needs.

The assessment is expanded and may be more helpful if the intensity of dyspnea is linked to a certain activity or level of activities. A baseline rating of dyspnea provides the healthcare provider, patient, and family a measure to compare with when assessing the effectiveness of medical and complementary treatments across the illness trajectory. The Medical Research Council (MRC)[34] or Baseline/Transitional Dyspnea Index (BDI/TDI)[35] are valid and reliable instruments that are brief and are used to estimate broad categories of activity that induce certain levels of shortness of breath for the patient. Changes in dyspnea with specific activities over months or years can be measured with more sensitive instruments, such as the Chronic Respiratory Questionnaire (CRQ)[36] dyspnea with activities scale, the University of California, San Diego Shortness of Breath Scale (SOBQ)[37] or the Pulmonary Functional Status and Dyspnea Questionnaire (PFSDQ).[38] In particular, the SOBQ or the PFSDQ can assist the provider to track the activities that the patient has abandoned because of breathlessness and support the patient in coping with the reduction in functioning level. In the early phases of advanced disease a multidimensional instrument like the Chronic Disease Questionnaire can determine the impact that the symptom is having on other components of the patient's quality of life, such as, mood, other symptoms and disruption of activities. In the chronically ill, dyspnea with changing activities, treatments, or emotional situations also can be monitored with a daily log.[39, 40]

Breathlessness is a subjective symptom that should be rated only by the patient. However, in acute or terminal disease if the patient is unable to communicate or report their level of breathlessness, behavioral responses can be used as 'proxy' variables to estimate the level of the patient's shortness of breath. Behavioral responses that are frequently observed when patients say they are breathless include increased respiratory rate, restlessness, diaphoresis, use of accessory respiratory muscles, tremulousness, gasping breaths, pallor, interrupted or 'staccato' speech, large staring eyes, professorial position or a frozen appearance, audible wheezing, and coughing and use of learned strategies including pursed lips breathing.[41]

Description and characteristics of instruments to assess dyspnea

Instruments that are commonly used in the clinical and research settings to measure dyspnea either evaluate dyspnea intensity exclusively or are multidimensional questionnaires that evaluate the impact of dyspnea on other domains of health-related quality of life. Extensive reviews of these instruments are published elsewhere.[42–48]

Unidimensional scales

Visual analogue scale

The visual analogue scale (VAS) is a vertical or horizontal line most commonly 100 cm in length with anchors to indicate extremes of the sensation. Subjects indicate their dyspnea intensity by pointing to or marking a line at the level of their dyspnea. Although investigators have used various end points it is recommended that anchors at the bottom and top should be 'No Breathlessness' and 'Worst Imaginable Breathlessness'. Concurrent validity with the modified Borg scale is high (r = >0.90) indicating that either of these can be used to rate dyspnea.[49, 50] The VAS is reproducible at the same level of exercise and at maximal exercise[51,52] and is sensitive to treatment effects.[53] The VAS has been labeled with and used to measure different sensations including shortness of breath, discomfort with breathing, and effort of breathing. It is important to discern the question that the patient is being asked since these sensations may not be strongly related and they may not have the same meaning to patients.[54] Although most clinicians use the vertical VAS, the correlation between a horizontal and vertical VAS is high at r = 0.97. [55]

Modified Borg scale for breathlessness (modified Borg)

The modified Borg scale is a 10 point category-ratio scale with a non-linear scaling scheme using descriptive terms to anchor responses.[56] This scale has strong and significant correlations with the VAS in COPD patients (r = 0.99)[49] with minute ventilation (r = 0.98), oxygen consumption during exercise (r = 0.95),[57] and moderate correlations with peak expiratory flow rates and SaO2 in emergency room patients.[58] Advantages of the modified Borg scale include that patients with acute dyspnea have reported they are satisfied with using the scale,[58] conceptually it is easier for older patients to use than the VAS that is 'open-ended', the descriptors may help patients in selecting the sensation intensity, and direct comparisons between individuals may be more valid. However, the sensitivity of the scale may be blunted by 'ceiling effects' triggered by the verbal descriptors, with patients tending to choose the numbers by the descriptors.

Numeric rating scale

The Numeric Rating Scale (NRS), a 0–10 scale, correlates well with the VAS and modified Borg scale.[59] If the patient prefers this type of scale it should be used, especially to compare intra-individual ratings even though it has not received the same amount of testing as the VAS and modified Borg scale.

Measurement of the affective responses to dyspnea

Both normal subjects[50] and patients with COPD who are exercising[54] or completing daily self-reports[43] can distinguish the intensity of their shortness of breath from the anxiety and/or distress it causes them. After treatment, patients have stated that the intensity of shortness of breath with exercise may be at the same level, but because they feel more in control of the symptom, they are less anxious about the symptom, and therefore, the same intensity of shortness of breath is less distressing for them. In addition, there is also evidence that patients with chronic illness may not change their rating of the level of the intensity of shortness of breath over time despite worsening of lung function[60] or advancing disease.[61] However, their anxiety or distress with the dyspnea may decrease after treatments such as pulmonary rehabilitation or exercise training.[62] Therefore, it is important that the anxiety or distress associated with dyspnea be measured in addition to the intensity. At this time there is little consensus as to the dimension of anxiety or distress that should be measured or the most valid method to measure anxiety or distress. VAS and Borg scales have been used to measure the distress of the symptom for the patient during exercise. Patients were asked to rate their response to the following questions: 'How anxious are you about your shortness of breath?' or 'How bothersome or distressing is your shortness of breath to you?'[62] Others were asked to complete daily self-report measures of breathing distress.[43] Other investigators have asked terminally ill cancer patients while at rest to rate their anxiety on a VAS anchored by 'no anxiety' and 'worst possible anxiety'.[63] Other investigators have measured 'state' anxiety, that is defined as 'situational anxiety' and measured by the State/Trait Anxiety Inventory,[64] during times that patients with asthma were acutely short of breath.[65] It is especially important that the affective response to breathlessness be measured as an outcome when the treatment is not expected to provide changes in physiological mechanisms or the intensity of dyspnea.

Breathlessness, Cough, and Sputum Scale

The Breathlessness, Cough, and Sputum Scale (BCSS) was developed to assess the severity of the three respiratory symptoms in clinical trials of patients with COPD.[66] Patients evaluate each symptom/item on a five point Likert-type scale, ranging from 0 to 4 with higher scores indicating a more severe manifestation of the symptom. A daily total score is expressed as the sum of the three item scores with a range from 0 to 12. The BCSS is internally consistent (alpha = 0.70 daily and 0.95–0.99 over time) and there is evidence of concurrent, convergent, divergent and discriminant validity.[67] The instrument was reproducible in a stable situation and responsive to change. A mean change in the BCSS total score >1.0 represents substantial symptomatic improvement, changes of approximately 0.6 can be interpreted as moderate and changes of 0.3 are considered small.[67]

Unidimensional instruments anchored to activities
Medical Research Council Breathlessness Scale (MRC)

This scale was originally developed by Fletcher in 1959.[34] Later it was adapted and labeled the ATS Grade of Breathlessness Scale. Although the MRC has been used extensively as a method to define or characterize the patient population, the testing of the MRC has been minimal. Earlier studies found the instrument to have test–retest and inter-rater reliability[68] and content validity;[69] however, the grades are not clearly discrete.[45] More recently it has gained favor as a simple tool that can be used to measure 'functional dyspnea'[70,71] because it was found to be predictive of health-related quality of life[72] and survival.[30] The MRC has five grades:

0: not troubled with breathlessness except with strenuous exercise
1: troubled by shortness of breath when hurrying or walking up a slight hill
2: walks slower than people of the same age due to breathlessness or has to stop for breath when walking at own pace on the level
3: stops for breath after walking ~100 m or after a few minutes on the level
4: too breathless to leave the house or breathless when dressing or undressing.

Oxygen cost diagram

The oxygen cost diagram (OCD) is a vertical line, usually 100 mm long, with a list of daily activities on both sides of the scale. Activities are listed from the bottom, those requiring low energy expenditure (e.g. sitting), to those activities likely to cause the most energy expenditure (brisk walking) at the top of the scale. Patients indicate on the line the activity during which their dyspnea would be severe enough that they would not be able to do any more of the activities listed above.[73] The point selected on the line is scored in millimeters. The reliability is reported as an intra-class correlation of 0.68[48] and it has a moderate correlation (r = 0.60) with the 12 minute walk.[73] The responsiveness of this instrument to treatments has not been reported.

Multidimensional indirect measures of dyspnea anchored to activities
Baseline/Transitional Dyspnea Index

The Baseline/Transitional Dyspnea Index (BDI/TDI) measures functional impairment (the degree to which activities of daily living are impaired), magnitude of effort (the overall effort exerted to perform activities), and the magnitude of task that provokes the breathing difficulty. The TDI measures changes in dyspnea rated by the interviewer comparing patient report with the baseline state. The focus is on the activity consequences of the individual's breathlessness.[35] Content validity was established by correlation of scores of the BDI with the MRC (r = −0.70 p <0.01) and the Oxygen Cost Diagram (OCD) (r = −0.54 p <0.01). Interobserver agreement (inter-rater reliability) between physician and pulmonary technician ranged across dimensions of 91 to 93 weighted percent agreement and a weighted kappa ranging from 0.66 to 0.73 demonstrating creditable agreement of the two observers.[35] The instrument is responsive to treatments including exercise training and rehabilitation programs,[74,75] inspiratory muscle training,[76] theophylline[77] and the TDI correlates with changes in the quality of life (SF36).[78] Most recently self-administered versions of the modified BDI and TDI were developed and compared to that of interviewers with high and significant correlations found between the interviewers and the self-administered versions.[79] Advantages include extensive testing and use in research studies, therefore, the patient's scores and outcomes can be compared to other studies. A disadvantage of this instrument is that although dyspnea is a subjective sensation, the healthcare provider scores this instrument rating the functional consequences of dyspnea for the patient.

Pulmonary Functional Status and Dyspnea Questionnaire

The Pulmonary Functional Status and Dyspnea Questionnaire (PFSDQ) is a self-administered instrument rating of dyspnea with 79 activities in six categories: self care, mobility, eating, home management, social, and recreational.[38] The more recently modified shorter version the PFSDQ-M measures dyspnea associated with 10 activities and includes a fatigue component.[80] Dyspnea is also measured as separate from activities with five items. The larger PFSDQ has high test–retest reliability on the dyspnea scale (0.94), internal consistency (alpha = 0.88 to 0.94)[38] and is responsive over time.[80] The shorter PFSDQ-M also has good test–retest reliability (r = 0.83) on the dyspnea scale and high internal consistency (alpha = 0.94) and is responsive to change after pulmonary rehabilitation.[60] The level of dyspnea for specific activities can be monitored over time and the instrument is sensitive to small changes in dyspnea with activities.

The University of California, San Diego Shortness of Breath Questionnaire

The University of California, San Diego Shortness of Breath Questionnaire (SOBQ) measures shortness of breath with daily activities. The questionnaire is self-administered and easy for the patient to understand. Patients rate their dyspnea associated with 21 activities of daily living from 0 = 'not at all' to 5 = 'maximally or unable to do because of breathlessness,' on a six-point scale.[81] Three additional questions ask about limitations caused by shortness of breath, fear of harm from overexertion, and fear of shortness of breath. SOBQ has a test-retest reliability of r = 0.94 over two days, good internal consistency (alpha = 0.91) and moderate correlation with 6MW (r = −0.47) and low correlation with percentage of predicted FEV1% (r = −0.28)[37] It has been responsive to pulmonary rehabilitation.[82]

The Pulmonary Functional Status Scale

The Pulmonary Functional Status Scale (PFSS) is a self-administered 53 item questionnaire that measures mental, physical, and social functioning.[83] Dyspnea ratings are obtained in relation to several activities and independent of activities and reflected in a dyspnea subscale. The PFSS has a test–retest reliability of 0.67 and internal consistency of 0.81,[84] and construct validity, including a moderate correlation with the 12 MW.[83] It has also been shown to be responsive to PR.[85]

The Cancer Dyspnea Scale

The Cancer Dyspnea Scale (CDS) is a 12-item, three factor (sense of effort/sense of anxiety/sense of discomfort) scale developed to assess the multidimensional nature of dyspnea in cancer patients. Although further improvements and validation are needed the Japanese version of the scale has some evidence of reliability and validity as a multidimensional instrument.[86]

Disease-specific quality of life instruments: instruments that measure dyspnea with activities and other components of quality of life

Chronic Respiratory Questionnaire

The Chronic Respiratory Questionnaire (CRQ) is a 20 item self-report questionnaire administered by an interviewer that measures four dimensions: dyspnea, fatigue, emotional function, and mastery of breathing.[36] The patient rates the level of dyspnea he/she has with five usual individual activities. The instrument requires a 15 minute interview, however, less time is required for repeated administrations. A paper and pencil version of the CRQ has been validated and can be used in place of the interview.[87] This questionnaire has been used extensively to measure health-related quality of life as an outcome for pulmonary rehabilitation, therefore, outcomes from one program can be compared with others. Internal consistency for all four scales ranged from $a = 0.71$ to 0.92 in this author's recent study with COPD patients,[88] however, other authors have reported lower internal consistency ($a = 0.53$) for the dyspnea scale most probably because the activities are individualized.[89] The questionnaire has acceptable reliability (test–retest r = 0.73)[89], has been responsive to therapy,[90] and a level of change that can be used to judge a clinically significant[91] Because the ratings for the dyspnea with activities scale are individualized, this dimension was found to have lower reliability in one study,[89] however it has high reliability in other studies.[36]

The St George Respiratory Questionnaire

The Saint George Respiratory Questionnaire (SGRQ) is a disease-specific quality of life self-administered questionnaire listing 53 questions measuring three areas of illness: symptoms, activity, and impact of disease on daily life. The symptoms category elicits information about four symptoms; cough, sputum, wheeze, and dyspnea. These are combined for the symptoms score, therefore dyspnea as a discrete symptom can not be measured.[92] Test–retest reliability of the questionnaire is r = 0.92[93] and the instrument is responsive to treatments,[94] and thresholds of significant clinical change are reported.[95] Advantages of this instrument are that it is self-administered, has been used extensively and has computerized scoring. One disadvantage of this instrument is that dyspnea is not measured as a separate symptom, therefore, the dyspnea response to therapy can not be measured separately.

Summary

The assessment of dyspnea includes a clinical appraisal of the symptom, measurement of different factors that may have an impact on the individual's perception of breathlessness, and evaluation of secondary physiological and behavioral responses to the symptom. This assessment is shaped by the acuity of the symptom; the patient's ability to rate the symptom and other related dimensions, such as activities or self-management strategies; the type and amount of the information needed for the diagnosis or treatment of the symptom; and the reason for the assessment, whether it is for clinical or research purposes. Early assessment of the symptom is preferred, since it provides a baseline from which to evaluate the effect of advancing disease or new treatments. Valid and reliable measurement instruments are available and should be used for measuring the intensity and distress of dyspnea at one time or over time, the level of dyspnea related to certain activities, or the multiple dimensions of the patient's health-related quality of life that may be affected by either acute or chronic breathlessness.

References

1. **American Thoracic Society.** Dyspnea. Mechanisms, assessment, and management: A consensus statement. *Am J Respir Crit Care Med* 1999; **159**: 321–40.
2. **Dudgeon D. Multidimensional assessment of dyspnea.** In: Portenoy RK, Bruera E, eds *Issues in Palliative Care Research*, pp. 83–96. New York: Oxford University Press, 2003.
3. **Swartz MH.** *Textbook of Physical Diagnosis: History and Examination*, 4th edn. Philadelphia: W. B. Saunders Company, 2002.
4. **Man GCW, Hsu K, Sproule BJ.** Effect of Alprazolam on exercise and dyspnea in patients with chronic obstructive pulmonary disease. *Chest* 1986; **906**: 832–6.
5. **Silvestri GA, Mahler DA.** Evaluation of dyspnea in the elderly patient. *Clin Chest Med* 1993; **14**(3): 393–404.
6. **Ferrin MS, Tino G. Acute dyspnea.** *American Association of Critical-Care Nurses Clin Issues* 1997; **8**(3): 398–410.
7. **Gift AG, Plaut SM, Jacox A.** Psychologic and physiologic factors related to dyspnea in subjects with chronic obstructive pulmonary disease. *Heart and Lung* 1986; **15**(6): 595–601.
8. **Hancox B, Whyte K.** *McGraw-Hill's Pocket Guide to Lung Function Tests.* Roseville NSW: McGraw-Hill, 2001.
9. **Lewis MI, Belman MJ.** Nutrition and the respiratory muscles. *Clin Chest Med* 1988; **9**(2): 337–47.
10. **Mahler DA, Wells CK.** Evaluation of clinical methods for rating dyspnea. *Chest* 1988; **93**(3): 580–6.
11. **Epler GR, Saber FA, Gaensler EA.** Determination of severe impairment (disability) in interstitial lung disease. *Am Rev Respir Dis* 1980; **121**: 647–59.
12. **Dudgeon DJ, Lertzman M, Askew GR.** Physiological changes and clinical correlations of dyspnea in cancer outpatients. *J Pain Symptom Manage* 2001; **21**(5): 373–9.
13. **Dudgeon D, Lertzman M.** Dyspnea in the advanced cancer patient. *J Pain Symptom Manage* 1998; **16**(4): 212–19.
14. **Bruera E, Schmitz B, Pither J, Neumann CM, Hanson J.** The frequency and correlates of dypsnea in patients with advanced cancer. *J Pain Symptom Manage* 2000; **19**(5): 357–62.
15. **Mahler DA, Weinberg DH, Wells CK, Feinstein AR.** The measurement of dyspnea. Contents, interobserver agreement, and physiologic correlates of two new clinical indexes. *Chest* 1984; **85**(6): 751–8.
16. **Singh SJ, Morgan MD, Hardman AE, Rowe C, Bardsley PA.** Comparison of oxygen uptake during a conventional treadmill test and the shuttle walking test in chronic airflow limitation. *Eur Respir J* 1994; **7**(11): 2016–20.
17. **Booth S, Adams L.** The shuttle walking test: a reproducible method for evaluating the impact of shortness of breath on functional capacity in patients with advanced cancer. *Thorax* 2001; **56**(2): 146–50.
18. **Simon PM, Schwartzstein RM, Weiss JW, Lahive K, Fencl V, Teghtsoonian M** *et al.* Distinguishable sensations of breathlessness induced in normal volunteers. *Am Rev Respir Dis* 1989; **140**: 1021–7.

19. Simon PM, Schwartzstein RM, Weiss JW, Fencl V, Teghtsoonian M, Weinberger SE. Distinguishable types of dyspnea in patients with shortness of breath. *Am Rev Respir Dis* 1990; 142: 1009–14.
20. Wilcock A, Crosby V, Hughes AC, Fielding K, Corcoran R, Tattersfield AE. Descriptors of breathlessness in patients with cancer and other cardiorespiratory diseases. *J Pain Symptom Manage* 2002; 23(3): 182–9.
21. O'Donnell DE, Chau LL, Bertley J, Webb KA. Qualitative aspects of exertional breathlessness in CAL: Pathophysiological mechanisms. *Am J Respir Crit Care Med* 1997; 155: 109–15.
22. O'Donnell DE, Chau LKL, Webb KA. Qualitative aspects of exertional dyspnea in interstitial lung disease. *J Appl Physiol* 1998; 84: 2000–09.
23. D'Arsigny C, Raj S, Abdollah H, Webb KA, O'Donnell DE. Ventilatory assistance improves leg discomfort and exercise endurance in stable congestive heart failure (CHF). *Am J Respir Crit Care Med* 1998; 157: A451.
24. Berry P. Compliance with the Joint Commission Standards. In: Organizations JCAHO, ed. *Approaches to Pain Managment: An Essential Guide for Clinical Leaders*, pp. 35–48. PMPP02SJ: Joint Commission; 2004.
25. Mahler DA, Harver A. A factor analysis of dyspnea ratings, respiratory muscle strength, and lung function in patients with chronic obstructive pulmonary disease. *American Review of Respiratory Disease* 1992; 145(2 Pt 1): 467–70.
26. Eakin EG, Kaplan RM, Ries A, Sassi-Dambron DE. Patients' self-reports of dyspnea: An important and independent outcome in chronic obstructive pulmonary disease. *Annals of Behavioral Medicine* 1996;18(2): 87–90.
27. Hajiro T, Nishimura K, Tsukino M, Ikeda A, Koyama H, Izumi T. Analysis of clinical methods used to evaluate dyspnea in patients with chronic obstructive pulmonary disease. *American Journal of Respiratory and Critical Care Medicine* 1998; 158(4): 1185–9.
28. Nguyen HQ, Altinger J, Carrieri-Kohlman V, Gormley JM, Stulbarg MS. Factor analysis of laboratory and clinical measurements of dyspnea in patients with chronic obstructive pulmonary disease. *J Pain Symptom Manage* 2003; 25(2): 118–27.
29. Jones PW, Baveystock CM, Littlejohns P. Relationships between general health measured with the sickness impact profile and respiratory symptoms, physiological measures, and mood in patients with chronic airflow limitation. *American Review of Respiratory Disease* 1989; 140(6): 1538–43.
30. Nishimura K, Izumi T, Tsukino M, Oga A. Dyspnea is a better predictor of 5-year survival than airway obstruction in patients with COPD. *Chest* 2002; 121: 1434–40.
31. Curtis JR, Deyo RA, Hudson LD. Pulmonary rehabilitation in chronic respiratory insufficiency. 7. Health-related quality of life among patients with chronic obstructive pulmonary disease. *Thorax* 1994; 49(2): 162–70.
32. Hardie GE, Janson S, Gold WM, Carrieri-Kohlman V, Boushey HA. Ethnic differences: word descriptors used by African-American and white asthma patients during induced bronchoconstriction. *Chest* 2000; 117(4): 935–43.
33. Schwartzstein RM. The language of dyspnea. In: Mahler DA, ed. *Dyspnea*, pp. 35–57. New York: Marcel Dekker, Inc.; 1998.
34. Fletcher CM, Elmes P, Fairbairn A, Wood C. The significance of respiratory symptoms and the diagnosis of chronic bronchitis in a working population. *BMJ* 1959; 257–66.

35. Mahler DA, Weinberg DH, Wells CK, Feinstein AR. The measurement of dyspnea. Contents, interobserver agreement, and physiologic correlates of two new clinical indexes. *Chest* 1984; **85**(6): 751–8.
36. Guyatt GH, Berman LB, Townsend M, Pugsley SO, Chambers LW. A measure of quality of life for clinical trials in chronic lung disease. *Thorax* 1987; **42**(10): 773–8.
37. Eakin EG, Resnikoff PM, Prewitt LM, Ries AL, Kaplan RM. Validation of a new dyspnea measure: the UCSD Shortness of Breath Questionnaire. University of California, San Diego. *Chest* 1998; **113**(3): 619–24.
38. Lareau SC, Carrieri-Kohlman V, Janson-Bjerklie S, Roos PJ. Development and testing of the Pulmonary Functional Status and Dyspnea Questionnaire (PFSDQ). *Heart and Lung* 1994; **23**(3): 242–50.
39. Janson-Bjerklie S, Shnell S. Effect of peak flow information on patterns of self-care in adult asthma. *Heart and Lung* 1988; **17**(5): 543–9.
40. Burman ME. Health diaries in nursing research and practice. *Image – the Journal of Nursing Scholarship* 1995; **27**(2): 147–52.
41. Carrieri-Kohlman V, Stulbarg MS. Dyspnea. In: Carrieri-Kohlman V, Lindsey A, West C, eds *Pathophysiological Phenomena in Nursing: Human Responses to Illness*, 3rd edn, pp. 57–90, 175–208. St Louis, Missouri: Saunders; 2003.
42. Pashkow P, Ades PA, Emery CF, Frid DJ, Houston-Miller N, Peske G, *et al.* Outcome measurement in cardiac and pulmonary rehabilitation. AACVPR Outcomes Committee. American Association of Cardiovascular and Pulmonary Rehabilitation. *Journal of Cardiopulmonary Rehabilitation* 1995; **15**(6): 394–405.
43. Meek PM, Lareau SC, Hu J. Are self-reports of breathing effort and breathing distress stable and valid measures among persons with asthma, persons with COPD, and healthy persons? *Heart and Lung* 2003; **32**: 335–346.
44. Carrieri-Kohlman V, Stulbarg MS. Dyspnea: assessment and management. In: Hodgkin JE, Celli BR, Connors GL, eds *Pulmonary Rehabilitation*, 3rd edn., 57–90. New York: Lippincott Wiliams and Wilkins; 2000.
45. Meek PM, Lareau SC. Critical outcomes in pulmonary rehabilitation: assessment and evaluation of dyspnea and fatigue. *J Rehabil Res Dev* 2003; **40**(5 Suppl 2): 13–24.
46. ATS. Dyspnea. Mechanisms, assessment, and management: a consensus statement. American Thoracic Society. *American Journal of Respiratory and Critical Care Medicine* 1999; **159**(1): 321–40.
47. ACCP/AACVPR PRGP. Pulmonary rehabilitation: joint ACCP/AACVPR evidence-based guidelines. ACCP/AACVPR Pulmonary Rehabilitation Guidelines Panel. American College of Chest Physicians. American Association of Cardiovascular and Pulmonary Rehabilitation (see comments). *Chest* 1997; **112**(5): 1363–96.
48. Mahler D, Guyatt G, Jones P. Clinical measurement of dyspnea. In: Mahler D, ed. *Dyspnea*, pp. 149–89. New York: Marcel Dekker; 1998.
49. Lush MT, Janson BS, Carrieri VK, Lovejoy N. Dyspnea in the ventilator-assisted patient. *Heart and Lung* 1988; **17**(5): 528–35.
50. Wilson RC, Jones PW. A comparison of the visual analogue scale and modified Borg scale for the measurement of dyspnoea during exercise. *Clin Sci* 1989; **76**: 277–82.
51. Muza SR, Silverman MT, Gilmore GC, Hellerstein HK, Kelsen SG. Comparison of scales used to quantitate the sense of effort to breathe in patients with chronic obstructive pulmonary disease. *American Review of Respiratory Disease* 1990; **141**: 909–13.

52. **Mador MJ, Kufel TJ.** Reproducibility of visual analog scale measurements of dyspnea in patients with chronic obstructive pulmonary disease. *American Review of Respiratory Disease* 1992;**146**: 82–7.

53. **Mahler DA, Faryniarz K, Lentine T, Ward J, Olmstead EM, O'Connor GT.** Measurement of breathlessness during exercise in asthmatics. Predictor variables, reliability, and responsiveness. *American Review of Respiratory Disease* 1991; **144**(1): 39–44.

54. **Carrieri-Kohlman V, Gormley JM, Douglas MK, Paul SM, Stulbarg MS.** Differentiation between dyspnea and its affective components. *West J Nurs Res* 1996; **18**(6): 626–42.

55. **Gift AG.** Validation of a vertical visual analogue scale as a measure of clinical dyspnea. *Rehabil Nurs* 1989; **14**(6): 323–5.

56. **Burdon JGW, Juniper EF, Killian KJ, Hargreave FE, Campbell EJM.** The perception of breathlessness in asthma. *American Review of Respiratory Disease* 1982; **126**: 825–8.

57. **Adams L, Chronos NRL, Guz A.** The measurement of breathlessness induced in normal subjects: validity of two scaling techniques. *Clin Sci* 1985; **69**: 7–16.

58. **Kendrick KR, Baxi SC, Smith RM.** Usefulness of the modified 0–10 Borg Scale in assessing the degree of dyspnea in patients with COPD and asthma. *J Emerg Nurs* 2000; **26**: 216–22.

59. **Gift AG, Narsavage G.** Validity of the numeric rating scale as a measure of dyspnea. *Am J Crit Care* 1998; **7**(3): 200–4.

60. **Lareau SC, Meek PM, Press D, Anholm JD, Roos PJ.** Dyspnea in patients with chronic obstructive pulmonary disease: does dyspnea worsen longitudinally in the presence of declining lung function? *Heart and Lung* 1999; **28**(1): 65–73.

61. **Roberts DK, Thorne SE, Pearson C.** The experience of dyspnea in late-stage cancer. Patients' and nurses' perspectives. *Cancer Nurs* 1993; **16**(4): 310–20.

62. **Carrieri-Kohlman V, Gormley JM, Douglas MK, Paul SM, Stulbarg MS.** Exercise training decreases dyspnea and the distress and anxiety associated with it. Monitoring alone may be as effective as coaching. *Chest* 1996; **110**(6): 1526–35.

63. **Dudgeon DJ, Lertzman M.** Dyspnea in the advanced cancer patient. *Journal of Pain and Symptom Management* 1998; **16**(4): 212–19.

64. **Spielberger L.** *STAI Manual.* Palo Alto: Psychologists Consultants Press; 1983.

65. **Gift AG.** Psychologic and physiologic aspects of acute dyspnea in asthmatics. *Heart and Lung* 1990; **19**(3): 252–7.

66. **Leidy NK, Rennard SI, Schmier J, Jones MK, Goldman M.** The breathlessness, cough, and sputum scale: the development of empirically based guidelines for interpretation. *Chest* 2003; **124**(6): 2182–91.

67. **Leidy NK, Schmier JK, Jones MK, Lloyd J, Rocchiccioli K.** Evaluating symptoms in chronic obstructive pulmonary disease: validation of the Breathlessness, Cough and Sputum Scale. *Respir Med* 2003; **97**(Suppl A): S59–70.

68. **Mahler DA, Wells CK.** Evaluation of clinical methods for rating dyspnea. *Chest* 1988; **93**(3): 580–6.

69. **Mahler DA, Rosiello RA, Harver A, Lentine T, McGovern JF, Daubenspeck JA.** Comparison of clinical dyspnea ratings and psychophysical measurements of respiratory sensation in obstructive airway disease. *American Review of Respiratory Disease* 1987; **135**(6): 1229–33.

70. **ATS/ERS.** Standards for the disgnosis and treatment of patients with COPD: a summary of of the ATS/ERS position paper. *Eur Respir J* 2004; **23**: 932–46.

71. Bestall JC, Paul EA, Garrod R, Garnham R, Jones PW, Wedzicha JA. Usefulness of the Medical Research Council (MRC) dyspnoea scale as a measure of disability in patients with chronic obstructive pulmonary disease. *Thorax* 1999; **54**(7): 581–6.

72. Hajiro T, Nishimura K, Tsukino M, Ikeda A, Oga A, Izumi T. A comparison of the level of dyspnea vs. disease severity in indicating the health-related quality of life of patients with COPD. *Chest* 1999; **116**: 1632–7.

73. McGavin CR, Artvinli M, Naoe H, McHardy GJR. Dyspnoea, disability and distance walked: comparison of estimates of exercise performance in respiratory disease. *BMJ* 1978; **2**: 241–3.

74. O'Donnell DE, McGuire M, Samis L, Webb KA. The impact of exercise reconditioning on breathlessness in severe chronic airflow limitation. *Am J Respir Crit Care Med* 1995: 2005–13.

75. Reardon J, Awad E, Normandin E, Vale F, Clark B, ZuWallack RL. The effect of comprehensive outpatient pulmonary rehabilitation on dyspnea. *Chest* 1994; **105**(4): 1046–52.

76. Harver A, Mahler DA, Daubenspeck JA. Targeted inspiratory muscle training improves respiratory muscle function and reduces dyspnea in patients wth chronic obstructive pulmonary disease. *Annals of Internal Medicine* 1989; **111**(2): 117–24.

77. Mahler DA, Matthay RA, Snyder PE, Wells CK, Loke J. Sustained-release theophylline reduces dyspnea in nonreversible obstructive airway disease. *American Review of Respiratory Disease* 1985; **131**: 22–5.

78. Mahler DA, Tomlinson D, Olmstead EM, Tosteson AN, O'Connor GT. Changes in dyspnea, health status, and lung function in chronic airway disease. *Am J Respir Crit Care Med* 1995; **151**(1): 61–5.

79. Mahler DA, Ward J, Fierro-Carrion G, Waterman LA, Lentine TF, Mejia-Alfaro R, *et al.* Development of self-administered versions of modified baseline and transition dyspnea indexes in COPD. *COPD: Journal of Chronic Obstructive Pulmonary Disease* 2004; **1**(2): 165–72.

80. Lareau SC, Meek PM, Roos PJ. Development and testing of the modified version of the pulmonary functional status and dyspnea questionnaire (PFSDQ-M). *Heart and Lung* 1998; **27**(3): 159–68.

81. Eakin E, Sassi-Dambron D, Ries A, Kaplan R. Reliability and validity of dyspnea measures in patients with obstructive lung disease. *Int J of Behav Med* 1995; **2**: 118–34.

82. Ries AL, Kaplan RM, Limberg TM, Prewitt LM. Effects of pulmonary rehabilitation on physiologic and psychosocial outcomes in patients with chronic obstructive pulmonary disease. *Ann Intern Med* 1995; **122**(11): 823–32.

83. Weaver TE, Richmond TS, Narsavage GL. An explanatory model of functional status in chronic obstructive pulmonary disease. *Nursing Research* 1997;**46**: 26.

84. Weaver TE, Narsavage GL. Physiological and psychological variables related to functional status in COPD. *Nursing Research* 1992; **43**: 286–91.

85. Normandin EA, McCusker C, Connors M, Vale F, Gerardi D, ZuWallack RL. An evaluation of two approaches to exercise conditioning in pulmonary rehabilitation. *Chest* 2002; **121**(4): 1085–91.

86. Tanaka K, Akechi T, Okuyama T, Nishiwaki Y, Uchitomi Y. Development and validation of the Cancer Dyspnea Scale: a multidimensional, brief, self-raing scale. *British Journal of Cancer* 2000; **82**: 800–05.

87. Guyatt GH, King DR, Feeny DH, Stubbing D, Goldstein RS. Generic and specific measurement of health-related quality of life in a clinical trial of respiratory rehabilitation. *Journal of Clinical Epidemiology* 1999; **52**(3): 187–92.

88. Stulbarg MS, Carrieri-Kohlman V, Demir-Deviren S, Nguyen HQ, Adams L, Tsang AH, *et al.* Exercise training improves outcomes of a dyspnea self-management program. *J Cardiopulm Rehabil* 2002; **22**(2): 109–21.

89. Wijkstra PJ, TenVergert EM, Van Altena R, Otten V, Postma DS, Kraan J, *et al.* Reliability and validity of the chronic respiratory questionnaire (CRQ). *Thorax* 1994; **49**(5): 465–7.

90. Guyatt GH, Townsend M, Pugsley SO, Keller JL, Short HD, Taylor DW, *et al.* Bronchodilators in chronic air-flow limitation: Effects on airway function, exercise capacity, and quality of life. *American Review of Respiratory Disease* 1987; **135**: 1069–74.

91. Jaeschke R, Singer J, Guyatt GH. Measurement of health status. Ascertaining the minimal clinically important difference. *Controlled Clin Trials* 1989; **10**(4): 407–15.

92. Jones PW, Quirk FH, Baveystock CM. The St George's Respiratory Questionnaire. *Respiratory Medicine* 1991; 85 Suppl B: 25–31; discussion 33–7.

93. Jones PW, Quirk FH, Baveystock CM, Littlejohns P. A self-complete measure of health status for chronic airflow limitation. The St. George's Respiratory Questionnaire. *American Review of Respiratory Disease* 1992; **145**(6): 1321–7.

94. Jones PW, Bosh TK. Quality of life changes in COPD patients treated with salmeterol. *American Journal of Respiratory and Critical Care Medicine* 1997; **155**(4): 1283–9.

95. Jones PW. Quality of life measurement for patients with diseases of the airways. *Thorax* 1991; **46**(9): 676–82.

3

Breathlessness in heart failure

David P. Dutka and Miriam J. Johnson

Introduction

Breathlessness is the cardinal symptom of heart failure. Its importance is highlighted by the fact that the severity of dyspnoea forms the basis of the New York Heart Association functional classification for heart failure. This has stood the test of time and continues to inform prognosis independently of left ventricular function. Despite the prognosis being as poor as certain types of cancer, heart failure is only recently spoken of as a terminal illness, and its sufferers being in need of palliative care.

It is appropriate to begin the discussion of breathlessness in heart failure by defining the clinical syndrome. This is not, however, a simple task and whereas the usual definitions focus on the limitations of the heart to act as a pump, it is clear that there is much more to the clinical syndrome of heart failure than just the impaired ability of the heart to pump blood from the veins to the arteries following oxygenation in the lungs. Although the haemodynamic disorders are important, abnormalities of other organs often dominate the clinical picture. For example, an increase in the volume of blood within the pulmonary circulation secondary to a decline in left ventricular performance results in both an increase in the work associated with breathing, and shortness of breath secondary to a reduction in the efficiency of the lungs. The fatigue and lethargy experienced by patients with significant heart failure, and which is initiated by the reduction in cardiac output, results in skeletal muscle myopathy that contributes not only to the exercise limitation of such patients but also to their dyspnoea. A number of vicious cycles result from the decline in cardiac output and the natural history of heart failure tends to be punctuated by periods of exacerbation as the balance between the compensatory and deleterious responses to the fall in cardiac output change.

Symptomatic heart failure is now thought to affect approximately 1–1.5 per cent of the population in developed countries, with a similar number having asymptomatic left ventricular dysfunction at echocardiography or other assessment of left ventricular function. The prevalence rises with age and abnormalities of left ventricular systolic function may be as high as 10 per cent in those over 80 years of age. Symptomatic limitation is central to the assessment of patients with heart failure. The New York Heart Association functional classification has stood the test of time and offers prognostic information independently of left ventricular function.[1] Breathlessness is a major factor limiting patients with heart failure and healthcare workers need to be aware of ways to alleviate this distressing symptom. This chapter will discuss both the pathophysiology of breathlessness in heart failure, and palliative clinical management options.

Clinical definition of heart failure

The traditional definition of heart failure has emphasized the clinical signs and symptoms that arise when the pump cannot satisfy the needs of the body, such as the dyspnoea and fatigue, although these do not relate to the heart itself. An alternative is that heart failure is a clinical syndrome in which heart disease reduces cardiac output and results in volume expansion, increased venous pressure and molecular abnormalities that cause progressive deterioration of the failing heart and premature myocardial cell death.[2,3] Increased understanding of the pathophysiological basis of heart failure is now directing therapy to optimize cardiac function. It should be remembered that even in the 1950s the clinical manifestations of heart failure were considered by many to be due largely to disordered renal function with consequent salt and water accumulation rather than a primary reduction in cardiac output. The availability of techniques such as echocardiography has enabled the signs and symptoms to be attributed to specific cardiac abnormalities. Heart failure is a complex clinical syndrome resulting from a variety of causes including coronary artery disease, hypertension, valvular disorders and cardiomyopathy. The following provides a summary of a more complex view:

- The failing heart causes a reduction of cardiac output and increase in venous pressure.
- This is accompanied by maladaptive responses leading to a vicious cycle of salt and water retention, skeletal muscle changes, and molecular and neurohormonal abnormalities.
- These abnormalities cause progressive deterioration of the failing heart, and premature myocardial cell death.
- As the condition worsens, these abnormalities also cause damage to other vital organs such as the kidneys, lungs and liver.
- There is a markedly impaired prognosis punctuated by significant periods of increased morbidity and a reduction in quality of life.

The failing heart

The human heart is not one pump, but two pumps arranged in series; the right and left ventricles. In the absence of a shunt, if less blood is pumped by one ventricle, less blood returns to the other. Reduced performance by either ventricle can modify the function of the other ventricle through the shared ventricular septum and through the pericardium. A heart that ejects poorly during systole does not fill normally during diastole and impaired filling results in impaired ejection. A vicious cycle is thereby established with increasing end-diastolic pressure and wall stress leading to not only ventricular dilatation but also afterload with an alteration in both systemic and pulmonary vascular resistance. It is now appreciated that the resultant neurohormonal activation is not only very important but also complex, and is now regarded as responsible for many of the clinical features seen in patients with advanced cardiac failure.[4-7] In response to a fall in cardiac output, neurohormonal activation results in an increase in ejection fraction, an increased capacity of the heart to fill during diastole, an increase in heart rate, and an increase in vascular resistance through constriction of both arteries and veins. In addition, blood volume is expanded through salt and water retention by the kidneys. In patients with a reduced cardiac output the precise balance between systolic and diastolic dysfunction is often difficult to determine and indeed neither can occur in isolation. It is important to appreciate that heart failure involves not only abnormalities of myocardial contraction but relaxation that is also an active and energy-consuming process. The external work done by the heart to eject blood under pressure into the great vessels accounts for only approximately one-fifth of the energy consumed by the heart and the majority is required to facilitate internal work that is performed in stretching elastic and viscous elements in the wall of the myocardium, particularly during diastole, and the biochemical reactions involved in such processes such as oxidative phosphorylation, excitation contraction, coupling and relaxation.

The failing heart and the lungs

In health, there is a linear increase in pulmonary blood flow from the apex to the base of the lung. An increase in left atrial pressure results in pulmonary venous hypertension, and a more uniform distribution of blood flow in the lungs,[8] via capillary distension and recruitment.[9] A modest elevation in pulmonary capillary wedge pressure can therefore be accommodated, without the development of pulmonary oedema. As left ventricular end-diastolic pressure increases, the rise in capillary hydrostatic pressure favours oedema formation in the interstitial compartment removed from the critical gas-exchanging regions thereby preserving gas exchange.[10–11] Vascular re-modelling therefore protects against the development of pulmonary oedema although patients may present later in the natural history of the disease with pulmonary oedema that represents a medical emergency.

Changes in skeletal muscle

The shortness of breath reported by patients with left ventricular dysfunction is due in large part to the increased work required to ventilate the congested lungs, which are stiffer and inelastic as a result of the increased blood volume within them. In health the work of breathing is barely perceived, but the elevation of left atrial and pulmonary venous pressure increases the respiratory effort required and the resulting difficulty in breathing is compounded by the weakness of the respiratory muscle.

Skeletal muscle exhibits histological and biochemical abnormalities in the patient with chronic heart failure and these changes develop early in the natural history of the condition leading to decreased muscle bulk and strength. The traditional view that fatigue is due to poorly perfused muscle is challenged in that patients can have abnormal muscles, but relatively normal blood flow. The 'muscle hypothesis' proposes a neural link – the ergoreflex, which connects ventilatory response to exercising muscle. The abnormal muscle results in an abnormally increased ventilatory response to a given exercise. The ergoreflex is enhanced in patients with chronic heart failure, causes increased sympathetic activity, and can be partially reduced by training.

Changes in pulmonary haemodynamics

In health the capillary endothelium and alveolar epithelium are attenuated, basement membranes are fused, and complex epithelial junctions exist such that oxygen transfer is optimized. As left ventricular function declines fluid accumulates in the interstitial compartment although lymphatic drainage is highly recruitable in humans and can increase clearance of lung water up to tenfold. The accumulation of interstitial fluid results in disruption of some or all layers of the alveolar capillary unit by the elevated capillary hydrostatic pressure and has been termed capillary stress failure. In humans, where the lungs have been subjected to chronically elevated pulmonary venous pressure, the capillary endothelial and alveolar epithelium basement membranes are thickened on electron microscopy; whilst these changes protect the alveoli by reducing the permeability of the alveolar capillary membrane to water, they impair gas exchange and result in dyspnoea.

Changes in pulmonary function

The administration of a diuretic, even to healthy subjects, suggests that pulmonary function is influenced to a considerable degree by the water content of the lung.[12] In patients with radiological evidence of pulmonary venous hypertension, the mechanical and gas exchanging properties of the lung are both limited. In a study of ten non-smoking patients with asymptomatic left ventricular dysfunction, volume loading with saline provoked airflow obstruction and a decrease in the alveolar capillary membrane conductance (DM),[13] and a similar obstructive defect has been described in patients with decompensated heart failure.[14] Diuretic treatment to reduce lung water improves spirometry and improves the FEV1 to FVC ratio although the effect on lung compliance has been more controversial.[15] Frank airway obstruction is uncommon in heart failure, although the syndrome of cardiac asthma associated with an increase in lung water and pulmonary oedema is well recognized clinically.[16–18]

Changes in the alveolar capillary membrane and gas exchange

The failing heart challenges the integrity of the lung capillaries by at least two factors: increased pressure and increased volume within the alveolar vasculature. The thickness of the alveolar capillary membrane is significantly increased in chronic heart failure mainly due to the deposition of collagen.[19,20] Similar findings have been reported in patients with mitral stenosis[21] and pulmonary venous hypertension.[22] Overall the anatomic changes that take place in the alveolar capillary unit lead to an increase resistance across the membrane and impaired gas transfer[23] that is inversely related to its diffusing capacity for carbon monoxide (DLCO). A reduction in DLCO may arise from a decrease in capillary blood volume or haemoglobin, or from an increase in the resistance of the alveolar capillary membrane to such diffusion. DLCO is commonly reduced in patients with severe heart failure and is unrelated to lung volume or the duration of heart failure.[24–27] A crucial question is whether these structural changes are the only reason for the excessive gas exchange impedance that occurs in patients with chronic heart failure or whether local, hormonal, cytotoxic or possibly even genetic factors impair alveolar fluid clearance and modify alveolar capillary membrane permeability. A number of putative neuroendocrine factors have been considered, including angiotensin II which promotes inappropriate apoptotic alveolar epithelial cell death[28] and also norepinephrine which induces alveolar epithelial apoptosis via a combination of alpha and beta adrenoreceptor stimulation.[29] Cytokines, in particular tumour necrosis factor alpha, have also been observed to alter the permeability of the membrane and to modify transalveolar fluid transport during hypoxia.[30,31]

An increase in the distance between the alveolar and capillary membranes will result in a change in diffusion capacity for carbon monoxide and in the alveolar capillary membrane conductance (DM). A reduction in DLCO that is proportional to the severity of symptomatic limitation in patients with chronic heart failure has been reported and the reduction is specifically dependent of the worsening of the DM component rather than changes in capillary blood volume.[13] A number of studies have emphasized that gas diffusion is impaired as a result of the reduction of global lung perfusion and in DM, that DM at rest and the relative changes during exercise strongly correlate with peak VO2 and that the DLCO is lower in patients with heart failure than in healthy subjects after maximal exercise.[32] Data from patients who have undergone cardiac transplantation suggest the reduction in membrane conduction may not be fully reversible.[33]

Heart failure and breathlessness

Fatigue and breathlessness on exertion are the key symptoms of heart failure, even in compensated and optimally treated patients. Although the mechanisms responsible for exercise intolerance are incompletely understood, cardiopulmonary exercise testing has facilitated the further understanding of a number of characteristic abnormalities. The reduction in exercise capacity may occur in patients with cardiac disease of any cause that compromises cardiac performance and is expressed as a reduction in peak oxygen uptake. This abnormality is not specific or diagnostic but the magnitude of the abnormality is of considerable prognostic importance and serves as a means of selecting and identifying patients for heart transplantation. Chronic heart failure is associated with an abnormally elevated ratio of ventilation to carbon dioxide production, and several factors including an early onset of metabolic acidosis during exercise contribute to an alteration in ventilatory equivalent for carbon dioxide on exercise.[34] The poor pulmonary perfusion associated with a reduced right ventricular performance may increase the dead space of the lungs disproportionately and again compromise efficient gas exchange.[35] Other abnormalities that contribute to the exercise intolerance of patients with chronic heart failure include pulmonary congestion which reduces the compliance of the lung, increases the work of breathing as discussed above, and also results in inefficiencies of gas exchange. However, despite all the above significant exertional arterial desaturation is uncommon in patients with heart failure (as opposed to patients with significant lung disease) and there is little evidence to support the hypothesis that hypoxia is the primary limiting factor. In addition, a variety of functional, metabolic and histological abnormalities have been described in both the peripheral and respiratory muscles of patients with heart failure and these may contribute to exercise intolerance.[23,36]

The central perception of dyspnoea

In general, an increase in [H+] production occurs at a low workload in patients with heart failure, with an increase in circulating lactate concentration that stimulates ventilation via ergoreceptors. The underlying ventilatory stimulus is, however, complex and whilst there is increased activity in brain stem neurons with exercise, hypoxia, hypercapnia and acidosis there is no clear relationship between these factors and the degree of breathlessness exhibited by the patient. Afferent feedback is incompletely understood and arises from both the lungs and chest wall. The former may contribute little as symptoms persist following lung transplantation (i.e. denervated lungs). The urge to breathe and perception of breathlessness may depend more on changes in the mechanical aspects of respiration increasing the activity of poorly defined central receptors.

Emotion is also important. Dyspnoea is often described as 'air hunger' and the perception of dyspnoea is heightened when patients believe it to be dangerous. This in turn exacerbates the situation and a vicious cycle ensues. Anxiety and depression are increasingly recognized in patients with heart failure.

The management of breathlessness in patients with heart failure

The following discussion assumes that the diagnosis of heart failure has been confirmed and medical therapy optimized. Excess fluid retention should be addressed with diuretics and angiotensin-converting enzyme inhibitors (or angiotensin II receptor antagonists), beta-blockers and spironolactone (or eplerenone) used as appropriate. Nitrates may be used to reduce preload. It is also worth noting that in many cases of advanced heart failure, hypotension and renal dysfunction may limit the use of optimum medical therapy and a compromise should be accepted. Symptomatic relief may become paramount, and it is not unusual for the patient to sacrifice the potential prognostic benefits of therapy for the short-term gain of reduced pulmonary and peripheral oedema.

Assessment

The cornerstone of any symptom control is assessment. It is easy, when faced with a distressed breathless patient to miss reversible factors. Coexistent pulmonary pathology such as chronic obstructive pulmonary disease (COPD) and asthma may be the main cause of the breathlessness, and the heart failure only a small component. There may be a chest infection that has either triggered acute decompensated heart failure, or is itself the prime cause of breathlessness. An intractable pleural effusion may be due to the failure, and require drainage, or it may signal another pathology such as bronchial carcinoma. Ascites and an engorged liver may restrict diaphragmatic movement.

General measures

Non-pharmacological techniques for managing breathlessness are described elsewhere in the book and are not discussed here. Although developed primarily in the field of COPD and lung cancer, the benefits seem to be transferable. It is always worth paying attention to seemingly small details of care: anecdotally, persuading elderly patients who have worn restrictive undergarments, such as corsets, for years may help to reduce the severity of breathlessness.

Pharmacological management

Oxygen

Oxygen is often the first treatment to be thought of by both patients and staff when faced with breathlessness and is well-established in the management of acute left heart failure in addition to diuretics and opioids. There is the assumption that it is also beneficial in chronic heart failure, but this does not fit with the evidence that, if anything, oxygen blood levels are increased in patients with chronic heart failure, and oxygen desaturation during exercise is not typical in compensated patients. There have been no studies specifically looking at the benefits of oxygen on the sensation of breathlessness in severe heart failure, although a few have commented on it as a secondary end-point. The studies are small, and only one randomized and controlled. Moore *et al.* looked at the benefits of 30 per cent and 50 per cent inspired oxygen in exercising 12 patients with heart failure and found that during exercise with oxygen-enriched air there was a significant increase in arterial oxygen saturation, total exercise duration was prolonged, carbon dioxide production was reduced and subjective dyspnoea scores rated lower on a visual analogue scale.[37] However this finding has not been confirmed.[38,39] Restrick, in a similar study, found that although 2 and 4l/min ambulatory oxygen increased resting arterial oxygen saturation compared with air, there was no significant difference in distance walked or perceived breathlessness.[38] Both of these studies were uncontrolled. In a randomized placebo controlled cross-over study of 16 patients, Russell et al. compared 21 per cent and 60 per cent inspired oxygen.[39] There was no reduction in minute ventilation or functional benefit with higher oxygen concentrations. The study did not look at the subjective assessment of breathlessness but did comment on the number of patients stopping because of breathlessness; all patients had the same reason for stopping during both exercise tests.[39]

Patients included in these studies had stable mild to moderate heart failure (NYHA II-III) and patients with unstable heart failure, concurrent respiratory disease or FEV_1 < 70 per cent were excluded. Thus it is difficult to extrapolate these results to patients with severe (NYHA IV) chronic heart failure, or those with unstable disease. Comorbidity with concurrent lung disease is common in many patients with heart failure and there may be some benefit to individual patients of oxygen therapy to symptomatically improve breathlessness. The practicalities of providing ambulatory oxygen should also be remembered in considering cost–benefit balance. Current recommendations therefore do not routinely include oxygen therapy, and decisions need to be made on an individual patient basis.

Opioids

Although morphine has been used for many years to relieve symptoms in acute left ventricular failure or myocardial ischaemia, there is still concern about its use in chronic heart failure by many because of the potential for respiratory depression – although paradoxically this does not appear to be a cause for concern in acute situations sufficient to prevent its use in these circumstances. There is also relatively little published literature supporting its use in chronic disease, and thus opioids tend to be reserved for use in advanced heart failure and may not be considered early in their illness where it could be a useful tool in the management of breathlessness. In chronic stable heart failure, there is only one report of two cases describing the use of nebulized morphine, a study on the effect of a single dose of dihydrocodeine on chemosensitivity and exercise tolerance, a study with the use of diamorphine prior to exercise, and more recently a pilot study using oral morphine for the relief of breathlessness in patients with heart failure.[40–43] This dearth of information about a potential useful palliative therapy has been recognized.[44] The beneficial effect is thought to be mediated through modulating the sensitivity of chemoceptors, rather than to the known minimal haemodynamic effects, or to respiratory depression.

The two single dose studies of diamorphine and dihydrocodeine respectively in patients with chronic heart failure suggest improvement in abnormal ventilatory patterns. The pilot study was a randomized placebo controlled cross-over study of 10 patients with NYHA III/IV symptoms.[43] Patients were recruited from a heart failure clinic and randomized to receive oral morphine or placebo. Patients were given 5mg of morphine four times a day in the active arm, or dose reduced to 2.5mg four times a day if the serum creatinine was greater than 200mcmol/l. Patients with a peak flow less than 150l/min or a serum creatinine greater than 300mcmol/l were excluded. On morphine, median breathlessness score (Visual Analogue Score 0 – 100mm) fell by 23mm (p = 0.022) by day 2, and this improvement was maintained. Sedation scores increased until day 3, reducing on day 4. Four patients reported constipation on morphine compared with one on placebo, but there were no other differences between the two arms in nausea, blood pressure, pulse or respiratory rate. The study concluded that oral morphine gave clinically significant improvement in breathlessness with few side-effects and good tolerability of chronic dosing. However questions remain regarding which patients will benefit, which is the best opioid (morphine is not the best opioid to use in renal failure) and the best regimen. Patients sometimes have fears relating to morphine and good communication skills are required to introduce opioids as a therapeutic option.

Beta-2 agonists

Many patients with heart failure will also have lung disease (asthma or chronic obstructive disease) and may take an inhaled beta-2 agonist. It has been suggested that such therapy might benefit patients with heart failure in the absence of significant lung disease because of the demonstrable increased airways resistance. Witte *et al.* have shown some benefit in breathlessness in 12 patients treated with inhaled salbutamol and the anticholinergic ipratropium (compared with 10 controls).[45] Breathlessness and airways resistance improved as did lung reactance and peak tidal volume during exercise although exercise capacity did not improve. The role of beta-2 agonists remains unclear; the benefits of beta blockade are now well established and should always be used in the absence of contraindications.

Benzodiazepines

The use of anxiolytic drugs, such as benzodiazepines, is another issue that causes concern to some clinicians. This is again due to fears of causing respiratory depression and oxygen desaturation as well as issues around addiction and tolerance. There are also more general concerns regarding the risks of giving sedative drugs to often frail and elderly patients with comorbidities.

Indeed the known increased risk of falling has to be considered. However, there appears little evidence to support the concerns regarding respiratory depression if used with care, and benzodiazepines such as lorazepam (which is also usefully absorbed sublingually for quicker onset of action) may be very useful in counteracting the panic and fear associated with acute episodes of severe breathlessness. It must be remembered that the respiratory depressive effects of opioids and benzodiazepines may be additive. In the light of a poor prognosis the issue of dependence and tolerance is less of an issue than in other patients with chronic anxiety. Depression is under-recognized and treated; careful choice of antidepressant is required due to the potential cardiac toxicity of these drugs. Tricyclics should be avoided and venlafaxine is relatively contra-indicated although selective serotonin reuptake inhibitors such as citalopram appear to be safe and well-tolerated.

Management of fatigue

Management of fatigue and breathlessness should go hand in hand as the two are inextricably linked in heart failure. The fatigue of heart failure is multi-factorial and potentially reversible factors should be sought and treated. Side-effects related to medication including hypokalaemia from loop diuretics, over-diuresis and the tiredness associated with beta-blockade are common. Timing and intensity of diuretic use may impinge on quality of sleep, and exacerbate a common problem contributing to impaired quality of life in patients with heart failure.

Normochromic normocytic anaemia (the so-called anaemia of chronic disease) is common in advanced heart failure and appears to reflect the severity of disease. It is also difficult to treat. Silverburg et al. treated 40 octegenarians with resistant severe heart failure and anaemia (Hb, 12 g/dL) with subcutaneous erythropoietin and intravenous iron.[46] They report a marked improvement in cardiac function, breathlessness, and fatigue, together with a reduction in hospitalisation. The authors suggested that anaemia was itself contributing to the progression of heart failure but more research is required to evaluate the cost effectiveness of such treatment.

Evidence is mounting that low intensity exercise programmes are safe and effective in patients with chronic stable heart failure in terms of improving symptoms of fatigue and breathlessness[47,48] and prognosis.[49] Patients often need reassurance as they may be very wary of inducing dyspnoea during physical exercise, believing it to precipitate further cardiac events. However rehabilitation programmes are an important and too often neglected part of optimal management. Encouraging patients to be more active can be very helpful with reduced social isolation and depression, and a management by a multidisciplinary team may be required to ensure optimum progress. Finally, both the patient and their carers may need time and assistance to adjust to their limitations and access provided to professionals with experience in simple cognitive behavioural techniques to promote problem solving and psychological self-help.

Factors contributing to dyspnoea in patients with heart failure

- Skeletal muscle changes leading to reduced muscle bulk (including respiratory muscles) and exaggerated ergoreflex. The increased stiffness of the lungs increases the work of breathing
- Increased arterial chemoceptor sensitivity
- These first two aspects contribute to an abnormal ventilatory response; there is an objective increase in ventilation for a given amount of carbon dioxide production. The degree of increase correlates with the severity of exercise limitation
- Increased anatomical dead space (oropharynx, trachea and bronchi) ventilation due to raised respiratory rates.
- Increased physiological dead space ventilation due to reduction of apical perfusion
- Airflow obstruction and wheezing in a setting of acute pulmonary oedema is well recognized clinically.[13,50] Some patients with left ventricular dysfunction exhibit an increase in bronchial responsiveness following Methacoline[51,52] but this finding has not been universal and the significance of these reports remain unclear[53–56]
- Diffusion abnormalities at the gas/air interface
- Anxiety and depression aggravating ventilatory abnormalities and perception of breathlessness
- Splinting of the diaphragm in the presence of significant ascites.

Summary

The aetiology of breathlessness in chronic heart failure is complex and poorly understood. The management of this troublesome symptom rests upon thorough assessment, attention to any reversible factors and palliation of any that are irreversible. Non-pharmacological approaches developed in non-cardiac breathlessness appear to be transferable, and exercise programmes look promising as a means of improving symptoms by maintaining and improving muscle bulk and making a contribution to improved morale. There is little published evidence on the use of opioids, but what there is indicates that they may be useful and that further research is justified and needed.

There needs to be more widespread acceptance that heart failure is a progressive and life-shortening condition, and a palliative care approach taking into account physical, psychological, social and spiritual factors should be implemented. In order to achieve this cardiology teams need to work closely with palliative care and primary (community) care to make use of resources and services such as hospice day centres, district/community nurses and psychosocial support for carers. Just as the concept of 'total pain', described by Dame Cicely Saunders, has altered the management of cancer pain, so the concept of 'total breathlessness' needs to permeate into cardiology and other clinics.

References

1. Rickenbacher PR, Trindade PT, Haywood GA, Vagelos RH, Schroeder JS, Willson K *et al.* Transplant candidates with severe left ventricular dysfunction managed with medical treatment: characteristics and survival. *J Am Coll Cardiol* 1996; 27(5): 1192–7.

2. Katz AM. Evolving concepts of heart failure: cooling furnace, malfunctioning pump, enlarging muscle. Part II: Hypertrophy and dilatation of the failing heart. *J Card Fail* 1998; 4(1): 67–81.

3. Katz AM. Evolving concepts of heart failure: cooling furnace, malfunctioning pump, enlarging muscle. Part I. *J Card Fail* 1997; 3(4): 319–34.

4. Hasking GJ, Esler MD, Jennings GL, Dewar E, Lambert G. Norepinephrine spillover to plasma during steady-state supine bicycle exercise. Comparison of patients with congestive heart failure and normal subjects. *Circulation* 1988; 78: 516–21.

5. Remes J, Tikkanen I, Fyhrquist F, Pyorala K. Neuroendocrine activity in untreated heart failure. *Br Heart J* 1991; 65 (5): 249–55.

6. Swedberg K, Eneroth P, Kjekshus J, Wilhelmsen L. Hormones regulating cardiovascular function in patients with severe congestive heart failure and their relation to mortality. CONSENSUS Trial Study Group. *Circulation* 1990; 82: 1730–6.

7. Sigurdsson A, Amtorp O, Gundersen T, Nilsson B, Remes J, Swedberg K. Neurohormonal activation in patients with mild or moderately severe congestive heart failure and effects of ramipril. The Ramipril Trial Study Group. *Br Heart J* 1994; 72(5): 422–7.

8. West JB, Dollery CT, Naimark A. Distribution of blood flow in isolated lung; relation to vascular and alveolar pressures. *J Appl Physiol* 1964; 19: 713–24.

9. Glazier JB, Hughes JM, Maloney JE, West JB. Measurements of capillary dimensions and blood volume in rapidly frozen lungs. *J Appl Physiol* 1969; 26(1): 65–76.

10. Broaddus VC, Wiener-Kronish JP, Staub NC. Clearance of lung edema into the pleural space of volume-loaded anesthetized sheep. *J Appl Physiol* 1990; 68(6): 2623–30.

11. Broaddus VC, Wiener-Kronish JP, Berthiaume Y, Staub NC. Removal of pleural liquid and protein by lymphatics in awake sheep. *J Appl Physiol* 1988; 64(1): 384–90.

12. Javaheri S, Bosken CH, Lim SP, Dohn MN, Greene NB, Baughman RP. Effects of hypohydration on lung functions in humans. *Am Rev Respir Dis* 1987; 135(3): 597–9.

13. Puri S, Dutka DP, Baker BL, Hughes JM, Cleland JG. Acute saline infusion reduces alveolar-capillary membrane conductance and increases airflow obstruction in patients with left ventricular dysfunction. *Circulation* 1999; **99**(9): 1190–6.

14. Light RW, George RB. Serial pulmonary function in patients with acute heart failure. *Arch Intern Med* 1983; **143**(3): 429–33.

15. Pepine CJ, Wiener L. Relationship of anginal symptoms to lung mechanics during myocardial ischemia. *Circulation* 1972; **46**(5): 863–9.

16. Rhodes KM, Evemy K, Nariman S, Gibson GJ. Relation between severity of mitral valve disease and results of routine lung function tests in non-smokers. *Thorax* 1982; **37**(10): 751–5.

17. Daganou M, Dimopoulou I, Alivizatos PA, Tzelepis GE. Pulmonary function and respiratory muscle strength in chronic heart failure: comparison between ischaemic and idiopathic dilated cardiomyopathy. *Heart* 1999; **81**(6): 618–20.

18. Dimopoulou I, Daganou M, Tsintzas OK, Tzelepis GE. Effects of severity of long-standing congestive heart failure on pulmonary function. *Respir Med* 1998; **92**(12): 1321–5.

19. Mathieu-Costello O, Willford DC, Fu Z, Garden RM, West JB. Pulmonary capillaries are more resistant to stress failure in dogs than in rabbits. *J Appl Physiol* 1995; **79**(3): 908–17.

20. Townsley MI, Fu Z, Mathieu-Costello O, West JB. Pulmonary microvascular permeability. Responses to high vascular pressure after induction of pacing-induced heart failure in dogs. *Circ Res* 1995; **77**(2): 317–25.

21. Kay JM, Edwards FR. Ultrastructure of the alveolar-capillary wall in mitral stenosis. *J Pathol* 1973; **111**(4): 239–45.

22. Smith RC, Burchell HB, Edwards JE. Pathology of the pulmonary vascular tree. IV. Structural changes in the pulmonary vessels in chronic left ventricular failure. *Circulation* 1954; **10**(6): 801–08.

23. Puri S, Baker BL, Dutka DP, Oakley CM, Hughes JM, Cleland JG. Reduced alveolar-capillary membrane diffusing capacity in chronic heart failure. Its pathophysiological relevance and relationship to exercise performance. *Circulation* 1995; **91**: 2769–74.

24. Naum CC, Sciurba FC, Rogers RM. Pulmonary function abnormalities in chronic severe cardiomyopathy preceding cardiac transplantation. *Am Rev Respir Dis* 1992; **145**(6): 1334–8.

25. Assayag P, Benamer H, Aubry P, de PC, Brochet E, Besse S *et al*. Alteration of the alveolar-capillary membrane diffusing capacity in chronic left heart disease. *Am J Cardiol* 1998; **82**(4): 459–64.

26. Davies SW, Bailey J, Keegan J, Balcon R, Rudd RM, Lipkin DP. Reduced pulmonary microvascular permeability in severe chronic left heart failure. *Am Heart J* 1992; **124**(1): 137–42.

27. Wilkinson PD, Keegan J, Davies SW, Bailey J, Rudd RM. Changes in pulmonary microvascular permeability accompanying re-expansion oedema: evidence from dual isotope scintigraphy. *Thorax* 1990; **45**(6): 456–9.

28. Filippatos G, Tilak M, Pinillos H, Uhal BD. Regulation of apoptosis by angiotensin II in the heart and lungs (Review). *Int J Mol Med* 2001; **7**(3): 273–80.

29. Dincer HE, Gangopadhyay N, Wang R, Uhal BD. Norepinephrine induces alveolar epithelial apoptosis mediated by alpha-, beta-, and angiotensin receptor activation. *Am J Physiol Lung Cell Mol Physiol* 2001; **281**(3): L624–30.

30. Hocking DC, Phillips PG, Ferro TJ, Johnson A. Mechanisms of pulmonary edema induced by tumor necrosis factor-alpha. *Circ Res* 1990; **67**(1): 68–77.

31. Fukuda N, Jayr C, Lazrak A, Wang Y, Lucas R, Matalon S *et al.* Mechanisms of TNF-alpha stimulation of amiloride-sensitive sodium transport across alveolar epithelium. *Am J Physiol Lung Cell Mol Physiol* 2001; **280**(6): L1258–65.

32. Guazzi M. Alveolar-capillary membrane dysfunction in heart failure: evidence of a pathophysiologic role. *Chest* 2003; **124**(3): 1090–102.

33. Niset G, Ninane V, Antoine M, Yernault JC. Respiratory dysfunction in congestive heart failure: correction after heart transplantation. *Eur Respir J* 1993. **6**(8): 1197–201.

34. Wasserman K. Diagnosing cardiovascular and lung pathophysiology from exercise gas exchange. *Chest* 1997; **112**(4): 1091–101.

35. Wasserman K, Zhang YY, Gitt A, Belardinelli R, Koike A, Lubarsky L *et al.* Lung function and exercise gas exchange in chronic heart failure. *Circulation* 1997; **96**(7): 2221–7.

36. Maehara K, Riley M, Galassetti P, Barstow TJ, Wasserman K. Effect of hypoxia and carbon monoxide on muscle oxygenation during exercise. *Am J Respir Crit Care Med* 1997; **155**(1): 229–35.

37. Moore DP, Weston AR, Hughes JM, Oakley CM, Cleland JG. Effects of increased inspired oxygen concentrations on exercise performance in chronic heart failure. *Lancet* 1992; **339**(8797): 850–3.

38. Restrick LJ, Davies SW, Noone L, Wedzicha JA. Ambulatory oxygen in chronic heart failure. *Lancet* 1992; **340**(8829): 1192–3.

39. Russell SD, Koshkarian GM, Medinger AE, Carson PE, Higginbotham MB. Lack of effect of increased inspired oxygen concentrations on maximal exercise capacity or ventilation in stable heart failure. *Am J Cardiol* 1999; **84**(12): 1412–16.

40. Farncombe M, Chater S. Case studies outlining use of nebulized morphine for patients with end-stage chronic lung and cardiac disease. *J Pain Sympton Manage* 1993; **8**(4): 221–5.

41. Williams SG, Wright DJ, Marshall P, Reese A, Tzeng BH, Coats AJ *et al.* Safety and potential benefits of low dose diamorphine during exercise in patients with chronic heart failure. *Heart* 2003; **89**(9): 1085–6.

42. Chua TP, Harrington D, Ponikowski P, Webb-Peploe K, Poole-Wilson PA, Coats AJ. Effects of dihydrocodeine on chemosensitivity and exercise tolerance in patients with chronic heart failure. *J Am Coll Cardiol* 1997; **29**(1): 147–52.

43. Johnson MJ, McDonagh TA, Harkness A, McKay SE, Dargie HJ. Morphine for the relief of breathlessness in patients with chronic heart failure–a pilot study. *Eur J Heart Fail* 2002; **4**(6): 753–6.

44. Fischer MD. Chronic heart failure and morphine treatment. *Mayo Clin Proc* 1998; **73**(2): 194.

45. Witte KK, Morice A, Cleland JG, Clark AL. The reversibility of increased airways resistance in chronic heart failure measured by impulse oscillometry. *J Card Fail* 2004; **10**(2): 149–54.

46. Silverberg DS, Wexler D, Blum M, Schwartz D, Keren G, Sheps D *et al.* Effect of correction of anemia with erythropoietin and intravenous iron in resistant heart failure in octogenarians. *Isr Med Assoc J* 2003; **5**(5): 337–9.

47. Beniaminovitz A, Lang CC, LaManca J, Mancini DM. Selective low-level leg muscle training alleviates dyspnea in patients with heart failure. *J Am Coll Cardiol* 2002; **40**(9): 1602–08.

48. McConnell TR, Mandak JS, Sykes JS, Fesniak H, Dasgupta H. Exercise training for heart failure patients improves respiratory muscle endurance, exercise tolerance, breathlessness, and quality of life. *J Cardiopulm Rehabil* 2003; **23**(1): 10–16.

49. Piepoli MF, Davos C, Francis DP, Coats AJ. Exercise training meta-analysis of trials in patients with chronic heart failure (ExTraMATCH). *BMJ* 2004; **328**(7433): 189.

50. Snashall PD, Chung KF. Airway obstruction and bronchial hyperresponsiveness in left ventricular failure and mitral stenosis. *Am Rev Respir Dis* 1991; **144**(4): 945–56.

51. Cabanes LR, Weber SN, Matran R, Regnard J, Richard MO, Degeorges ME *et al.* Bronchial hyperresponsiveness to methacholine in patients with impaired left ventricular function. *N Engl J Med* 1989; **320**(20): 1317–22.

52. Eichacker PQ, Seidelman MJ, Rothstein MS, LeJemtel T. Methacholine bronchial reactivity testing in patients with chronic congestive heart failure. *Chest* 1988; **93**(2): 336–8.

53. Evans SA, Kinnear WJ, Watson L, Hawkins M, Cowley AJ, Johnston ID. Breathlessness and exercise capacity in heart failure: the role of bronchial obstruction and responsiveness. *Int J Cardiol* 1996; **57**(3): 233–40.

54. Nishimura Y, Maeda H, Hashimoto A, Tanaka K, Yokoyama M. Relationship between bronchial hyperreactivity and symptoms of cardiac asthma in patients with non-valvular left ventricular failure. *Jpn Circ J* 1996; **60**(12): 933–9.

55. Chua TP, Lalloo UG, Worsdell MY, Kharitonov S, Chung KF, Coats AJ. Airway and cough responsiveness and exhaled nitric oxide in non-smoking patients with stable chronic heart failure. *Heart* 1996; **76**(2): 144–9.

56. Cabanes LR, Weber SN, Matran R, Regnard J, Richard MO, Degeorges ME *et al.* Bronchial hyperresponsiveness to methacholine in patients with impaired left ventricular function. *N Engl J Med* 1989; **320**(20): 1317–22.

4

Dyspnea in chronic obstructive pulmonary disorder

Michelle M. Peters and Denis E. O'Donnell

Dyspnea, the perception of respiratory discomfort, is the primary symptom of chronic obstructive pulmonary disease (COPD) and is an important contributor to the poor quality of life in this population. Dyspnea is the result of a complex interaction of mechanical, physiological, metabolic, neurological, and psychosocial factors. In this chapter, we will briefly consider the pathophysiology of COPD during rest and exercise since this is necessary to understand the origin of the symptom. We will then examine the relationship between dyspnea and the well-described derangements of ventilatory mechanics and gas exchange in COPD. Finally, we will review possible neurophysiological underpinnings of this multidimensional symptom.

Pathophysiology of COPD

COPD is characterized by complex and diverse pathophysiological and clinical manifestations. Persistent inflammation of the small and large airways, the lung parenchyma, and its vasculature occur in highly variable combinations between patients. Expiratory flow limitation is the pathophysiological hallmark of COPD.[1,2] This arises because of intrinsic airway factors that increase airway resistance (i.e. mucosal inflammation/edema, airway remodeling and secretions), and extrinsic airway factors (i.e. reduced airway tethering from emphysema).[1,2] Emphysematous destruction, particularly in patients with diffuse pan-acinar emphysema, also reduces elastic lung recoil and thus, the driving pressure for expiratory flow, further compounding flow limitation (Figure 4.1). Expiratory flow limitation with dynamic collapse of the airways compromises the ability of patients to expel air during both forced and quiet expiration.[2-4] Therefore, during expiration while breathing at rest, many alveolar units continue to empty even after the onset of inspiration. In other words, inspiration begins before expiration is complete and lung volume fails to decline to the natural relaxation volume of the respiratory system at end expiration,

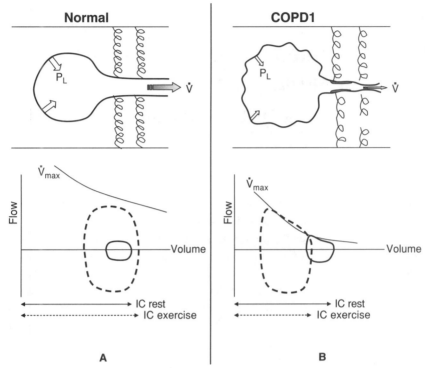

Figure 4.1 Schematic representations of alveolar units in health (A) and in COPD (B). In COPD expiratory flow limitation (EFL) occurs because of the combined effects of increased airway resistance and reduced lung recoil: alveolar emptying is therefore critically dependent on expiratory time, which if insufficiently long, results in lung over-inflation (reduction in IC). The presence of EFL is suggested in COPD by the encroachment of tidal expiratory flows on the forced maximal expiratory flow envelope over the tidal operating lung volume range. In contrast to health, hyperinflation occurs in COPD during exercise as indicated by the shift in EELV to the left (i.e., reduced IC). P_L = lung recoil pressure; V' = flow; V'max = maximal expiratory flow; IC = inspiratory capacity.

resulting in lung hyperinflation. End expiratory lung volume (EELV) is, therefore, significantly larger in people with COPD than in health (Figure 4.2).

When breathing rate acutely increases (and expiratory time diminishes) during exercise there is further dynamic lung hyperinflation (DH) as a result of air trapping. This phenomenon has serious mechanical and sensory consequences. Dynamic hyperinflation results in increased 'elastic' loading of the inspiratory muscles, which are already burdened with increased resistive work. In other words, a COPD patient breathing close to total lung capacity (TLC) must exert a much greater effort to generate a given tidal volume (V_T) than in health.[1] Moreover, acute-on-chronic hyperinflation compromises the ability

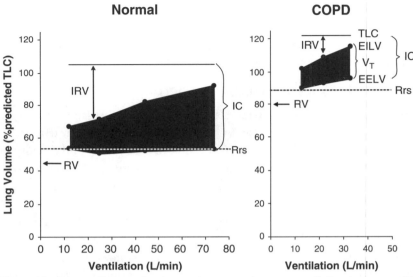

Figure 4.2 Changes in operating lung volumes are shown as ventilation increases with exercise in COPD and in age-matched healthy subjects. End-expiratory lung volume (EELV) increases above the relaxation volume of the respiratory system (Rrs) in COPD, as reflected by a decrease in inspiratory capacity (IC), while EELV in health either remains unchanged or decreases. 'Restrictive' constraints on tidal volume (V_T, solid area) expansion during exercise are significantly greater in the COPD group from both below (increased EELV) and above (reduced IRV as EILV approaches TLC). EILV = end-inspiratory lung volume; IRV = inspiratory reserve volume; AV = residual volume; TLC = total lung capacity.

of the inspiratory muscles, particularly the diaphragm, to increase pressure generation in response to the increased drive to breathe during exercise. Fast breathing rates during exercise, which are associated with early mechanical restriction of tidal volume expansion, rebound to cause even further DH, creating a vicious cycle.[6]

Increased ventilatory demand during exercise

The effects of the mechanical derangements in COPD outlined above are often amplified by concomitantly increased ventilatory demand. The primary stimulus for increased submaximal ventilation is a high physiological deadspace (V_D/V_T) that fails to decline with exercise as a result of worsening ventilation–perfusion abnormalities.[5–8] Other contributing factors are:

1 early metabolic (lactic) acidosis due to deconditioning,
2 critical hypoxemia,

3 high metabolic cost of breathing,
4 lower set points for arterial carbon dioxide ($PaCO_2$), and
5 other sources of ventilatory stimulation (i.e., anxiety and increased sympathetic system stimulation).[5–10]

Gas exchange abnormalities in COPD

Arterial hypoxemia during exercise commonly occurs in patients with severe COPD as a result of shunting and a fall in mixed venous oxygen tension on low ventilation–perfusion lung units.[7–10] In severe COPD, both the ability to increase lung perfusion and to distribute inspired ventilation throughout the lungs during exercise is compromised. In more advanced COPD, arterial hypoxemia during exercise occurs as a result of alveolar hypoventilation.[11,12] An increase in arterial CO_2 during exercise in COPD has been variously attributed to reduced central respiratory drive, altered breathing patterns to minimize respiratory discomfort, excessive inspiratory muscle loading relative to capacity, and inspiratory muscle fatigue.[13–15] The extent of exercise hypercapnia cannot be predicted by measurement of forced expiratory volume ($FEV_{1.0}$), resting $PaCO_2$, V_D/V_T or tests of chemosensitivity.[10–15] Greater dynamic mechanical constraints on the expansion of tidal volume in the setting of a fixed high physiological deadspace, is associated with carbon dioxide retention as VCO_2 increases during exercise.[16]

Mechanisms of dyspnea in COPD
Chemoreceptors

There are both peripheral and centrally located chemoreceptors capable of sensing changes in PaO_2, $PaCO_2$, and pH. These receptors play an important role in the control of breathing. Given that oxygen uptake and excretion of carbon dioxide are among the most important functions of the respiratory system, it would not be unreasonable to assume that dyspnea is the result of increased chemoreceptor activity in the setting of hypoxia or hypercapnia. Indeed, this assumption was prevalent in the early twentieth century. At that time, dyspnea was believed to be the result of one of two processes: 'want of oxygen' and 'carbon dioxide retention'.[17] Numerous studies have demonstrated that healthy subjects report being dyspneic when hypercapnia is experimentally produced.[13,17,18]

Dyspnea and hypercapnia

Hypercapnia is a powerful dyspneogenic stimulus in health.[18–22] Many studies, which have demonstrated a relationship between hypercapnia and dyspnea in health, did not control for the attendant increases in ventilation and respiratory muscle activation. When ventilation and muscle activation are controlled, the results of the research in this area are somewhat contradictory. Campbell et al.[23] observed that patients paralyzed with curare did not complain of air hunger after inhaling carbon dioxide. On the other hand, Banzett et al.,[24] found that patients with high level quadriplegia and almost total respiratory muscle paralysis reported air hunger with increasing levels of carbon dioxide, in the absence of any increase in ventilation. Most recently, Gandevia et al.[25] demonstrated that healthy subjects who were completely paralyzed with high doses of atracurium still reported severe dyspnea in response to a relatively mild hypercapnia change of 4 mmHg. Notwithstanding Campbell's earlier results, it would seem that the existing evidence favors a direct central role for carbon dioxide in the pathogenesis of dyspnea and, in particular, the perception of air hunger.

The role of hypercapnia in dyspnea causation in COPD remains unknown. There is significant overlap in the relationship between arterial carbon dioxide and dyspnea intensity in this population. Patients with advanced COPD often tolerate acute elevation of carbon dioxide to high levels, presumably reflecting effective buffering. Traditionally, patients who retain carbon dioxide are thought to be less breathless than those with a similar forced expiratory volume ($FEV_{1.0}$) who maintain the carbon dioxide in the normal range (i.e., 'pink puffers').[26–34] It remains unclear, however, whether this apparent disparity in symptom intensity is the result of differences in ventilatory mechanics, chemosensitivity or both. The bulk of evidence indicates that even patients with compensated hypercapnic respiratory acidosis have a preserved, or amplified, central respiratory drive when compared with emphysematous patients with normal arterial CO_2.[26–32] Many of the early studies that examined ventilatory responses to carbon dioxide re-breathing in COPD did not specifically measure dyspnea intensity and did not account for the simultaneous changes in mechanics (i.e., dynamic hyperinflation) that were occurring.[26–34] It is possible that mechanical factors, particularly 'high-end mechanics' resulting from dynamic hyperinflation and breathing close to TLC, contribute importantly to respiratory discomfort and that increases in chemical drive merely accentuate the dynamic mechanical abnormalities, which intensifies dyspnea by disrupting neuromechanical coupling. Neuromechanical uncoupling occurs when there is a mismatch or disparity between central drive to breathe and the mechanical response of the respiratory system. Information concerning the latter is instantaneously provided via incoming signals from receptors in the airways, lungs and chest wall.

Dyspnea and hypoxia

The effects of arterial hypoxia on dyspnea are complex and poorly understood.[18,35–39] The response to induced hypoxemia is also quite variable and appears to be closely related to the attendant increases in ventilation. In COPD, the level of arterial oxygen desaturation during activity correlates poorly with the intensity of dyspnea and the responses to supplemental oxygen are highly variable and cannot be predicted from pulmonary function or resting arterial oxygen saturation on room air.[35–41] Critical arterial hypoxemia (PaO_2 <60 mmHg) acutely stimulates peripheral chemoreceptors, whose afferent activity may directly reach consciousness, however the evidence to support this is presently inconclusive. Additionally, the resultant ventilatory stimulation, with increased central motor output and respiratory muscle activation, may contribute to breathing discomfort.[42,43] Hypoxic effects on the cardiac pump and pulmonary vasculature may also have negative sensory consequences that are currently poorly understood.[40,41]

In the exercising subject, the sensory effects of hypoxia are even more complex.[44–46,19–20] Low arterial oxygenation will alter the metabolic milieu and the level of sympathetic activation at the peripheral muscle level and consequently, influence ventilatory and sensory responses during exercise. Hypoxia may contribute to ventilatory muscle fatigue, which would require greater motor activation and effort for a given muscle contraction.[43,22] This perception of heightened inspiratory effort may contribute to respiratory discomfort.[42,43] The relative contribution of these multiple sensory inputs that arise as a consequence of hypoxia is difficult, if not impossible, to determine with precision.

Respiratory mechanoreceptors

Three different classes of sensory receptors have been identified in the lung.[21] Slowly adapting stretch receptors are located principally in large airways and respond to increases in lung volume.[21] Rapidly adapting receptors (also known as irritant receptors) are present in the airway epithelium and respond to a wide range of stimuli, including particulate irritants, direct stimulation of the airways, and pulmonary congestion. Juxtapulmonary (J) receptors (also known as c-fibers) are located throughout the lung and are stimulated by mechanical and chemical stimuli.[21] There have been several attempts to implicate pulmonary receptors, particularly J-receptors, in the sensation of dyspnea. For example, inhaled lidocaine has been shown to reduce breathlessness associated with bronchoconstriction, but not breathlessness caused by external loading.[47] Raj *et al.*[48] injected lobeline (a j-receptor stimulant) into 26 normal subjects, 12 of whom consequently reported a sensation similar to dyspnea.

Almost all of the afferent signals from pulmonary receptors are ultimately carried to the central nervous system (CNS) via the vagus nerve. Several studies have examined the effects of vagal nerve block or vagotomy on respiratory sensation.[49,50] Guz *et al.*[49] found that the dyspnea associated with breath-holding was decreased following injection of lidocaine around both vagus nerves, however, patients were still able to perceive differences in external loading. Several studies attempting to block vagal activity via different methods have shown inconsistent effects on dyspnea associated with pulmonary diseases such as emphysema[50] or interstitial lung disease.[51] The results of the above studies suggest that although peripheral receptors may contribute to the sensation of dyspnea in some situations, they are not involved in all causes of dyspnea.

Afferent information from receptors, located in the chest wall and respiratory muscles, may serve to modulate the perception of dyspnea. Fowler.[52] demonstrated that at the end of breath-holding, being allowed to breathe decreased dyspnea even though the inhaled gas mixture actually caused a further drop in PaO_2 and rise in $PaCO_2$. In patients with chronic lung disease, the application of vibration to the inspiratory intercostals during inspiration and the expiratory intercostals during expiration decreased resting dyspnea[53] Conversely, voluntarily limiting chest wall movement has been shown to increase the dyspnea associated with hypercapnia.[54]

Respiratory muscles and effort

Several investigators have suggested that dyspnea may reflect greater respiratory muscle activity or effort and that the sensation of dyspnea arises from awareness of the efferent motor command from the central nervous system to the respiratory muscles.[43] It has been hypothesized that this awareness arises from a corollary discharge from respiratory neurons in the brainstem and motor cortex, to the sensory cortex. The sense of muscle effort reflects the magnitude of this corollary discharge and is dependent not only on the absolute magnitude of the load, but also on the relative magnitude of the load compared to the maximum capacity of the muscle.[25,42,43] For example, the act of moving a light load may be perceived as requiring significant effort if muscle weakness is present. With regards to the respiratory muscles, inspiratory effort is proportional to the intrathoracic pressures generated during tidal breathing (which can be measured by esophageal balloon) and the peak pressures generated during a maximum inspiratory effort. This can be expressed as a ratio ($Pes : Pi_{max}$).

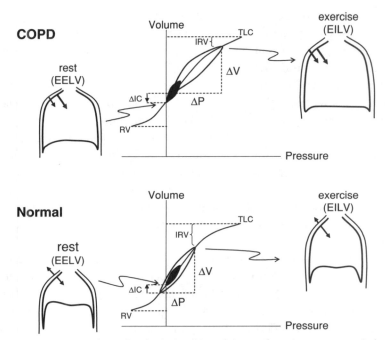

Figure 4.3 Pressure–volume (P–V) relationships of the total respiratory system in health and in COPD. Tidal pressure–volume curves during rest (filled area) and exercise (open area) are shown. Note that in COPD, because of resting and dynamic hyperinflation (a further decreased IC), exercise tidal volume (V_T) encroaches on the upper, alinear extreme of the respiratory system's P-V curve where there is increased elastic loading. In COPD the ability to further expand V_T is reduced, i.e., inspiratory reserve volume (IRV) is diminished. In contrast to health, the combined recoil pressure of the lungs and chest wall in hyperinflated patients with COPD is inwardly directed during both rest and exercise: this results in an inspiratory threshold load (ITL) on the inspiratory muscles.

Patients with a wide variety of lung diseases experience dyspnea, which can be attributed, in part, to increased effort of breathing.[60] Obstructive lung diseases, interstitial lung diseases and pulmonary vascular diseases are all associated with (varying degrees of) increased physiologic dead space (V_D/V_T). Consequently, greater ventilation (and greater respiratory effort) is required to maintain adequate gas exchange. Altered lung mechanics are also important contributors to respiratory workload in COPD. Patients with obstructive lung disease are predisposed to hyperinflation. Further acute-on-chronic DH will force ventilation to occur at a less compliant region of the pressure-volume curve and reduce inspiratory muscle strength (Pi_{max}), both of which will increase respiratory muscle effort (Figure 4.3).

Unfortunately, the perception of respiratory muscle effort is not always synonymous with dyspnea, which as suggested by its definition, has a distressing or uncomfortable aspect. An abundance of studies on respiratory muscle loading have shown that external loads can be sensed, but it is important to acknowledge that this sensation was not universally reported as distressing or uncomfortable.[60] Furthermore, carefully controlled chemoreceptor and mechanoreceptor studies, such as those discussed above,[55] have shown that dyspnea may occur even in the absence of increased respiratory effort.

Neuromechanical dissociation

It is evident from the brief review provided above, that there is no afferent receptor solely responsible for the sensation of dyspnea. It is also clear that awareness of efferent signals (respiratory effort) is also not sufficient for the experience of dyspnea. Several attempts have been made to incorporate both afferent and efferent information into a comprehensive theory of dyspnea.

Campbell and Howell[56] hypothesized that dyspnea was the result of an altered relationship between 'the demand for, and effort of, breathing'. They used the term 'length: tension inappropriateness' to describe this altered relationship. 'Length' actually refers to the change in lung volume, while 'tension' refers to the respiratory muscle tension required to produce that change. According to this hypothesis, conditions whereby increased respiratory muscle activity is required to produce a given amount of ventilation would be expected to produce dyspnea. Schwartzstein et al.[57] expanded Campbell and Howell's original hypothesis by incorporating the concept that dyspnea was the result of a 'dissociation' or discrepancy between the ventilatory drive and the degree of ventilation produced.

The most recent refinement of Campbell and Howell's original hypothesis is termed neuromechanical dissociation.[58] This refinement suggests that the potential sources of the afferent signal included not only the respiratory muscles, but also the multitude of different receptors throughout the respiratory system. In health, there is appropriate coupling (matching) between efferent motor signals and afferent feedback (Figure 4.4). Dyspnea is believed to be the result of the dissociation between amplitudes of the central efferent discharge and afferent sensory inputs (feedback) from peripheral mechanoreceptors. The magnitude of the efferent signal is determined, in part, by metabolic requirements such as carbon dioxide production and oxygen utilization, and by respiratory muscle function (magnitude of efferent signal will increase in presence of respiratory muscle weakness). The afferent signal is an amalgam of sensory information related to respiratory pressures, lung and chest wall motion, and airflow. In the example of interstitial lung disease, the

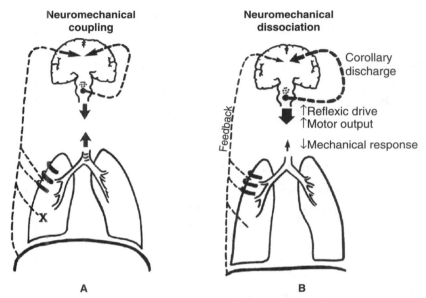

Figure 4.4 In health (A) there is appropriate coupling (matching) between efferent motor signals and afferent feedback. In COPD (B) dyspnea is believed to be the result of the dissociation between amplitudes of the central efferent discharge and afferent sensory inputs (feedback) from peripheral mechanoreceptors. This dissociation becomes amplified during exercise, when there is a further increase in efferent discharge (in response to metabolic demands) without an appropriate afferent response, which is due to the mechanical constraints produced by lung restriction.

source of this dissociation is the derangement of ventilatory mechanics, which arises from decreased lung compliance and, in some cases, expiratory flow limitation.[59] These derangements are associated with a diminished afferent response. Efferent discharge is also greater than normal because increased ventilation is required to ensure adequate removal of carbon dioxide in the setting of increased physiologic dead space. This dissociation becomes amplified during exercise, when there is a further increase in efferent discharge (in response to metabolic demands) without an appropriate afferent response, which is due to the mechanical constraints produced by lung restriction. The concept of neuromechanical dissociation has also proven to be useful in explaining the increased levels of exertional dyspnea observed in COPD and will be discussed below.[60]

The theory of neuromechanical dissociation (NMD) is difficult to prove because we currently lack the ability to accurately measure the amplitude of central drive and afferent inputs from peripheral receptors. A number of studies, however, support the notion that NMD may form the basis, at least in part, for the perception of dyspnea.[60-65] When tidal volume expansion is constrained in healthy humans, either voluntarily or by externally imposed mechanical impedance (e.g., chest wall strapping) in the setting of an increased chemical drive to breathe, severe dyspnea is provoked. Combined chest wall strapping and dead-space loading in healthy subjects during exercise cause intense dyspnea that is qualitatively and quantitatively similar to that experienced by patients with COPD at the peak of exercise i.e., unsatisfied inspiration.[66] Dyspnea intensity during exercise in COPD was found to correlate well with the high ratio of inspiratory muscle effort (measured by esophageal pressure) to tidal volume, which is a crude index of NMD. To the extent that esophageal pressure swings do not reflect the amplitude of neural drive in the setting of abnormal mechanic impedances, the calculated effort : displacement ratio is an underestimation of the true NMD. Relief of dyspnea in COPD patients who adopted a leaning forward position was shown by Sharp et al.[67] to be associated with a more efficient conversion of electrical activation of the diaphragm to force generation by this muscle in this position. Recent studies have demonstrated that exertional dyspnea relief following bronchodilator treatment in COPD was associated with improved dynamic ventilatory mechanics, i.e., increased inspiratory capacity (IC) and increased dynamic inspiratory reserve volume (IRV) (Figure 4.5).[68-71] Pharmacological lung

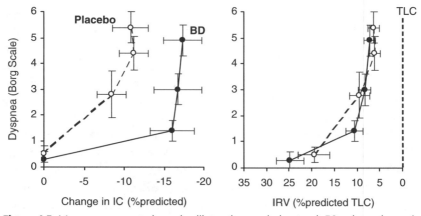

Figure 4.5 Mean responses to bronchodilator therapy (salmeterol, 50 μg) are shown in 10 patients with COPD. Post-bronchodilator (BD), resting inspiratory capacity (IC) increased by 0.40 ± 0.08 L (p = 0.001). Post-BD during exercise, patients were able to tolerate significantly larger decreases in IC before exceeding an IRV 'threshold' (i.e., IRV <20% predicted TLC or <1 L) and developing intolerable dyspnea. Under both conditions, increased dyspnea was closely associated with a reduced IRV. Data from (76).

volume reduction at rest results in a delay in reaching the threshold for intolerable dyspnea during incremental hyperinflation imposed by exercise or by mechanical limitation using an airway closure analog.[68,72] Thus, the dyspnea/IRV relationship during both of these interventions was unaltered by prior bronchodilatation and lung deflation. The reduced resting EELV means a delay in reaching a critically low IRV where NMD approaches the maximal level, thus intolerable dyspnea is delayed.

Relieving dyspnea: a physiological rationale

The NMD theory of dyspnea provides a useful construct for the development of therapeutic strategies in COPD. Thus, interventions that reduce central drive, improve the mechanical/muscular response for a given drive or achieve both these effects in combination should alleviate dyspnea. Opioids, oxygen therapy and exercise training (via reduced metabolic acidosis) all reduce central drive – the reduced ventilatory requirement has salutary effects in mechanically compromised patients.[68–71] Pharmacological and surgical lung volume reduction improves the mechanical response of the respiratory system for a given drive.[72–75,77–80] Combination treatments that both reduce central drive and improve dynamic mechanics should, theoretically, have greater impact on dyspnea but this remains to be studied.

Managing dyspnea in COPD

Recent national guidelines have recommended a dyspnea/disability driven paradigm for managing COPD.[81–83] Thus, therapy is escalated on an individual basis with the goal being maximum possible symptom relief. Education and smoking cessation are the first steps in symptom management (Figure 4.6) and are regarded as one of the best strategies to reduce mortality in COPD patients. Treatment with bronchodilators is another initial approach to therapy as they provide symptomatic relief by improving airway function, enhancing lung emptying, and therefore, reducing lung hyperinflation.[73–75,84] By improving ventilatory mechanics in this manner, a greater ventilatory output can be achieved for a given neural drive (i.e., enhanced neuromechanical coupling). Should patients remain symptomatic in spite of optimized bronchodilator therapy, exercise training, preferably in a supervised setting, is the next important step.[81–83] Exercise training improves peripheral muscle function and reduces ventilatory demand, as well as improving the strength and endurance of the ventilatory muscles.[10,68,85] A reduction in ventilation in flow-limited patients results in attendant decreases in dynamic lung hyperinflation during exercise. Exercise training, therefore, reduces ventilatory drive and improves ventilatory muscle pump function and mechanics, which collectively enhances

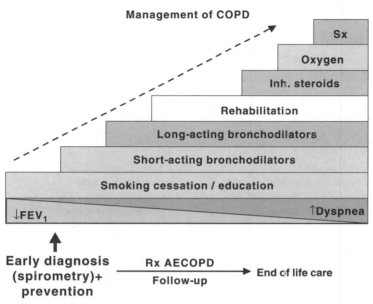

Figure 4.6 A stepwise approach to the management of chronic obstructive pulmonary disease (COPD). As symptoms worsen, there is an escalation of therapy in order to provide the maximum possible symptom relief. FEV1 = Forced expiratory volume in 1 s; Inh = Inhaled; Rx AECOPD = Treatment of acute exacerbations of COPD; Sx = Surgery (lung volume reduction surgery and transplantation).

neuromechanical coupling. For selected individuals, oxygen therapy is an additional consideration. Patients with a resting arterial oxygen of < 55 mmHg or a PaO_2 between 55 and 60 mmHg or who have evidence of pulmonary hypertension or other end organ damage, should receive continuous oxygen. [81–83] Recent studies have confirmed that even normoxic or mildly hypoxic patients benefit from ambulatory oxygen in terms of improved dyspnea and exercise endurance.[44,69–71] Reduced lung hyperinflation, as a result the reduction in ventilatory drive, is an important contributing factor to symptom improvement during oxygen therapy. Oxygen therapy may be a useful dyspnea-relieving intervention in patients with advanced mechanical derangements, but who have relative preservation of gas exchange capabilities.[69–71] Surgical lung volume reduction therapy should be reserved for patients with advanced symptomatic COPD who meet stringent surgical criteria (Table 4.1) and who remain breathless despite maximal bronchodilator therapy and rehabilitation.[77–79,86] In the terminal phases of their illness, opiate therapy is often offered to patients with COPD to ameliorate dyspnea and the associated distress. Reduced ventilatory drive appears to be the main mechanism of benefit during opiate administration.[87]

Table 4.1 Selection criteria for lung volume reduction surgery.

Indications	Contraindications
Disability from emphysema (not from bronchitis or asthma) despite maximal medical treatment	Comorbid disease (i.e. operation prohibitive risk or life expectancy less than 2 years
Age less than 75 to 80 years	Severe obesity or cachexia
Abstinence from smoking more than four months	Severe coronary artery disease
FEV$_1$ <40% predicted	Active smoker
TLC > 120% predicted	Alpha-1 antitrypsin deficiency
RV >175% predicted	Extensive pleural symphysis
Hyperinflation particularly with upper lobe dominance by computed tomography scan (heterogeneous distribution)	Chest wall deformity
	PaCO$_2$ >50 to 60 mmHg
	PAP >35 mmHg (mean)
	FEV$_1$ <20% predicted and homogeneous distribution or D$_L$CO <20% predicted

D$_L$CO = diffusing capacity for carbon monoxide; FEV$_1$ = forced expired volume in 1 second; PaCO$_2$ = partial pressure of arterial carbon dioxide; PAP = pulmonary arterial pressure; RV = residual volume; TLC = total lung capacity. Guidelines from the Canadian Thoracic Society, 2003.

In order to maximize symptom relief in COPD patients, a stepwise individualized approach, which escalates as the disease progresses, is required (Figure 4.6). This integrated and comprehensive approach culminates in meaningful improvements in dyspnea and exercise endurance (Figure 4.7).

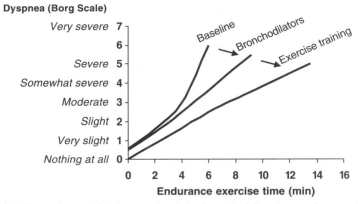

Figure 4.7 Plots of exertional dyspnea intensity (Borg Scale) against endurance time using a constant work rate exercise test illustrate the cumulative effects of a stepwise approach to therapy in (COPD). An integrative approach can provide marked improvements in symptom relief and exercise endurance.

Summary

Our knowledge of the pathophysiological mechanisms of dyspnea in COPD continues to grow. Correlative analysis has shown that the intensity of dyspnea during exercise is closely associated with a number of interrelated physiological variables including the extent of dynamic hyperinflation, ventilation (relative to capacity), inspiratory effort (relative to maximum) and the effort : displacement ratio. The validity of these associations are supported by studies that have shown that dyspnea relief following a number of therapeutic interventions was found to be closely associated with reductions in DH, ventilation and inspiratory effort and an increased ability to expand V_T.

The neurophysiological underpinnings of dyspnea in COPD remain speculative. There is currently little evidence that peripheral sensory afferent inputs from the respiratory system directly give rise to breathing discomfort in COPD. Their primary role appears to be to provide precise, instantaneous, integrated feedback on the dynamic mechanical output of the ventilatory system in relation to neural drive. Similarly, there is inconclusive evidence that acute alterations in chemical stimuli (hypercapnia or hypoxia) directly influence dyspnea intensity, independent of the attendant simultaneous changes in dynamic mechanics and ventilatory muscle activation. The sense of heightened inspiratory effort is pervasive in COPD during exercise and likely contributes to this multidimensional symptom. Finally, the neuromechanical dissociation hypothesis is intuitively appealing and states that exertional dyspnea in COPD is not only a function of the amplitude of central neural drive, but is also importantly modulated by peripheral sensory feedback from multiple mechanoreceptors throughout the respiratory system. Modern pharmacologic and non-pharmacologic interventions effectively ameliorate dyspnea by enhancing neuromechanical coupling, even in patients with advanced COPD.

References

1. **Pride NB, Macklem PT.** Lung mechanics in disease. In: AP Fishman, ed. *Handbook of Physiology*, Section 3, Vol III, Part 2: The Respiratory System, pp. 659–92. American Physiological Society, Bethesda, MD, 1986.
2. **Hyatt RE.** Expiratory flow limitation. *J Appl Physiol* 1983; **55**: 1–8.
3. **O'Donnell DE, Sanii R, Anthonisen NR, Younes M.** The effect of airway dynamic compression on breathing pattern and respiratory sensation in severe chronic obstructive pulmonary disease. *Am Rev Respir Dis* 1987; **135**: 912–18.
4. **Lever DG, Pride NB.** Flow volume curves and expiratory pressures during exercise in patients with chronic airflow obstruction. *Scand J Respir Dis* 1971; **42**(suppl): 23–7.
5. **O'Donnell DE, Webb KA.** Exercise. In: PMA Calverley, W. MacNee, NB Pride, SI Rennard eds *Chronic Obstructive Pulmonary Disease*, London: Arnold pp. 243–69. 2003.

6. O'Donnell DE. Ventilatory limitations in chronic obstructive pulmonary disease. *Med Sci Sports Exer* 2001; **33**: S647–55.

7. Barbera JA, Roca J, Ramirez J, Wagner PD, Usetti P, Rodriquez-Roisin R. Gas exchange during exercise in mild chronic obstructive pulmonary disease: correlation with lung structure. *Am Rev Respir Dis* 1991; **144**: 520–5.

8. Dantzker DR, D'Alonzo GE. The effect of exercise on pulmonary gas exchange in patients with severe chronic obstructive pulmonary disease. *Am Rev Respir Dis* 1986; **134**: 1135–9.

9. Dillard TA, Piantadosi S, Rajagopal KR. Prediction of ventilation at maximal exercise in chronic airflow obstructive. *Am Rev Respir Dis* 1985; **132**: 230–5.

10. O'Donnell DE, McGuire M. Samis L, Webb KA. Effects of general exercise training on ventilatory and peripheral muscle strength and endurance in chronic airflow limitation. *Am J Respir Crit Care Med* 1998; **157**: 1489–97.

11. Begin P, Grassino A. Inspiratory muscle dysfunction and chronic hypercapnia in chronic obstructive pulmonary disease. *Am Rev Respir Dis* 1991; **143**: 905–12.

12. Borrows B, Earle RH. Course and prognosis of chronic obstructive lung disease: a prospective study of 200 patients. *N Engl J Med* 1969; **280**: 397–404.

13. Altose MD, McCauley WC, Kelsen SG, Cherniack NS. Effects of hypercapnia and inspiratory flow-resistive loading on respiratory activity in chronic airways obstruction. *J Clin Invest* 1977; **59**: 500–7.

14. Light RW, Mahutte CK, Brown SE. Etiology of carbon dioxide retention at rest and during exercise in chronic airflow obstruction. *Chest* 1988; **84**: 61–7.

15. DeTroyer A, Leeper JB, McKenzie D, Gandevia S. Neural drive to the diaphragm in patients with severe COPD. *Am J Respir Crit Care Med* 1997; **155**: 1335–40.

16. O'Donnell DE, D'Arsigny C, Fitzpatrick M, Webb KA. Exercise hypercapnia in advanced COPD: The role of lung hyperinflation. (Accompanying editorial by J. Dempsey, 634–5). *Am J Respir Crit Care Med* 2002; **166**: 663–8.

17. Meakins J. The cause and treatment of dyspnoea in cardio-vascular disease. *BMJ* 1923; **1043**: 1045.

18. Adams L, Lane R, Shea SA, Cockroft A, Guz A. Breathlessness during different forms of ventilatory stimulation: a study of mechanisms in normal subjects and respiratory patients. *Clin Sci* 1985; **69**: 663–72.

19. Bledsoe SW, Hornbein TF. Central chemoreceptors and the regulation of their chemical environment. In: TF Hornbein ed. *Regulation of Breathing*, pp. 347–406. Marcel Dekker, New York, 1981.

20. Manning HL, Shea SA, Schwartzstein RM, Lansing RW, Brown R, Banzett RB. Reduced tidal volume increases air 'hunger' at fixed PCO_2 in ventilated quadriplegics. *Respir Physiol* 1992; **90**: 19–30.

21. Zechman FR Jr, Wiley RL. Afferent inputs to breathing: respiratory sensation: In: AP Fishman, ed. *Handbook of Physiology*, pp. 449–74, Section 3, Vol II, Part 2: The Respiratory System. Bethesda, MD: American Physiological Society, 1986.

22. Gandevia SC. The perception of motor commands on effort during muscular paralysis. *Brain* 1982; **105**: 151–95.

23. Campbell EJM, Godfrey S, Clark TJH, Freedman S, Norman J. The effect of muscular paralysis induced by tubocurarine on the duration and sensation of breath-holding during hypercapnia. *Clin Sci* 1969; **36**: 323–8.

24. Banzett RB, Lansing RW, Reid MB, Brown R. 'Air hunger' arising from increasing PCO_2 in mechanically ventilated quadriplegics. *Respir Physiol* 1989; **76**: 53–68.

25. Gandevia SC, Killian K, McKenzie DK, Crawford M, Allen GM, Gorman RB, Hales JP. Respiratory sensations, cardiovascular control, kinaesthesia and transcranial stimulation during paralysis in humans. *J Physiol* 1993; **470**: 85–107.

26. Cherniack RM, Snidal DP. The effect of obstruction to breathing on the ventilatory response to CO_2. *J Clin Invest* 1956; **35**: 1286–90.

27. DeTroyer A, Leeper JB, McKenzie DK, Gandevia SC. Neural drive to the diaphragm in patients with severe COPD. *Am J Respir Crit Care Med* 1997; **155**: 1335–40.

28. Lourenco RV, Miranda JM. Drive and performance of the ventilatory apparatus in chronic obstructive lung disease. *N Engl J Med* 1968; **279**: 53–9.

29. Gorini MD, Spinelli A, Duranti R, Gigliotti F, Scano G. Neural respiratory drive and neuromuscular coupling in patients with chronic obstructive pulmonary disease (COPD). *Chest* 1990; **98**: 1179–86.

30. Scano G, Spinelli A, Duranti R, *et al.* Carbon dioxide responsiveness in COPD patients with and without chronic hypercapnia. *Eur Respir J* 1995; 878–85.

31. Lopata M, Onal E, Cromydas G. Respiratory load compensation in chronic airway obstruction. *J Appl Physiol* 1985; **59**: 1947–54.

32. Costello R, Deegan P, Fitzpatrick M, McNicholas WT. Reversible hypercapnia in chronic obstructive pulmonary disease: a distinct pattern of respiratory failure with a favorable prognosis. *Am J Med* 1997; **102**: 239–44.

33. Gorini M, Misuri G, Corrado A, *et al.* Breathing pattern and carbon dioxide retention in severe chronic obstructive pulmonary disease. *Thorax* 1996; **51**: 677–83.

34. Haluszka J, Chartrand KA, Grassino A, Milic-Emili J. Intrinsic PEEP and arterial PCO_2 in stable patients with chronic obstructive pulmonary disease. *Am Rev Respir Dis* 1990; **141**: 1194–7.

35. Lane R, Adams L, Guz A. The effects of hypoxia and hypercapnia on perceived breathlessness during exercise in humans. *J Physiol (Lond)* 1990; **429**: 579–93.

36. Swinburn CR, Wakefield JM, Jones PW. Relationship between ventilation and breathlessness during exercise in chronic obstructive airways disease is not altered by prevention of hypoxemia. *Clin Sci* 1984; **67**: 515–19.

37. Stein DA, Bradley BL, Miller W. Mechanisms of oxygen effects on exercises in patients with chronic obstructive pulmonary disease. *Chest* 1982; **81**: 6–10.

38. Libby DM, Biscoe WA, King TKC. Relief of hypoxia-related bronchoconstriction by breathing 30 percent oxygen. *Am Rev Respir Dis* 1981; **123**: 171–5.

39. Agusti AGN, Barbera JA, Roca J, Wagner PD, Guitart R, Rodriguez-Roisin R. Hypoxic pulmonary vasoconstriction and gas exchange during exercise in chronic obstructive pulmonary disease. *Chest* 1990; **97**: 268–75.

40. Matthay RA, Berger HJ, Davies RA, *et al.* Right and left ventricular exercise performance in chronic obstructive pulmonary disease: radionuclide assessment. *Ann Int Med* 1980; **93**: 234–9.

41. Mahler DA, Brent BN, Loke J, Zaert BL, Matthay RA. Right ventricular performance and central hemodynamics during upright exercise in patients with chronic obstructive pulmonary disease. *Am Rev Respir Dis* 1984; **130**: 722–9.

42. El-Manshawi A, Killian KJ, Summers E, Jones NL. Breathlessness and exercise with and without resistive loading. *J Appl Physiol* 1986; **61**: 896–905.

43. Gandevia SC, Killian KJ, Campbell EJM. The effect of respiratory muscle fatigue on respiratory sensations. *Clin Sci* 1981; **60**: 463–6.

44. O'Donnell DE, D'Arsigny C, Webb KA. Effects of hyperoxia on ventilatory limitation during exercise in advanced chronic obstructive pulmonary disease. *Am J Respir Crit Care Med* 2001; **163**: 892–8.

45. Webb KA, D'Arsigny C, O'Donnell DE. Exercise response to added oxygen in patients with COPD and variable gas exchange abnormalities. *Am J Respir Crit Care Med* 2001; **163**: A169.
46. Chronos N, Adams L, Guz A. Effect of hyperoxia and hypoxia on exercise-induced breathlessness in normal subjects. *Clin Sci* 1988; **74**: 531–7.
47. Taguchi O, Kikuchi Y, Hida W, Iwase N, Satoh M, Chonan T, Takishima T. Effects of bronchoconstriction and external resistive loading on the sensation of dyspnea. *J Appl Physiol* 1991; **71**: 2183–90.
48. Raj H, Singh VK, Anand A, Paintal AS. Sensory origin of lobeline-induced sensations: a correlative study in man and cat. *J Physiol* 1995; **482**: 235–46.
49. Guz A, Noble MIM, Widdicombe JG, Trenchard D, Mushin WW, Makey AR. The role of vagal and glossopharyngeal afferent nerves in respiratory sensation, control of breathing and arterial pressure regulation in conscious man. *Clin Sci* 1966; **30**: 161–70.
50. Bradley GW, Hale T, Pimble J, Rowlandson R, Noble MIM. Effect of vagotomy on the breathing pattern and exercise ability in emphysematous patients. *Clin Sci* 1982; **62**: 311–19.
51. Winning AJ, Hamilton RD, Guz A. Ventilation and breathlessness on maximal exercise in patients with interstitial lung disease after local anesthetic aerosol inhalation. *Clin Sci* 1988; **74**: 275–81.
52. Fowler WS. Breaking point of breath-holding. *J Appl Physiol* 1954; **6**: 539–45.
53. Sibuya M, Yamada M, Kanamaru A, Tanaka K, Suzuki H, Noguchi E, Altose MD, Homma I. Effect of chest wall vibration on dyspnea in patients with chronic respiratory disease. *Am J Respir Crit Care Med* 1994; **149**: 1235–40.
54. Chonan T, Mulholland MB, Cherniak NS, Altose MD. Effects of voluntary constraining of thoracic displacement during hypercapnia. *J Appl Physiol* 1987; **63**: 1822–8.
55. Banzett RB, Lansing RW, Reid MB, Brown R. 'Air hunger' arising from increasing PCO2 in mechanically ventilated quadriplegics. *Respir Physiol* 1989; **76**: 53–68.
56. Campbell EJM, Howell JBL. The sensation of breathlessness. *Br Med Bull* 1963; **18**: 36–40.
57. Schwartzstein RM, Simon PM, Weiss JW, Fencl V, Weinberger SE. Breathlessness induced by dissociation between ventilation and chemical drive. *Am Rev Respir Dis* 1989; **139**: 1231–7.
58. O'Donnell DE, Webb KA. Exertional breathlessness in patients with chronic airflow limitation: the role of hyperinflation. *Am Rev Respir Dis* 1993; **148**: 1351–7.
59. Marciniuk DD, Sridhar G, Clemens RE, Zintel TA, Gallagher CG. Lung volumes and expiratory flow limitation during exercise in interstitial lung disease. *J Appl Physiol* 1994; **77**: 963–73.
60. O'Donnell DE, Chau LKL, Bertley JC, Webb KA. Qualitative aspects of exertional breathlessness in chronic airflow limitation: pathophysiologic mechanisms. *Am J Respir Crit Care Med* 1997; **155**: 109–15.
61. Fowler WS. Breaking point of breath-holding. *J Appl Physiol* 1954; **6**: 539–45.
62. Xu F, Taylor RF, McLarney T, Lee L-Y, Frazier DT. Respiratory load compensation. 1 Role of the cerebrum. *J Appl Physiol* 1993; **74**: 853–8.
63. Chonan T, Mulholland MB, Cherniack NS, Altose MD. Effect of voluntary constraining of thoracic displacement during hypercapnia. *J Appl Physiol* 1987; **63**: 1822–8.
64. Campbell EJM, Howell JBL. The sensation of breathlessness. *Br Med Bull* 1963; **18**: 36–40.

65. Schwartzstein RM, Simon PM, Weiss JW, Fencl V, Weinberger SE. Breathlessness induced by dissociation between ventilation and chemical drive. *Am Rev Respir Dis* 1989; **139**: 1231–7.

66. O'Donnell DE, Hong HH, Webb KA. Effects of chest wall restriction and deadspace loading on dyspnea and exercise tolerance in healthy normals. *J Appl Physiol* 2000; **88**: 1859–69.

67. Sharp JT, Druz WS, Moisan T, Foster J, Machnach W. Postural relief of dyspnea in severe COPD. *Am Rev Respir Dis* 1980; **122**: 201–11.

68. O'Donnell DE, McGuire M, Samis L, Webb KA. The impact of exercise reconditioning on breathlessness during hyperoxia in chronic airflow limitation. *Am J Respir Crit Care Med* 1995; **152**: 2005–13.

69. O'Donnell DE, Bain DJ, Webb KA. Factors contributing to relief of exertional breathlessness during hyperoxia in chronic airflow limitation. *Am J Respir Crit Care Med* 1997; **155**: 530–5.

70. Light RW, Muro JR, Sato RI, Stansbury DW, Fischer CE, Brown SE. Effects of oral morphine on breathlessness and exercise tolerance in patients with chronic obstructive pulmonary disease. *Am Rev Respir Dis* 1989; **139**: 126–33.

71. Somfy A, Porszasz J, Lee SM, Casaburi R. Dose-response effect of oxygen on hyperinflation and exercise endurance in non-hypoxemic COPD patients. *Eur Respir J* 2001; **18**: 77–84.

72. O'Donnell DE, Voduc N, Fitzpatrick M, Webb KA. Effect of salmeterol on the ventilatory response to exercise in COPD. *Eur Respir J* 2004; **24**: 86–94.

73. O'Donnell DE, Lam M, Webb KA. Spirometric correlates of improvement in exercise performance after anticholinergic therapy in COPD. *Am J Respir Crit Care Med* 1999; **160**: 542–9.

74. Belman MJ, Botnick WC, Shin JW. Inhaled bronchodilators reduce dynamic hyperinflation during exercise in patients with chronic obstructive pulmonary disease. *Am J Respir Crit Care Med* 1996; **153**: 967–75.

75. O'Donnell DE, Fleuge T, Gerken F, Hamilton A, Make B, Magnusson H. Effect of tiotropium on dynamic hyperinflation, dyspnea and exercise tolerance in patients with COPD. *Eur Resp J* 2004; **23**(6): 832–40.

76. O'Donnell DE, Webb KA. Pharmacological volume reduction delays the threshold for intolerable dyspnea during acute hyperinflation in COPD. *Am J Respir Crit Care Med* 2003; **167**(7): A293.

77. Young J, Fry-Smith A, Hyde C. Lung volume reduction surgery (LVRS) for chronic obstructive pulmonary disease (COPD) with underlying severe emphysema. *Thorax* 1999; **54**: 779–89.

78. Martinez FJ, De Oca MM, Whyte RI, Stetz J, Gay SE, Celli BR. Lung-volume reduction improves dyspnea, dynamic hyperinflation, and respiratory muscle function. *Am J Respir Crit Care Med* 1997; **155**: 1984–90.

79. Tschernko EM, Gruber EM, Jaksch P, *et al.* Ventilatory mechanics and gas exchange during exercise before and after lung volume reduction surgery. *Am J Respir Crit Care Med* 1998; **158**: 1424–31.

80. Shade DJ, Cordova F, Lando Y, *et al.* Relationship between resting hypercapnia and physiologic parameters before and after lung volume reduction surgery in severe chronic obstructive pulmonary disease. *Am J Respir Crit Care Med* 1999; **159**: 1405–1.

81. O'Donnell DE, Aaron S, Bourbeau J, *et al.* Canadian Thoracic Society Recommendations for the Management of COPD. *Cdn Resp J* 2003, May–June supplement.

82. Celli BR, MacNee W, *et al.* Standards for the diagnosis and treatment of patients with COPD: A summary of the ATS/ERS position paper. *Eur Resp J* 2004; **23**: 932–46.
83. *Management of Chronic Obstructive Pulmonary Disease in Adults in Primary and Secondary Care.* Clinical Guidelines 12. NHS National Institute for Clinical Excellence; 2004. http://thorax.bmjjournals.comcontent/vo159/suppl_1, www.nice.org.uk/ CG012fullguideline.
84. O'Donnell DE, Forkert L, Webb KA. Evaluation of bronchodilator responses in patients with 'irreversible' emphysema. *Eur Respir J* 2001; **18**: 914–20.
85. Lacasse Y, Wing E, Guyatt GH, King D, Cook DJ, Goldstein RS. Meta-analysis of respiratory rehabilitation in chronic obstructive pulmonary disease. *Lancet* 1996; **348**: 1115–19.
86. Laghi F, Jurban A, Topeli A, Fahey PH, Garrity F Jr, Archids JM, DePinto DJ, Edwards LC, Tobin MJ. Effect of lung volume reduction surgery on neuromechanical coupling of the diaphragm. *Am J Respir Crit Care Med* 1998; **157**: 475–83.
87. Light RW, Muro JR, Sato RI, Stansbury DW, Fischer CE, Brown SE. Effects of oral morphine on breathlessness and exercise tolerance in patients with chronic obstructive pulmonary disease. *Am Rev Respir Dis* 1989; **139**: 126–33.

5

Breathlessness in advanced cancer

Deborah Dudgeon

Introduction

Dyspnea is a very common symptom that is often unrecognized in patients with cancer. Breathlessness can result in significant morbidity with patients experiencing marked impairment in their quality of life. Dyspnea in patients with cancer is typically chronic with most patients experiencing episodes of heightened shortness of breath. This acute breathlessness is often accompanied by anxiety, fear, panic, and a sensation of impending death.[1] Typically breathlessness is triggered by exertion or less commonly by emotion, resulting in patients restricting their activity and isolating themselves socially.[1–3] In a study of late stage cancer patients, Roberts and associates found that 62 per cent of patients with dyspnea had been short of breath for a duration exceeding three months. Various activities intensified breathlessness for these patients: climbing stairs – 95.6 per cent; walking slowly – 47.8 per cent; getting dressed – 52.2 per cent; talking or eating – 56.5 per cent, and at rest – 26.1 per cent. The patients universally responded by decreasing their activity to whatever degree would relieve their shortness of breath. Unfortunately, the majority of the patients had received no direct medical or nursing assistance with their breathlessness, leaving them to cope in isolation.[2] Others have found that dyspnea interfered with not only physical activities but also with patients' mood, relationships, and enjoyment of life.[4] In a study that examined 'will to live' in terminally ill cancer patients, Chochinov and colleagues found that as death approached, breathlessness was the most important variable that influenced a person's will to live.[5] Edmonds and colleagues found that the presence of dyspnea was associated with an increased severity of spiritual distress and weakness in the patient and more distress in the caregivers and staff. Patients with breathlessness were also more likely to die in the hospital than at home.[6]

Unfortunately, despite the prevalence, severity and impact on people's lives, studies have found that, unlike pain that significantly decreases after palliative intervention, dyspnea is more refractory to treatment[7,8] and can increase in intensity in the last days of life.[9] In a multinational study of terminal sedation, dyspnea was found to be the most common problem requiring sedation in one of the four regions studied and the second most prevalent in another.[10] To more effectively manage breathlessness a greater understanding of the epidemiology, pathophysiology and syndromes commonly encountered by patients with cancer is required.

Epidemiology

A study of an outpatient general cancer population found that 46 per cent reported breathlessness and 15 per cent described the intensity as moderate to severe.[11] This number was thought to be conservative as only four per cent of the patients had a diagnosis of lung cancer and in an international study of 1840 cancer patients in seven hospices in Europe, the United States, and Australia, the prevalence of dyspnea was highest in patients with lung cancer (46 per cent).[12] The frequency and severity of dyspnea increase with progression of the disease and/or when death is approaching. Edmonds and colleagues found that, at referral, 39 per cent of patients who were managed by home palliative care teams in Ireland were breathless,[6] whereas during the last six weeks of life of the terminally ill cancer patients studied by Reuben and Mors, 70 per cent suffered from dyspnea with 28 per cent rating it as moderate to severe.[13] Muers and Round had previously noted that breathlessness was a complaint at presentation in 60 per cent of 298 patients with non-small cell lung cancer and in nearly 90 per cent just prior to death.[14] One half of this group described their breathlessness as moderate or severe. In another study of patients with lung cancer, Edmonds and colleagues found that 78 per cent were breathless in the final year of life and 60 per cent described the intensity as very distressing.[15] Lutz and colleagues found that 73 per cent of patients with locally advanced lung cancer seen in a community radiation oncology facility presented with dyspnea. The overall severity and frequency was worse in the group who survived less than three months.[16]

Dyspnea was the fourth most common symptom in patients who presented to the Emergency Department of M.D. Anderson Cancer Center with a prevalence of 11.1 per cent. Sixty-eight per cent of these patients had uncontrolled disease with a median survival after the initial visit of 12 weeks. Thirty-one per cent of lung cancer patients died within two weeks versus 15 per cent of others (p = 0.029). Fifty-three per cent of the breast cancer patients died within six months of their initial visit.[17] When the characteristics of this group of patients were further analyzed a respiratory rate >28/minute, pulse ≥110 beats/minute, uncontrolled progressive disease and a history of metastases were found to be statistically significant predictors ($\alpha \leq 0.05$) of death within two weeks, with a relative risk of 21.93. The authors suggested that, in a group of cancer patients with acute dyspnea, using these factors might make it possible to identify patients in whom death is imminent and therefore perhaps appropriately limit treatment.[18]

Factors associated with dyspnea

Few studies have examined the factors associated with dyspnea in patients with cancer.[11,13,17,19–24] Some of these have found that dyspnea in cancer patients has diverse etiologies, commonly with more than one factor contributing to the breathlessness.[17,20] In one study the prevalence of dyspnea was strongly related to the number of risk factors a patient had.[11] Most studies have found that lung or pleural involvement with cancer is associated with the presence of dyspnea.[11,13,17,19,20] Escalante and associates found that the most common cause of shortness of breath in a group of patients presenting to an emergency room: in lung cancer patients was their underlying disease (64 per cent); in breast cancer patients, pleural effusions (31 per cent); and in other cancers, lung metastases (20 per cent).[17] Dudgeon and colleagues found that shortness of breath was significantly more common among cancer patients with a history of smoking, asthma, or chronic obstructive pulmonary disease, lung irradiation, or a history of exposure to asbestos, coal dust, cotton dust, or grain dust.[11] They also found that hilar, mediastinal, and rib metastases were all significantly associated with the dyspnea level; and surprisingly, the presence of mediastinal metastases was more highly associated with dyspnea than was the presence of lung metastases.[11]

The general debility of terminal cancer,[13] respiratory muscle weakness,[20–22] and the presence of the hyperventilation syndrome[19] have also been found to be associated with the presence of dyspnea in cancer patients. Interestingly neither the level of oxygen saturation, air flow obstruction, nor the type or severity of abnormal spirometry predicted the presence or severity of dyspnea.[20–22]

In 171 consecutive outpatients with lung cancer, Tanaka and colleagues showed that psychological distress, the presence of organic causes, cough, and pain were significantly correlated with total dyspnea as measured by the Cancer Dyspnea Scale.[24] In this study heart rate was significantly correlated with the 'sense of effort' subscale and psychological distress and pain were significantly correlated with the 'sense of anxiety' factor.

A number of studies in cancer patients have shown that anxiety is significantly correlated with the intensity of dyspnea.[19–22,24] These correlations are significant but low, with anxiety explaining only 9 per cent of the variance in the intensity of dyspnea. Tanaka and colleagues also found significant correlations with the Hospital Anxiety and Depression Scale (HADS) depression scores.[24] When they combined the HADS anxiety and depression scores the correlation coefficient was r = 0.63 (p <0.01), explaining 36 per cent of variance in the intensity of dyspnea.

Pathophysiology

Pathophysiological mechanisms of dyspnea can be categorized as: impaired ventilation; increased ventilatory demand, or a combination of these two mechanisms.[25] This classification is helpful in determining the cause of dyspnea as it reflects spirometry and other pulmonary function tests. Table 5.1 outlines the pathophysiological mechanisms of dyspnea with the potential clinical causes in a person with cancer.

Impaired ventilation

Restrictive ventilatory deficit

The principal diagnostic features of a restrictive ventilatory defect are a concurrent reduction in both forced expiratory volume in 1 minute (FEV_1) and vital capacity (FVC), decreased total lung capacity (TLC) and residual volume (RV), and often decreased diffusing capacity as well. A restrictive ventilatory defect results from decreased distensibility of the lung parenchyma, pleura, or chest wall or from a reduction in the maximum force exerted by the respiratory muscles.

Obstructive ventilatory deficit

The hallmarks of an obstructive ventilatory deficit are a reduced FEV_1/FVC and an increase in TLC, residual volume (RV), and functional residual capacity (FRC). An obstructive ventilatory deficit refers to impedance to the flow of air. Both structural and functional changes can lead to progressive narrowing of the airways. Tumor, mucus, inflammation, or edema can lead to external compression or obstruction within the lumen of the airway. Bronchoconstriction results from increased bronchomotor tone from the release of histamine, leukotrienes, and other mediators.

Increased ventilatory demand

An increase in ventilatory demand can occur when there is interruption of perfusion of the lung secondary to thrombo- or tumor emboli, vascular obstruction, or chemo- or radiation therapy. Other conditions that increase ventilatory demand are: severe deconditioning with subsequent early and

Table 5.1 Pathophysiological and clinical mechanisms of dyspnea in the cancer patient

1. Impaired ventilation
  (a) Restrictive ventilatory deficit
    (i) Pleural or parenchymal disease
       – primary or metastatic
       – pleural effusion
    (ii) Reduced movement of diaphragm
       – ascites
       – hepatomegaly
    (iii) Reduced chest wall compliance
       – pain
       – hilar/mediastinal involvement
       – chest wall invasion with tumour
       – deconditioning
       – neuromuscular
       – neurohumoral
    (iv) Respiratory muscle weakness
       – phrenic nerve paralysis
       – cachexia
       – electrolyte abnormalities
       – steroid use
       – deconditioning

  (b) Obstructive ventilatory deficit
    (i) Tumour obstruction
    (ii) Asthma
    (iii) COPD

  (c) Mixed obstructive/restrictive disease (any combination of factors)

2. Increased ventilatory demand
  (a) Increased physiologic dead space
    (i) Thromboemboli
    (ii) Tumour emboli
    (iii) Vascular obstruction
    (iv) Radiation therapy
    (v) Chemotherapy

  (b) Severe deconditioning

  (c) Hypoxemia – anemia

  (d) Change in VCO_2 or arterial PCO_2 set point

  (e) Increased neural reflex activity

  (f) Psychological causes
    – anxiety
    – depression

accelerated rise in blood lactate levels[26]; hypoxemia from anemia and other causes; changes in V_{CO2} or arterial P_{CO2} set points; increased neural reflex activity: and psychological causes such as anxiety and depression.

Causes and management of dyspnea

The causes of dyspnea in the cancer patient fall into four clinical categories: direct tumor effects, indirect tumor effects, treatment-related causes, and problems unrelated to the cancer (Table 5.2).

Table 5.2 Causes of dyspnea in cancer patients

Dyspnea due directly to cancer	Dyspnea due to cancer treatment
Pulmonary parenchymal involvement (primary or metastatic)	Surgery
	Radiation pneumonitis/fibrosis
Lymphangitic carcinomatosis	Chemotherapy-induced pulmonary disease
Intrinsic or extrinsic airway obstruction by tumor	Chemotherapy-induced cardiomyopathy
Pleural effusion	Radiation-induced pericardial disease
Pericardial effusion	**Dyspnea Unrelated to Cancer**
Ascites	Chronic obstructive pulmonary disease
Hepatomegaly	Asthma
Phrenic nerve paralysis	Congestive heart failure
Multiple tumor microemboli	Interstitial lung disease
Pulmonary leukostasis	Pneumothorax
Superior vena cava syndrome	Anxiety
Dyspnea due indirectly to cancer	Chest wall deformity
Cachexia	Obesity
Electrolyte abnormalities	Neuromuscular disorders
Anemia	Pulmonary vascular disease
Pneumonia	
Pulmonary aspiration	
Pulmonary emboli	
Neurological paraneoplastic syndromes	

Reprinted with Dudgeon D, Rosenthal S. Management of dyspnea and cough in patients with cancer. In: Cherny NI, Foley KM, eds. *Hematology/Oncology Clinics of North America: Pain and Palliative Care*, Vol. 10 (1). Philadelphia: W. B. Saunders Co., 1996; 157–71 with permission from Elsevier.

Direct tumor effects

The causes of dyspnea due directly to cancer include parenchymal involvement by tumor (primary or metastatic), lymphangitic carcinomatosis, extrinsic or intrinsic obstruction of airways by tumor, pleural tumor, pleural effusion, pericardial effusion, ascites, hepatomegaly, phrenic nerve paralysis, superior vena cava obstruction, multiple tumor microemboli, and pulmonary leukostasis.

If the tumour itself is causing shortness of breath, then chemotherapy, external beam radiation, or surgery should be considered if appropriate to the stage of disease and the overall condition of the patient. Patients can present with acute respiratory distress if they develop an exacerbating illness on top of the malignant airway narrowing. A 50 per cent reduction in the cross-sectional area of the trachea usually results in dyspnea only with exertion, whereas narrowing of the lumen to less than 25 per cent produces dyspnea and stridor at rest.[27] In an appropriate situation, nebulized racemic epinephrine and intravenous steroids will help reduce the inflammation and edema associated with the obstruction. Ventilation with Heliox may provide further relief by minimizing ventilatory airflow turbulence. These measures will provide temporary improvement in symptoms, allowing preparation for an urgent rigid bronchoscopy to evaluate and possibly treat the obstruction.[27] Airway obstruction can be reduced or eliminated with tracheobronchial stenting, laser ablation and/or bronchial irradiation, electrocautery, cryotherapy, and photodynamic therapy.[27–29] Corticosteroids offer temporary relief from dyspnea associated with lymphangitic carcinomatosis, superior vena cava syndrome, and extrinsic airway obstruction caused by the tumour. Surgical interventions are described in detail in Chapter 10.

Pleural effusion

Virtually any type of cancer can cause an abnormal accumulation of fluid in the pleural space, but over 75 per cent of all malignant pleural effusions are due to only four tumor types: lung cancer, breast cancer, ovarian cancer and lymphoma.[30] The diagnosis of a malignant pleural effusion signifies a short survival with a median of only four months. If an individual with a known malignancy has a pleural effusion, cancer is probably the cause but other possibilities include: congestive heart failure, pneumonia, pulmonary embolus with infaction, postradiation changes, tuberculosis, and vasculitis. If the cause of the effusion is unknown, and the person's situation and stage of disease warrants, a diagnostic thoracentesis to identify malignant cells in the fluid is the first step in evaluation. Approximately 50 per cent of malignant effusions are diagnosed on initial cytology, with an additional 10 per cent on the second cytologic examination[30]

Patients with pleural effusions usually complain of progressive dyspnea, cough, or, less often, pleuritic chest pain. Physical examination reveals the classic findings of: dullness to percussion, decreased breath sounds, decreased tactile fremitus, egophony, decreased chest wall expansion and if large enough tracheal deviation to the opposite side. A chest X-ray confirms the diagnosis.

Treatment options for malignant pleural effusion depend on the patient's degree of breathlessness, response to therapeutic thoracentesis, extent of disease and prognosis, effectiveness of systemic therapy, and patient perform-ance status.[31] If systemic therapy is ineffective or inappropriate then local therapy should be considered.

At the time of initial diagnostic or therapeutic tap of the pleural effusion, the removal of 1000 to 1500 ml of pleural fluid will help predict response to further therapies.[32] If symptoms are not relieved and the lung does not re-expand, then further thoracenteses or insertion of a chest tube are unlikely to be of any benefit and treatment should include medications to relieve symptoms. In 97 per cent of cases, fluid re-accumulates within one month after thoracentesis alone.[33] Repeated thoracenteses increase the risk for pneumothorax, empyema, and pleural fluid loculation, and therefore should be limited to people with a short life span. Traditionally, tube thoracostomy is performed with large bore chest tubes that are connected to wall suction requiring hospitalization, limit-ing mobility with substantial discomfort and expense. Recent studies have shown the effectiveness of small bore catheters and indwelling small pleural catheters in the outpatient setting.[34–37] Instillation of any one of several sclerosing agents into the pleural space after adequate drainage by tube thor-acostomy creates a chemical pleuritis that obliterates the pleural space and prevents reaccumulation of the pleural fluid. As pleurodesis is often painful, intrapleural lidocaine is administered prior to the instillation of the sclerosing agent to reduce local pain. Patients should also be pre-medicated and have adequate analgesic available post procedure. In patients who are not candidates for pleurodesis because pleural apposition cannot be achieved because of conditions such as a trapped lung from tumor encasement or thick fibrous plaques, indwelling pleural catheters are an option.[38]

Pericardial effusion

Metastatic disease involving the heart is discovered in up to 20 per cent of autopsied cancer patients, but clinically significant cardiac involvement is much less common. Pericardial involvement is most frequently encountered in patients with cancers of the lung, breast, gastrointestinal tract, melanoma, lymphoma, and leukemia. Malignancy is the most common cause of cardiac tamponade (16–41 per cent),[39] but radiation, drugs, infection, hypothyroidism, autoimmune disorders, and other nonmalignant etiologies underlie 50 per cent of symptomatic pericardial disease in patients with cancer.[40] Pleural effusions accompany the pericardial effusion in more than 50 per cent of patients.[41]

The clinical significance of a pericardial effusion is determined by the rate of fluid accumulation, the compliance of the pericardium, the mass of the myocardium, and the total blood volume.[42] Malignant effusions tend to accumulate rapidly, causing orthopnea, chest pain, and exertional dyspnea. Physical findings may include tachycardia, peripheral edema, hypotension, soft heart sounds, significant pulsus paradoxus, elevated jugular venous pressure, and pericardial friction rub. These findings are often not present and the diagnosis of pericardial effusion is frequently not suspected from physical examination.[41]

Characteristic electrocardiographic findings (low QRS voltage, T-wave changes, and electrical alternans) and an enlarged cardiac silhouette on a chest X-ray should raise the suspicion of pericardial effusion. Echocardiography is the most useful diagnostic test to detect the presence of pericardial fluid and the degree of myocardial dysfunction. Computed tomography (CT) can detect as little as 50 ml of fluid and provides further information if echocardiographic results are inconclusive.[41]

In one study more than 80 per cent of patients derived significant clinical benefit from pericardiocentesis despite the fact that echocardiographic evidence of right atrial and right ventricular collapse was only present in 42 and 62 per cent respectively. The authors recommended that pericardiocentesis should not be withheld from symptomatic patients simply because of the absence of echocardiographic findings of tamponade.[43] When pericardial tamponade with hemodynamic compromise is present, and treatment appropriate, an emergent pericardiocentesis is indicated with aggressive intravenous fluid support and administration of a sympathomimetic agent to temporize.[39] Hemodynamic improvement usually occurs with removal of 50 to 100 ml of pericardial fluid. Continuous drainage can be achieved by placement of an indwelling pigtail catheter or creation of a pericardial window, or percutaneous balloon pericardotomy.[44,45] Total pericardectomy is seldom performed today for malignant pericardial effusions, as operative risks range from 17–30 per cent. Pericardial drainage can be followed by instillation of a sclerozing agent to obliterate the pericardial space.[45] Definitive management for malignant pericardial effusion remains controversial as to whether initial treatment should be surgical or medical, as recent reviews suggest the results are equivalent.[41] Radiation or systemic chemotherapy should be considered if the tumour is responsive to either and it is otherwise appropriate.[46] Pericardioperitoneal shunts have also been used for palliation of malignant pericardial effusions.[47]

Superior vena cava syndrome

Obstruction of the superior vena cava may result from invasion of the venous wall by tumour or from occlusion due to extrinsic compression or intraluminal thrombus.[48] The diagnosis of superior vena cava syndrome is essentially clinical, based on characteristic symptoms and physical signs. Patients will typically complain of breathlessness that is worsened by lying flat, a sensation of fullness in the head, and cough. The physical findings are: periorbital edema, increased venous markings on the chest, delayed venous return when the person's arm is raised above the level of the heart, increased JVP, and orthopnea and flushing with recumbancy. An infused CT scan of the chest is the diagnostic imaging technique of choice; it helps confirm the diagnosis, determine the extent of the tumour, and visualize the actual occlusion.

The treatment of superior vena cava syndrome depends on the etiology, the severity of symptoms, the patient's prognosis, and the underlying malignancy. Chemotherapy, in patients with a good performance status and prognosis, is the treatment of choice for chemo-sensitive malignancies such as small cell carcinoma of the lung and lymphomas; those cases caused by less sensitive cancers require mediastinal irradiation.

Corticosteroids are recommended as they may decrease any inflammatory reaction that is contributing to the superior vena cava obstruction. Diuretics should be used with caution, if at all, as a decrease in vascular volume may precipitate shock if venous return to the heart is reduced further.[49] Diuretics may also increase the risk of thrombosis. Tissue plasminogen activator or other thrombotic agents such as streptokinase or urokinase are a options for intraluminal clot in the appropriate clinical setting.[49,50]

Dyspnea due to cancer treatment

Surgery

Pneumonectomy or lobectomy can result in shortness of breath in patients with pre-existing impairment of pulmonary function.

Radiation therapy

Thoracic irradiation can cause two clinical syndromes: radiation pneumonitis which occurs 6–12 weeks following treatment and radiation fibrosis 6–12 months later.[51] Clinically significant radiation effects on the lung occur in up to 10 per cent of treated patients. The degree of lung damage is determined by the radiation dose, the volume of lung irradiated, and presence of comorbid lung disease.[52] Concomitant chemotherapy with certain drugs and steroid withdrawal may also exacerbate the process.[51,53]

Symptomatic radiation pneumonitis ranges in severity from a mild cough with fever and breathlessness to severe respiratory distress and death.[54] It is know thought that acute radiation-induced pneumonitis is a bilateral lymphocytic alveolitis. Chest radiography may show an infiltrate with well-defined borders that correspond to the radiation field, although not in all patients.[52,54] Radiation fibrosis develops in areas of previous pneumonitis as a consequence of repair initiated by the tissue injury and the local release of cytokines.[54] Radiation fibrosis is usually asymptomatic except in patients with underlying pulmonary functional impairment or severe radiation pneumonitis.[51] Thoracic irradiation can also cause pleural effusions, spontaneous pneumothoraces, pericardial effusions, and acute airway obstruction.[51]

Corticosteroids are the mainstay of treatment for radiation pneumonitis. In more severe cases, oxygen and even ventilatory support may be required. Gross suggested dose ranges of 60 to 100 mg daily of prednisone following diagnosis and then after several weeks a gradual taper, observing for signs of radiation pneumonitis flare.[51] Pulmonary fibrosis secondary to radiation may require supportive oxygen, bronchodilators, expectorants, steroids, and possibly a penicillamine.[55]

Systemic therapy

Numerous pharmacological agents used to treat cancer can cause pulmonary damage but the most frequent offenders are: bleomycin, carmustine (BCNU), busulfan, and high dose cyclophosphamide. There are three patterns of pulmonary injury: chronic pneumonitis/fibrosis, acute hypersensitivity lung disease, and non-cardiogenic pulmonary edema. Risk factors for the development of pulmonary toxicity include cumulative dose, age, previous or subsequent thoracic radiotherapy, high concentrations of inspired oxygen, concomitant or subsequent use of other chemotherapeutic agents, steroid withdrawal, and pre-existing lung disease.[53,56]

Chronic pneumonitis, pulmonary fibrosis, and hypersensitivity lung disease caused by chemotherapeutic agents are treated with corticosteroids and symptomatic interventions. A short trial of high dose steroids can help to confirm or rule out the diagnosis of pneumonitis in cases without obvious infectious etiologies. Dyspnea should start to resolve within 48 hours of initiating steroid treatment.[57] Non-cardiogenic pulmonary edema caused by chemotherapeutic agents is treated in the same manner as pulmonary edema of other etiologies.[56]

Dyspnea indirectly due to cancer

Cancer causes dyspnea indirectly as a consequence of malnutrition, mineral and electrolyte deficiencies, infection, anemia, pulmonary emboli, aspiration, neurological paraneoplastic syndromes and severe deconditioning. If appropriate to the person's stage of disease, prognosis, and wishes these underlying causes of dyspnea should be treated appropriately.

Muscle weakness

Studies have demonstrated an association between dyspnea and respiratory[20–22] and generalized[13,58] muscle weakness in the advanced cancer patient. Both types of muscle weakness could be a result of severe deconditioning but other factors that could affect muscle function are hypocalcemia, hypokalemia, hypomagnesemia, severe hypophosphatemia, malnutrition, and possibly the cancer itself.[59,60] Although no studies have been conducted in cancer patients, there is evidence in COPD patients that re-feeding, exercise reconditioning, and anabolic steroids improve exercise tolerance.[61–63]

Infection

Patients with cancer are at an increased risk of pneumonia due to immunosuppression from the disease or its treatment, and also from the tumour causing mucosal erosion or a mass effect resulting in an abscess, fistula, or obstruction.

Pulmonary emboli

The association of cancer with venous thrombosis and pulmonary embolism has been recognized for many years.[64,65] The mechanisms by which cancers predispose to thromboembolism include stasis and immobility, compression or direct invasion of the venous system by the tumour, and interactions between the tumor cells and the coagulation system, the fibrinolytic system, platelets, and the endothelium.[65] Typically patients with acute pulmonary embolic disease describe a single or multiple episodes of acute shortness of breath. Less commonly, multiple small emboli produce pulmonary hypertension with no history of acute episodes.[66] It is possible that an episode of acute shortness of breath just prior to death is a result of a large pulmonary embolus.

Dyspnea unrelated to the cancer

Risk factors for dyspnea unrelated to cancer include: pre-existing chronic obstructive lung disease (COPD), cardiovascular disease, asthma, interstitial lung disease, pneumothorax, anxiety, chest wall deformity, obesity, neuromuscular disorders, and pulmonary vascular disease.

The treatment of breathlessness from COPD, cardiovascular disease, neuro-muscular disorders are outlined in Chapters 3, 4, and 6.

Pharmacological management

Opioids A recent systematic review examined the effectiveness of oral or parenteral opioids for the management of dyspnea.[67] The authors identified 18 randomized double-blind, controlled trials comparing the use of any opioid drug against placebo for the treatment of breathlessness in patients with any illness (only two studies conducted with cancer patients met the inclusion criteria for review (1 parenteral, 1 nebulized).

In the studies[68–75] involving the non-nebulized route of administration there was statistically strong evidence for a small effect of oral and parenteral opioids for the treatment of breathlessness.[67]

In cancer patients, three trials, one open, uncontrolled trial[76] and two placebo-controlled crossover trials[74,77] significantly improved dyspnea after a single bolus dose of morphine.

One study described the use of a continuous intravenous infusion of morphine for severe dyspnea in patients with terminal lung cancer.[78] Six of eight patients obtained good relief of their breathlessness, however, carbon dioxide levels rose steadily over the course of the infusion in five of seven patients and seven of eight patients died while receiving morphine infusions.

Boyd and colleagues studied the effectiveness of slow release morphine preparations on dyspnea in 15 cancer patients in an open uncontrolled study.[79] Thirteen opioid-naive patients received 10 mg twice a day and two already on opioids a 30 per cent dose increase. Assessments were made before, at 48 hours, and at 7 to 10 days. Only nine patients were able to complete all three assessments. The mean dyspnea VAS (visual analogue scale) score decreased over the time, but failed to reach statistical significance with $p = 0.06$. Patients' respiratory rate was not significantly affected. Sedation significantly increased at 48 hours, but had resolved by 7 to 10 days.

Allard and colleagues[80] studied the effectiveness of supplemental doses of opioids to improve breathlessness in terminally ill cancer patients who were already receiving regular doses of opioids. They found patients received almost equal benefit from a supplemental equivalent of 25 or 50 per cent of their 4-hourly oral or subcutaneous regular opioid dose. The authors also found that the supplemental dose was more effective in patients with initial dyspnea intensities of a mild to moderate range. This was an observation that had previously been made by Cohen and colleagues, who had suggested that continuous infusions may be more effective for patients with severe dyspnea.[81] This needs to be tested in further trials.

Opioid receptors are located throughout the respiratory tract and it is hypothesized that if the receptors are interrupted directly, lower doses, with fewer systemic side-effects, would be required to control breathlessness.[82] The recent systemic review[67] identified nine randomized double-blind, controlled trials comparing the use of nebulized opioids or placebo for the control of breathlessness.[83–91] The authors concluded that there was no evidence that nebulized opioids were more effective than nebulized saline in relieving breathlessness.[67]

At this time the evidence supports the safe use of oral and parenteral opioids for control of dyspnea. Appendix A outlines medical guidelines regarding the initiation and titration of opioids for the management of dyspnea. When using the guidelines it is important to use clinical judgment and make adjustments as appropriate for a given patient.

Sedatives and tranquilizers Chlorpromazine decreases breathlessness without affecting ventilation or producing sedation in healthy subjects.[92] There are conflicting results from trials studying the effectiveness of promethazine, a phenothiazine antihistamine, in reducing dyspnea.[92–94] In an open-labeled trial McIver and colleagues found chlorpromazine effective for relief of dyspnea in advanced cancer.[95]

In a double-blind, placebo controlled, randomized trial, Light and colleagues studied the effectiveness of morphine alone, morphine and promethazine, and morphine and prochlorperazine for the treatment of breathlessness in COPD patients.[71] The combination of morphine and promethazine significantly improved exercise tolerance without worsening dyspnea compared to placebo, morphine alone, or the combination of morphine and prochlorperazine.[71] Ventafridda and colleagues have also found the combination of morphine and chlorpromazine to be effective.[96] Appendix A outlines when phenothiazines could be considered as an adjunct to opioids in the management of dyspnea.

There are conflicting results from clinical trials conducted to determine the effectiveness of anxiolytics for the treatment of chronic breathlessness.[97,98] None of these trials was conducted in cancer patients. Anecdotal evidence supports the use of anxiolytics for episodes of acute breathlessness.

Appendix A outlines guidelines for the management of dyspnea in palliative cancer patients. These guidelines were developed by a multidisciplinary team and are based on literature that is referenced in this chapter. When using the guidelines it is important to use clinical judgment and determine their appropriateness for a given patient.

Non-pharmacological management

Non-pharmacological approaches are very appropriate for the management of breathlessness in the cancer patient. Please see Chapter 11 for an excellent summary.

Summary

Dyspnea is a very common symptom in patients with cancer. Despite breathlessness' profound effect on people's quality of life it is often unrecognized, and therefore people often receive little assistance in managing this distressing symptom. Effective management requires an understanding of the epidemiology, pathophysiology, common syndromes and treatment options. More research is necessary to further optimize the available treatment options.

References

1. O'Driscoll M, Corner J, Bailey C. The experience of breathlessness in lung cancer. *European Journal of Cancer Care* 1999; **8**(1): 37–43.
2. Roberts DK, Thorne SE, Pearson C. The experience of dyspnea in late-stage cancer. Patients' and nurses' perspectives. *Cancer Nursing* 1993; **16**(4): 310–20.
3. Brown ML, Carrieri V, Janson-Bjerklie S, Dodd MJ. Lung cancer and dyspnea: The patient's perception. *Oncol Nurs Forum* 1986; **13**(5): 19–24.
4. Tanaka K, Akechi T, Okuyama T, Nishiwaki Y, Uchitomi Y. Prevalence and screening of dyspnea interfering with daily life activities in ambulatory patients with advanced lung cancer. *J Pain Symptom Manage* 2002; **23**(6): 484–9.
5. Chochinov MH, Tataryn D, Clinch JJ, Dudgeon D. Will to live in the terminally ill. *Lancet* 1999; **354**(9181): 816–19.
6. Edmonds P, Higginson I, Altmann D, Sen-Gupta G, McDonnell M. Is the presence of dyspnea a risk factor for morbidity in cancer patients? *J Pain Symptom Manage* 2000; **19**(1): 15–22.
7. Dudgeon D, Harlos M, Clinch JJ. The Edmonton Symptom Assessment Scale (ESAS) as an Audit Tool. *J Palliat Care* 1999; **15**(3): 14–19.
8. Higginson I, McCarthy M. Measuring symptoms in terminal cancer: are pain and dyspnoea controlled? *J Royal Soc Med* 1989; **82**: 264–7.
9. Mercadante S, Casuccio A, Fulfaro F. The course of symptom frequency and intensity in advanced cancer patients followed at home. *J Pain Symptom Manage* 2000; **20**(2): 104–12.
10. Fainsinger R, Waller A, Bercovici M, Bengston K, Landman W, Hosking M *et al.* A multicentre international study of sedation for uncontrolled symptoms in terminally ill patients. *Palliat Med* 2000; **14**(4): 257–65.
11. Dudgeon DJ, Kristjanson L, Sloan JA, Lertzman M, Clement K. Dyspnea in cancer patients: prevalence and associated factors. *J Pain Symptom Manage* 2001; **21**(2): 95–102.
12. Vainio A, Auvinen A. Prevalence of symptoms among patients with advanced cancer: an international collaborative study. *J Pain Symptom Manage* 1996; **12**(1): 3–10.
13. Reuben DB, Mor V. Dyspnea in terminally ill cancer patients. *Chest* 1986; **89**: 234–6.

14. Muers MF, Round CE. Palliation of symptoms in non-small cell lung cancer: a study by the Yorkshire Regional Cancer Organisation thoracic group. *Thorax* 1993; **48**: 339–43.
15. Edmonds P, Karlsen S, Khan S, Addington-Hall J. A comparison of the palliative care needs of patients dying from chronic respiratory diseases and lung cancer. *Palliat Med* 2001; **15**: 287–95.
16. Lutz ST, Norrell R, Bertucio C, Kachnic L, Johnson C, Arthur D *et al.* Symptom frequency and severity in patients with metastatic or locally recurrent lung cancer: A prospective study using the lung cancer symptom scale in a community hospital. *J Palliat Med* 2001; **4**(2): 157–65.
17. Escalante CP, Martin CG, Elting LS, Cantor SB, Harle TS, Price KJ *et al.* Dyspnea in cancer patients. etiology, resource utilization, and survival – implications in a managed care world. *Cancer* 1996; **78**(6): 1314–19.
18. Escalante CP, Martin CG, Elting LS, Price KJ, Manzullo EF, Weiser MA *et al.* Identifying risk factors for imminent death in cancer patients with acute dyspnea. *J Pain Symptom Manage* 2000; **20**(5): 318–25.
19. Heyse-Moore LH. On Dyspnoea in Advanced Cancer [dissertation]. Southampton, UK: Southampton University, 1993.
20. Dudgeon D, Lertzman M. Dyspnea in the advanced cancer patient. *J Pain Symptom Manage* 1998; **16**(4): 212–19.
21. Dudgeon DJ, Lertzman M, Askew GR. Physiological changes and clinical correlations of dyspnea in cancer outpatients. *J Pain Symptom Manage* 2001; **21**(5): 373–9.
22. Bruera E, Schmitz B, Pither J, Neumann CM, Hanson J. The frequency and correlates of dypsnea in patients with advanced cancer. *J Pain Symptom Manage* 2000; **19**(5): 357–62.
23. Dudgeon DJ, Webb KA, O'Donnell DE. Unexplained dyspnea and exercise intolerance in patients with cancer: physiological correlates. *American Society of Clinical Oncology* 2001; 303b: 20.
24. Tanaka K, Akechi T, Okuyama T, Nishiwaki Y, Uchitomi Y. Factors correlated with dyspnea in advanced lung cancer patients: Organic causes and what else? *J Pain Symptom Manage* 2002; **23**(6): 490–500.
25. O'Donnell DE. Exertional breathlessness in chronic respiratory disease. In: Mahler D, ed. *Dyspnea*, pp. 97–147. New York: Marcel Dekker Inc., 1998.
26. American Thoracic Society. Dyspnea. Mechanisms, assessment, and management: a consensus statement. *Am J Respir Crit Care Med* 1999; **159**: 321–40.
27. Wood DE. Management of malignant tracheobronchial obstruction. *Surgical Clinics of North America* 2002; **82**: 621–42.
28. Lee P, Kupeli E, Mehta AC. Therapeutic bronchoscopy in lung cancer. Laser therapy, electrocautery, brachytherapy, stents, and photodynamic therapy. *Clin Chest Med* 2002; **23**(1): 241–56.
29. Wood DE, Liu Y, Vallieres E, Karmy-Jones R, Mulligan MS. Airway stenting for malignant and benign tracheobronchial stenosis. *Annals of Thoracic Surgery* 2003; **76**: 167–74.
30. Martel MK, Sahijdak WM, Ten Haken RK, Kessler ML, Turrisi AT. Fraction size and dose parameters related to the incidence of pericardial effusions. *Int J Radiation Oncology Biol Phys* 1998; **40**(1): 155–61.
31. Sahn SA. Management of malignant pleural effusions. *Monaldi Archives for Chest Disease* 2001; **56**(5): 394–9.
32. Lynch TJ. Management of malignant pleural effusions. *Chest* 1993; 4(Supplement): 385S–389S.

33. Anderson CB, Philpott GW, Ferguson TB. The treatment of malignant pleural effusions. *Cancer* 1974; **33**(4): 916–22.

34. Rauthe G, Sistermanns J. Recombinant tumour necrosis factor in the local therapy of malignant pleural effusion. *Eur J Cancer* 1997; **33**(2): 226–31.

35. Grodzin CJ, Balk RA. Indwelling small pleural catheter needle thoracentesis in the management of large pleural effusions. *Chest* 1997; **111**(4): 981–8.

36. Patz EFJr. Malignant pleural effusions. Recent advances and ambulatory sclerotherapy. *Chest* 1998; **113**(1 Suppl): 74S–77S.

37. Brubacher S, Gobel BH. Use of the Pleurx pleural catheter for the management of malignant pleural effusions. *Clinical Journal of Oncology Nursing* 2003; **7**(1): 1–4.

38. Ohm C, Park D, Vogen M, Bendick P, Welsh R, Pursel S *et al.* Use of an indwelling pleural catheter compared with thorascopic talc pleurodesis in the management of malignant pleural effusions. *The American Surgeon* 2003; **69**(3): 198–202.

39. Press OW, Livingston R. Management of malignant pericardial effusion and tamponade. *JAMA* 1987; **257**(8): 1088–92.

40. Missri J, Schechter D. When pericardial effusion complicates cancer. *Hosp Pract* 1988; **23**(4): 277–86.

41. Shepherd FA. Malignant pericardial effusion. *Current Opinion in Oncology* 1997; **9**(2): 170–4.

42. Miles DW, Knight RK. Diagnosis and management of malignant pleural effusion. *Cancer Treat Rev* 1993; **19**: 151–68.

43. Cooper JP, Oliver RM, Currie P, Walker JM, Swanton RH. How do the clinical findings in patients with pericardial effusions influence the success of aspiration? *British Heart Journal* 1995; **73**: 351–4.

44. Vaitkus PT, Hermann HC, LeWinter MM. Treatment of malignant pericardial effusion. *JAMA* 1994; **272**(1): 59–64.

45. Chong HH, Plotnick GD. Pericardial effusion and tamponade: evaluation, imaging modalities, and management. *Comprehensive Therapy* 1995; **21**(7): 378–85.

46. Mangan CM. Malignant pericardial effusions: pathophysiology and clinical correlates. *Oncol Nurs Forum* 1992; **19**(8): 1215–23.

47. Wang N, Feikes JR, Mogensen T, Vyhmeister EE, Bailey LL. Pericardioperitoneal shunt: an alternative treatment for malignant pericardial effusion. *Annals of Thoracic Surgery* 1994; **57**(2): 289–92.

48. Jones LA. Superior vena cava syndrome: an oncologic complication. *Semin Oncol Nurs* 1987; **3**(3): 211–15.

49. Haapoja IS, Blendowski C. Superior vena cava syndrome. Case study. *Semin Oncol Nurs* 1999; **15**(3): 183–9.

50. Gray BH, Olin JW, Graor RA. Safety and efficacy of thrombolytic therapy for superior vena cava syndrome. *Chest* 1991; **99**: 54–9.

51. Gross NJ. Pulmonary effects of radiation therapy. *Ann Int Med* 1977; **86**(1): 81–92.

52. Monson JM, Stark P, Reilly JJ, Sugarbaker DJ, Strauss GM, Swanson SJ *et al.* Clinical radiation pneumonitis and radiographic changes after thoracic radiation therapy for lung carcinoma. *Cancer* 1998; **82**(5): 842–50.

53. Castellino RA, Glatstein E, Turbow MM, Rosenberg S, Kaplan HS. Latent radiation injury of lungs or heart activated by steroid withdrawal. *Ann Int Med* 1974; **80**(5): 593–9.

54. Abratt RP, Morgan GW. Lung toxicity following chest irradiation in patients with lung cancer. *Lung Cancer* 2002; **35**: 103–9.

55. Movsas B, Raffin TA, Epstein AH, Link CJJr. Pulmonary radiation injury. *Chest* 1997; **111**(4): 1061–76.
56. Cooper JAD, Jr., White DA, Matthay RA. Drug-induced pulmonary disease. *Am Rev Respir Dis* 1986; **133**: 321–40.
57. Ash-Bernal R, Browner I, Erlich R. Early detection and successful treatment of drug-induced pneumonitis with corticosteroids. *Cancer Invest* 2002; **20**(7 and 8): 876–9.
58. Dudgeon DJ, O'Donnell DE, Day A, Webb KA, McBride I, Dillon K. Mechanisms of exertional dyspnea in patients with cancer: a case-matched control study. *Journal of Palliative Care* 2002; **18**(3): 207.
59. Lewis MI, Belman MJ. Nutrition and the respiratory muscles. *Clin Chest Med* 1988; **9**(2): 337–47.
60. Rochester DF, Arora NS. Respiratory muscle failure. *Med Clin North Am* 1983; **67**(3): 573–97.
61. Whittaker JS, Ryan CF, Buckley PA, Road JD. The effects of refeeding on peripheral and respiratory muscle function in malnourished chronic obstructive pulmonary disease patients. *Am Rev Respir Dis* 1990; **142**: 283–8.
62. O'Donnell DE, McGuire M, Samis L, Webb KA. The impact of exercise reconditioning on breathlessness in severe chronic airflow limitation. *Am J Respir Crit Care Med* 1995; **152**: 2005–13.
63. Schols AM, Soeters PB, Mostert R, Pluymers RJ, Wouters EF. Physiologic effects of nutritional support and anabolic steroids in patients with chronic obstructive pulmonary disease. A placebo-controlled randomized trial. *Am J Respir Crit Care Med* 1995; **152**(4:1): 1268–74.
64. Prandoni P, Lensing AWA, Buller HR, Cogo A, Prins MH, Cattelan AM *et al.* Deep-vein thrombosis and the incidence of subsequent symptomatic cancer. *N Engl J Med* 1992; **327**(16): 1128–33.
65. Silverstein RL, Nachman RL. Cancer and clotting – Trousseau's warning. *N Engl J Med* 1992; **327**(16): 1163–4.
66. Scully RE, Mark EJ, McNeely WF, McNeely BU. Case record of the Massachusetts General Hospital (Case 30–1987). *N Engl J Med* 1987; **317**(4): 225–35.
67. Jennings AL, Davies A, Higgins JPT, Broadley K. Opioids for the palliation of breathlessness in terminal illness (Cochrane Review). In: The Cochrane Library [4]. 2001. Oxford: Update Software.
68. Woodcock AA, Johnson MA, Geddes DM. Breathlessness, alcohol and opiates. *N Engl J Med* 1982; **306**: 1363–4.
69. Woodcock AA, Gross ER, Gellert A, Shah S, Johnson M, Geddes DM. Effects of dihydrocodeine, alcohol, and caffeine on breathlessness and exercise tolerance in patients with chronic obstructive lung disease and normal blood gases. *N Engl J Med* 1981; **305**(27): 1611–16.
70. Poole PJ, Veale AG, Black PN. The effect of sustained-release morphine on breathlessness and quality of life in severe chronic obstructive pulmonary disease. *Am J Respir Crit Care Med* 1998; **157**(6 Pt 1): 1877–80.
71. Light RW, Stansbury DW, Webster JS. Effect of 30 mg of morphine alone or with promethazine or prochlorperazine on the exercise capacity of patients with COPD. *Chest* 1996; **109**(4): 975–81.
72. Johnson MA, Woodcock AA, Geddes DM. Dihydrocodeine for breathlessness in 'pink puffers'. *BMJ* 1983; **286**: 675–77.

73. Eiser N, Denman WT, West C, Luce P. Oral diamorphine: lack of effect on dyspnoea and exercise tolerance in the 'pink puffer' syndrome. *Eur Respir J* 1991; 4(8): 926–31.

74. Bruera E, MacEachern T, Ripamonti C, Hanson J. Subcutaneous morphine for dyspnea in cancer patients. *Ann Int Med* 1993; 119(9): 906–7.

75. Chua TP, Harrington D, Ponikowski P, Webb-Peploe K, Poole-Wilson PA, Coats AJ. Effects of dihydrocodeine on chemosensitivity and exercise tolerance in patients with chronic heart failure. *Journal of the American College of Cardiology* 1997; 29(1): 147–52.

76. Bruera E, Macmillan K, Pither J, MacDonald RN. Effects of morphine on the dyspnea of terminal cancer patients. *J Pain Symptom Manage* 1990; 5(6): 341–4.

77. Mazzocato C, Buclin T, Rapin CH. The effects of morphine on dyspnea and ventilatory function in elderly patients with advanced cancer: A randomized double-blind controlled trial. *Annals of Oncology* 1999; 10(12): 1511–14.

78. Cherniack NS, Altose MD. Mechanisms of dyspnea. *Clin Chest Med* 1987; 8(2): 207–14.

79. Boyd KJ, Kelly M. Oral morphine as symptomatic treatment of dyspnoea in patients with advanced cancer. *Palliat Med* 1997; 11: 277–81.

80. Allard P, Lamontagne C, Bernard P, Tremblay C. How effective are supplementary doses of opioids for dyspnea in terminally ill cancer patients? A randomized continuous sequential clinical trial. *J Pain Symptom Manage* 1999; 17(4): 256–65.

81. Cohen MH, Johnston Anderson A, Krasnow SH, Spagnolo SV, Citron ML, Payne M *et al.* Continuous intravenous infusion of morphine for severe dyspnea. *South Med J* 1991; 84(2): 229–34.

82. Zebraski SE, Kochenash SM, Raffa RB. Lung opioid receptors: pharmacology and possible target for nebulized morphine in dyspnea. *Life Sciences* 2000; 66(23): 2221–31.

83. Beauford W, Saylor TT, Stansbury DW, Avalos K, Light RW. Effects of nebulized morphine sulfate on the exercise tolerance of the ventilatory limited COPD patient. *Chest* 1993; 104(1): 175–78.

84. Davis CL, Hodder C, Love S, Shah R, Slevin M, Wedzicha J. Effect of nebulised morphine and morphine 6-glucuronide on exercise endurance in patients with chronic obstructive pulmonary disease. *Thorax* 1994; 49: 393P.

85. Davis CL, Penn K, A'Hern R, Daniels J, Slevin M. Single dose randomised controlled trial of nebulised morphine in patients with cancer related breathlessness. *Palliative Medicine* 1996; 10(1): 64–5.

86. Harris-Eze AO, Sridhar G, Clemens RE, Zintel TA, Gallagher CG, Marciniuk DD. Low-dose nebulized morphine does not improve exercise in interstitial lung disease. *Am J Respir Crit Care Med* 1995; 152: 1940–5.

87. Jankelson D, Hosseini K, Mather LE, Seale JP, Young IH. Lack of effect of high doses of inhaled morphine on exercise endurance in chronic obstructive pulmonary disease. *Eur Respir J* 1997; 10(10): 2270–4.

88. Leung R, Hill P, Burdon JGW. Effect of inhaled morphine on the development of breathlessness during exercise in patients with chronic lung disease. *Thorax* 1996; 51(6): 596–600.

89. Masood AR, Reed JW, Thomas SHL. Lack of effect of inhaled morphine on exercise-induced breathlessness in chronic obstructive pulmonary disease. *Thorax* 1995; 50(6): 629–34.

90. Noseda A, Carpiaux JP, Markstein C, Meyvaert A, de Maertelaer V. Disabling dyspnoea in patients with advanced disease: lack of effect of nebulized morphine. *Eur Respir J* 1997; 10(5): 1079–83.

91. Young IH, Daviskas E, Keena VA. Effect of low dose nebulised morphine on exercise endurance in patients with chronic lung disease. *Thorax* 1989; **44**: 387–90.
92. O'Neill PA, Morton PB, Stark RD. Chlorpromazine – a specific effect on breathlessness? *Br J Clin Pharmacol* 1985; **19**: 793–7.
93. Woodcock AA, Gross ER, Geddes DM. Drug treatment of breathlessness: contrasting effects of diazepam and promethazine in pink puffers. *BMJ* 1981; **283**: 343–6.
94. Rice KL, Kronenberg RS, Hedemark LL, Niewoehner DE. Effects of chronic administration of codeine and promethazine on breathlessness and exercise tolerance in patients with chronic airflow obstruction. *Br J Dis Chest* 1987; **81**: 287–92.
95. McIver B, Walsh D, Nelson K. The use of chlorpromazine for symptom control in dying cancer patients. *J Pain Symptom Manage* 1994; **9**(5): 341–5.
96. Ventafridda V, Spoldi E, De Conno F. Control of dyspnea in advanced cancer patients. *Chest* 1990; **98**: 1544–5.
97. Man GCW, Hsu K, Sproule BJ. Effect of alprazolam on exercise and dyspnea in patients with chronic obstructive pulmonary disease. *Chest* 1986; **90**(6): 832–6.
98. Eimer M, Cable T, Gal P, Rothenberger LA, McCue JD. Effects of clorazepate on breathlessness and exercise tolerance in patients with chronic airflow obstruction. *J Fam Pract* 1985; **21**(5): 359–62.

Appendix

DYSPNEA MANAGEMENT GUIDELINES FOR PALLIATIVE CARE PATIENTS

Considerations:
- Identify and treat common exacerbating medical conditions underlying dyspnea or shortness of breath, e.g. COPD, CHF, pneumonia.
- Drug treatments listed are not intended to represent a comprehensive treatment. Other treatments should be considered such as fan, open window etc.
- Evaluate impact of anxiety and fear on dyspnea and treat appropriately.
- Use Edmonton Symptom Assessment Scale (ESAS) and Oxygen Cost Diagram to measure outcome.

Level of dyspnea	Treatment
Mild dyspnea **ESAS (0–3)** • Usually can sit and lie quietly • May be intermittent or persistent • Worsens with exertion • No anxiety or mild anxiety during shortness of breath • Breathing not observed as laboured • No cyanosis	• Ensure access to fresh air or use a fan directing cold air on the face. • Start humidified oxygen prn if the patient is hypoxic (SaO$_2$<92%) or if deemed helpful by the patient. (Up to 6L/min by nasal prongs.) • If the patient is not taking an opioid, initiate short-acting morphine 2.5–5.0 mg PO q4h & 2.5 mg PO q2h prn for breakthrough **OR** hydromorphone 0.5–1.0 mg PO q4h & 0.5 mg PO q2h prn. for breakthrough (if the SC route is needed, divide the PO dose by half.) • Titrate up by 25% every 3 to 5 doses until dyspnea is relieved. (See titration guide.) • If the patient is taking an opioid with q4h dosing, increase this dose by 25%. • If the patient is taking a long-acting opioid, change back to q4h dosing and increase this dose by 25% (see conversion guide), **alternatively**, increase both the long-acting and breakthrough dose by 25%. • Titrate short-acting opioid by 25% every 3 to 5 doses until dyspnea is relieved. (See titration guide.) • If significant opioid side effects are present (e.g. nausea, drowsiness, myoclonus), consider switching to another opioid (see conversion tables), and re-titrate.
Moderate dyspnea **(ESAS 4–6)** • Usually persistent • May be new or chronic • Shortness of breath worsens if walking or with exertion; settles partially with rest • Pauses while talking every 30 seconds • Breathing mildly laboured	• Ensure access to fresh air or use a fan directing cold air on the face. • Start humidified oxygen prn if the patient is hypoxic (SaO$_2$<92%) or if deemed helpful by the patient. (Up to 6L/min by nasal prongs.) • If the patient is NOT taking an opioid, initiate short-acting morphine 2.5–5.0 mg PO q4h & 2.5 mg PO q1h prn **OR** hydromorphone 0.5 – 1.0 mg PO q4h & 0.5 mg PO q1h prn. (If the SC route is needed, divide the PO dose by half, and the prn dose can be as frequent as q30minutes). • Titrate the dose by 25% every 2–3 doses until dyspnea is relieved. (See titration guide.) • If the patient is taking an opioid with q4h dosing, increase the dose by 25%, (this applies to SC or PO dosing) and continue with breakthrough dosing at 50% of the regular dose q1h prn (or q30 minutes prn if it is SC). • If the patient is taking a long-acting opioid, change back to q4h dosing and increase this dose by 25%, (see conversion guide), **alternatively**, increase both the long-acting and breakthrough doses by 25%. Give breakthrough q1h prn. • Titrate the dose by 25% every 2–3 doses until dyspnea is relieved. (See titration guide.) • If opioids provide only a limited effect, consider adding chlorpromazine 12.5 or 25 mg q4–6h PO or methotrimeprazine 2.5–5.0 mg PO/SC q4–6h as an adjuvant. • If significant opioid side effects are present (e.g. nausea, drowsiness, myoclonus), consider switching to another opioid (see conversion tables), and re-titrate.

Progressive severe dyspnea (ESAS 7–10)
 	
• Often acute on chronic
• Worsening over days/weeks
• Anxiety present
• Often awakes suddenly with shortness of breath
• +/– cyanosis
• +/– onset of confusion
• Laboured breathing awake and asleep
• Pauses while talking q 5–15 seconds
	• Start humidified oxygen, up to 6L/min by nasal prongs or even higher flow rate with mask, as tolerated (even if not hypoxic). Consider nebulized saline 1–3 mL by mask, prn.
	• If the patient is NOT taking an opioid, initiate short-acting opioid. Consider:
	    Oral: Morphine 5–10 mg PO q4h & 5 mg PO q1h prn ***OR*** hydromorphone 1.0–2.0 mg PO q4h & 1.0 mg PO q1h prn ***OR***
	    Subcutaneous: Morphine 2.5–5 mg SC q4h & 2.5 mg SC q30min prn ***OR*** hydromorphone 0.5–1.0 mg SC q4h & 0.5 mg SC q30min prn.
	• Titrate dose by 25% every 1–2 doses until dyspnea is relieved. (See titration guide.)
	• If the patient is taking an opioid with q4h dosing, increase the regular and breakthrough doses by 25%. Change frequency of the breakthrough to q1h prn if PO and q30min prn if SC.
	• If the patient is taking a long-acting opioid, switch back to q4h dosing and increase this dose by 25%. (See conversion guide.) **Do Not** try to manage severe dyspnea with a long-acting opioid. Change the breakthrough dose to half of the regular dose, either q1h prn PO or q30min prn SC.
	• Titrate the dose by 25% increments every 1–2 doses until dyspnea is relieved. (See titration guide.)
	• If opioids provide a limited effect only, consider adding chlorpromazine 12.5 or 25 mg q4–6h PO or methotrimeprazine 2.5–5.0 mg PO/SC q4–6h as an adjuvant.
	• If unmanageable opioid-limiting side effects are present (e.g. nausea, drowsiness, myoclonus), consider switching to another opioid (see conversion tables), and re-titrate.

Acute exacerbation or very severe dyspnea • Sudden onset (minutes to hours) • High anxiety and fear • Agitation with very laboured respirations • Air hunger • Pauses while talking or unable to speak • Exhausted • Total concentration on breathing • Cyanosis usually • May be cold/clammy • +/– respiratory congestion • +/– acute chest pain • +/– diaphoresis • +/– confusion	• Start humidified oxygen, up to 6L/min by nasal prongs or even higher flow rate with mask, face tent if tolerated (even if not hypoxic). **If the patient is NOT taking an opioid:** • If IV access is present, stat morphine 5–10 mg IV q10 minutes until settled. • If NO IV access is available, stat morphine 5–10 mg SC q20-30 minutes until settled. When settled: morphine 10-20 mg PO q4h and q1h prn **OR** morphine 5 – 10 mg SC or IV q4h and q 30 to 60 minutes prn and titrate vigilantly. **If the patient is taking an opioid and has IV access:** • Stat opioid administration, dosed as follows: • If taking a PO opioid, give the same dose *IV*, and repeat q10 minutes until settled (e.g. if on 15 mg PO q4h usually, then give 15 mg IV q10 minutes until settled). • If taking a SC opioid, give double the SC dose *IV*, as often as, q10 minutes until settled. When settled: continue q4h dosing with breakthrough q30–60 minutes prn (will likely need a higher dose than previous) and titrate vigilantly. **If the patient is taking an opioid and has no IV access:** • Stat opioid administration, dosed as follows: • If taking a PO opioid, give the usual PO dose SC q 20–30 minutes until settled (e.g. if usually takes 15 mg PO q4h, then give 15 mg SC q20–30 minutes until settled). • If taking a SC opioid, give the usual dose (or double it) q20–30 minutes until settled (e.g. if on 15 mg SC q4h usually, then give 15–30 mg SC q20–30 minutes until settled). When settled: continue q4h dosing with breakthrough q30–60 minutes prn (will likely need a higher dose than previous) and titrate vigilantly. To treat agitation: For all patients, consider methotrimeprazine 5 mg PO/SC q4–6h prn and titrate to a maximum of 25 mg q4–6h prn. For all patients, if significant anxiety is present, consider lorazepam 0.5–1.0 mg PO/IV/SC/SL q30min prn for anxiety. (Carefully!) If the patient is already taking a higher dose of lorazepam or another benzodiazepine, then dose appropriately. Monitor for paradoxical agitation or excessive somnolence. For all patients with very congested breathing, consider glycopyrrolate 0.1–0.2 mg SC q4h prn or scopolamine 0.3–0.6 mg SC q2–3h prn.

Some reminders
- It is usually best to use one opioid only.
- If the patient has been prescribed a fentanyl patch, then another opioid will be used for breakthrough.
- Some patients will be taking multiple opioids and care must be taken when determining the total opioid dose in the past 24 hours.

Titration Guide

General principles:
1. Calculate the total opioid dose taken by the patient in 24 hours (regular q4h dose x 6 **PLUS** the total number of breakthrough doses given x breakthrough dose).
2. Divide this 24-hour total by 6 for the equivalent q4h dose.
3. Divide the newly calculated q4h dose by 2 for the breakthrough dose.
4. Use clinical judgement regarding symptom control as to whether to round up or down the obtained result (both breakthrough and regular dosing). Remember to consider available doses (in the case of PO medications especially).
5. If the patient is very symptomatic, a review of how many breakthrough doses have been given in the past few hours might be more representative of his/her needs.

Example:
A patient is ordered morphine 20 mg q4h PO and 10 mg PO q2h prn, and has taken 3 breakthrough doses in the past 24 hours.
1. Add up the amount of morphine taken in the past 24 hours:
   6 x 20 mg of regular dosing, plus 3 x10 mg prn doses equals a total of 150 mg morphine in 24 hours
2. Divide this total by 6 to obtain the new q4h dose:
   150 divided by 6 = 25 mg q4h
3. Divide the newly calculated q4h dose by 2 to obtain the new breakthrough dose:
   25 mg divided by 2 = 12.5 mg q1-2h prn
4. If this dose provided reasonable symptom control, then order 25 mg PO q4h, with 12.5 mg PO q1–2h prn. (It would also be reasonable to order 10 mg or 15 mg PO q2h for breakthrough.)

Conversion Guide
(To convert from long-acting preparations to short-acting preparations)

General principles in converting from *long-acting* to *short-acting* preparations (for the same drug).
1. Add up the total amount of opioid used in the past 24 hours, including breakthrough dosing.
2. Divide this total by 6 to obtain equivalent q4h dosing.
3. Divide the q4h dose by 2 to obtain breakthrough dosing.
4. Use clinical judgement to adjust this dose up or down depending on symptom control.
5. Consider available tablet sizes when calculating doses.

Example:
A patient is ordered a long-acting morphine preparation at a dose of 60 mg PO q12h, with 20 mg PO q4h for breakthrough, and has taken 4 breakthrough doses in 24 hours.
1. Add up the amount of opioid taken in 24 hours:
   2 X 60 mg of long-acting morphine plus 4 X 20mg of breakthrough is 200 mg of morphine in 24 hours
2. Divide this total by 6 to obtain the equivalent q4h dosing:
   200 divided by 6 is approximately 33 mg PO q4h
3. Divide this q4h dose by 2 for the breakthrough dose
   33 mg divided by 2 is 16.5 mg
4. If the patient had reasonable symptom control with the previous regimen, then a reasonable order would be:
   30 mg PO q4h and 15 mg q1–2h PO prn

EQUIANALGESIC CONVERSIONS			
DRUG	**SC**	**PO**	**Ratio**
Morphine	10 mg	20 mg	2:1 = PO:SC
Codeine	120 mg	200 mg	12:1 (codeine: morphine)
Oxycodone	N/A	10-15 mg	1:2 (oxycodone: morphine)
Hydromorphone	2 mg	4 mg	1:5 (hydromorphone: morphine)

Reproduced with permission from 'Dyspnea Management Guidelines for Palliative Care', pp. 26-36 in Kingston, Frontenac, Lennox and Addington (KFL and A) Palliative Care Integration Project: Symptom Management Guidelines, 2003 August.

A note on guidelines

Although the principles of dyspnoea management, particularly non-pharmacological care, should not differ greatly from institution to institution, the drugs easily available and the sorts of patients cared for might be different. In the UK midazolam (only for parenteral use) is used more frequently before chlorpromazine or levomepromazine and the doses of the former tend to be more conservative. Evidence is scarce for all the drugs used in palliative care and practice varies.

Examples of drugs used in UK

- For dyspnoea and low level anxiety: midazolam 5–10 mg subcutaneously over 24 hours with diamorphine 5–10 mg over 24 hours (if opioid-naive) or convert from their opioid dose.
- Or use oral levomepromazine 6.25–12.5 mg nocte or subcutaneously over 24 hours.
- Midazolam and levomepromazine can be used at higher doses if required.
- Generally 20–30mg in 24 hours will produce some sedation, above this patients will generally be drowsy or fully sedated (60 mg in 24 hours).

6

Breathlessness in neurological disease

Fliss Murtagh, Rachel Burman and
Polly Edmonds

Introduction

While some aspects of breathlessness in neurological disease are common to the different neurological diseases, other aspects are either specific to the disease process or need to be given special consideration in the context of the particular disease. This chapter therefore addresses first the pathophysiology of breathlessness as it relates to neurological disease, then explores a common approach to breathlessness for this group of diseases, and finally addresses more specific considerations under each disease type, focusing on the more common diseases, or those where breathlessness may be particularly challenging to manage.

It is important to remember that neurological disease itself often limits mobility, precluding the early presentation of exertional dyspnoea, in advance of dyspnoea at rest. For this reason, clinicians need a higher index of suspicion for respiratory dysfunction in neurological diseases, and to be proactive in identifying breathlessness and other respiratory symptoms early.

Although breathlessness is usually considered a single sensation, it may well include several distinguishable sensations occurring together.[1] In a study comparing sensations of breathlessness in different diseases, the features more commonly described in neurological disease included gasping, inability to take a breath in fully, heavy or effortful breathing, smothering or suffocating feelings, shallow breathing and an inability to get enough air.[2] While these descriptors cannot be a clinical guide to the causes of breathlessness, they nevertheless give us some insight into the considerable distress and impact that breathlessness in neurological disease can bring.

The pathophysiology of breathlessness as it relates to neurological disease

The pathophysiology of breathlessness is described more fully in Chapter 1. While it is clear that multiple pathophysiological mechanisms are involved, some aspects of the complex mechanisms that control breathing and induce breathlessness are more critical for patients with neurological disease. Of the four main pathophysiological processes involved (increased afferent input from chemoreceptors, increased afferent input from upper airway and pulmonary receptors, increased sense of respiratory effort, and afferent mismatch), it is the increased sense of respiratory effort and the afferent mismatch that are key factors in neurological disease.

In patients with disorders such as amyotrophic lateral sclerosis or myasthenia gravis, the mechanical properties of the respiratory system may be normal, but the weakened respiratory muscles require greater neural drive for activation.[3] This has been demonstrated in patients with myasthenia gravis, who show greater electromyography activity, and higher airway pressures, as compared to controls.[4] This greater neural drive increases sense of respiratory effort, and hence induces dyspnoea. The sense of effort is related to the ratio of the pressure generated by respiratory muscles to the maximum pressure-generating capacity of those muscles.[5] Whenever there is muscle weakness, fatigue or paralysis, the maximum pressure-generating capacity is reduced, which increases the central motor command to the respiratory muscles, raises the sense of respiratory effort, and so induces dyspnoea. The greater neural drive may also add to 'mismatch' between the outgoing motor command, and incoming afferent information. It is as if the brain almost 'expects' a certain pattern of ventilation and afferent feedback according to particular circumstances, and 'mismatch' occurs when the expected and the actual patterns do not coincide. This mismatch further contributes to the sensation of dyspnoea.

Respiratory muscle weakness is a very frequent finding in neurological disease, and contributes directly to the increased sense of respiratory effort, as weak muscles need more neural drive to produce the required effect, as described above. Respiratory muscle weakness is also associated with an increased risk of respiratory infection, which complicates and further compromises respiratory function.

The general debility associated with many neurological diseases is likely to add to respiratory muscle weakness, although evidence for the role of debility in respiratory muscle weakness stems in part from non-neurological conditions. For example, in COPD patients it has been clearly shown that respiratory muscle strength is closely associated with body weight and lean body mass.[6]

Assessment of breathlessness in neurological disease

The assessment of patients with advanced neurological disease will vary depending on stage of the illness and prognosis, but should be geared to assessing the severity of the symptom and identifying potentially reversible or treatable underlying causes. There are several important factors to identify in assessment:

- When does the breathlessness occur? On moderate exertion, e.g. stairs; on minimal exertion, e.g. washing, dressing, eating or talking; at rest?
- Is there associated anxiety, or panic attacks? Can these be distinguished from the sensation of breathlessness?
- Can the patient sleep? Elicit fear of dying associated with insomnia; effect of sleeping position – worse on lying flat?
- Are there other symptoms, e.g. presence of morning headaches, daytime somnolence, fatigue, lethargy and difficulty concentrating that might be suggestive of CO_2 retention in chronic respiratory failure?
- Are there any symptoms suggestive of the presence of bulbar symptoms: difficulty coughing and/or expectorating tenacious secretions, thereby exacerbating anxiety/panic/breathlessness and/or a sensation of choking?
- Does the breathlessness have practical implications for patient, e.g. effect of disability on activities of daily living; use of or requirement for aids; presence of carers or other support during day and night?

Alternative and potentially reversible causes of breathlessness should also be sought where possible, such as infection (particularly if associated with aspiration), anaemia, and acute exacerbation of comorbid conditions, such as chronic obstructive pulmonary disease (COPD) or heart failure. Patients with neurological diseases are particularly susceptible to infection – immobility, aspiration, poor cough reflex, respiratory muscle weakness and malnutrition are all factors that contribute to this.

In patients with neurological disease, it is important to identify respiratory failure as a cause of breathlessness. Chronic respiratory failure secondary to neuromuscular disorders usually occurs in association with motor neurone disease/amyotrophic lateral sclerosis (MND/ALS) or muscular dystrophies.[7] Other neurological conditions also involve the respiratory muscles and can rarely lead to respiratory failure, such as multiple sclerosis, myotonic dystrophy, mitochondrial myopathy, limb girdle syndromes and inflammatory myopathies.[7] Many MND/ALS patients with respiratory muscle weakness will also have bulbar symptoms. Assessments by a speech and language therapist and a physiotherapist are therefore very helpful, particularly where aspiration and difficulty expectorating sputum are exacerbating the breathlessness.

Respiratory failure can be identified by an assessment of arterial blood gases; this will usually be characterised by a low PaO_2 (<8 kPa) in the context of a normal/low (type 1) or raised (>7.5 kPa, type 2) $PaCO_2$. In chronic neurological conditions, respiratory failure is usually type 2; acutely the hydrogen ion $[H^+]$ concentration in the blood will rise, resulting in a respiratory acidosis; a chronically raised $PaCO_2$ is compensated by renal retention of bicarbonate and the $[H^+]$ returns towards normal, representing a primary respiratory acidosis with compensatory metabolic alkalosis.

Arterial oxygen saturation (SaO_2) can be continuously monitored using an oximeter with either ear or finger probes. The oximeter measures the differential absorption of light by oxy- and deoxyhaemoglobin and measures saturation to within 5 per cent that obtained by blood gas analysis.

In the assessment of patients with MND/ALS, the measurement of respiratory muscle strength has been shown to have prognostic value. In a series of 81 patients with ALS, measurement of respiratory muscle strength using nasal sniff pressure was more sensitive than vital capacity and static inspiratory mouth pressures in patients without significant bulbar involvement.[8] In patients with significant bulbar involvement, tests of respiratory muscle strength did not predict hypercapnia.

Sleep-disordered breathing is correlated with respiratory muscle strength and so measurement of SaO_2 overnight can help identify patients with early respiratory failure.

General management strategies

Management should focus on treating reversible underlying causes when these can be identified and are appropriate, e.g. using antibiotics for a chest infection. The effectiveness of specific interventions should be evaluated on an individual basis and repeated as appropriate when symptom relief has been obtained. Where there are no obvious treatable factors, or for patients with poor performance status and/or very short prognosis, the focus should be on symptom management.

General measures

Explanation and reassurance

Patients and carers should receive as full an explanation as possible of the factors contributing to their breathlessness and possible management strategies. Breathlessness is a symptom frequently accompanied by fear and anxiety; these components should be identified to help understand the patient's whole experience of breathlessness. A calm, cohesive, team-orientated approach is particularly useful in allaying patient and carer anxiety. Allowing patients to explore fears and difficulties associated with breathlessness, and to identify losses with respect to activity levels and lifestyle, may assist in the relief of the patients' distress.

Environment

Attention to a breathless patient's home or inpatient environment can improve quality of life. Factors that can be helpful include:

- Easy access to fresh air, where possible, and a fan.
- Some breathless patients need to be upright in order to be comfortable, and find it difficult to sleep in a bed. Aids such as a mattress variator to raise the head of the bed or V-shaped pillow may improve comfort, but some patients will need to sleep in a chair. Adjustable chairs can be very useful in these circumstances.
- Breathless patients with significant anxiety also need to be looked after in a calm environment with carers available for reassurance and support.

Specific measures

Physiotherapy

This can be helpful in aiding patients to expectorate thick, tenacious airway secretions.

Anxiety management

- It is important to differentiate anxiety from breathlessness.
- Anxiety and panic attacks are best managed by a non-pharmacological approach encompassing relaxation and breathing control techniques.[9]
- Although the evidence to support their use in breathlessness is conflicting,[10] in our clinical experience some patients will benefit from using medium-acting benzodiazepines, e.g. lorazepam 0.5–1mg sublingually, for coexisting anxiety, particularly where their prognosis is short and non-pharmacological approaches for anxiety are more difficult to use.
- In our clinical experience, longer acting benzodiazepines, such as diazepam (2–5mg), may be useful where there are high levels of anxiety and especially at night, where breathlessness and fear contribute to insomnia.
- In patients with symptomatic respiratory failure, where symptomatic retention of CO_2 may limit the use of benzodiazepines, anxiolytics that cause do not cause respiratory sedation may be helpful:
  - Nabilone is an anxiolytic with bronchodilator and respiratory stimulant activity.[11] There is little objective data to support its use in

breathlessness, but clinical experience suggests that it can be useful to relieve anxiety and breathlessness for patients with type 2 respiratory failure. Local experience with nabilone suggests that it is started at doses of 0.1mg nocte, and the dose gradually titrated to minimize unpleasant psychomimetic effects, up to doses of 0.25mg twice a day.

- Similarly, buspirone is a drug that stimulates respiration; clinical experience at doses up to 20mg four times a day suggests efficacy in some patients.

Oxygen

The role of oxygen in reducing breathlessness is controversial. The majority of studies in COPD suggest that oxygen is of symptomatic benefit at rest and on exertion,[12] although care must be taken in patients with hypercapnia.

In patients with neurological disorders associated with respiratory muscle weakness, low-flow oxygen, whilst relieving hypoxia, may increase the $PaCO_2$ and therefore should be administered with caution.[13] In this group of patients, formal assessment of respiratory function should be undertaken with a view to suitability for non-invasive ventilation (NIV).

Opioids

There is currently no evidence to support the use of opioids for the systematic relief of breathlessness specifically in patients with advanced neurological diseases. However a recent systematic review of the use of opioids for the management of breathlessness, which included patients with COPD and chronic heart failure, showed that oral and parenteral opioids reduce breathlessness in advanced disease. In some studies opioid use was limited by opioid-related adverse effects, such as nausea and constipation, but clinically significant respiratory depression did not occur.[14]

It would seem reasonable to postulate therefore that in patients with advanced neurological disease and symptomatic breathlessness a trial of low dose opioids may be indicated. It is our practice to limit the use of opioids to patients whose breathlessness is not reversible or managed by other interventions, in view of the high rate of opioid-related adverse effects in opioid-naive patients.[14] Appropriate patients can be started on low dose morphine, e.g. 2.5mg 4 hourly and the dose carefully titrated to response.

Management of thick secretions

Patients with respiratory muscle and bulbar weakness often develop upper respiratory tract and oropharyngeal secretions that are difficult to expectorate and that patients are unable to swallow. The accumulation of these secretions can lead to patients describing a feeling of choking. In the first instance, anti-secretory agents such as hyoscine (delivered by a transdermal patch 1mg/ 3 days) or glycopyrronium 0.6–1mg three times a day given via a gastrostomy can be helpful.

Where the secretions become thick and tenacious, anecdotal reports suggest that mucolytic agents, such as carbocisteine (mucodyne) 750mg three times a day (available in the U.K) can be helpful in this situation. Nebulized hypertonic saline may also be used to thin viscous sputum. The potential problem with the use of mucolytic agents, however, is the production of copious liquid sputum that a weak patient is still not able to expectorate and may aspirate.

In some cases suction may be required to clear secretions, but the procedure is often uncomfortable and distressing for patients and they and relatives may become psychologically focused on the need for suction. Secretions can usually be managed medically; in the terminal phases when patients' conscious level decreases, effective re-positioning and the judicious use of anti-secretory agents is usually adequate.

Management of breathlessness in the terminal phase

Many patients are frightened by uncontrolled breathlessness in the terminal phase. Even in this setting it is useful to differentiate clinically between breathlessness and terminal agitation, as this will affect the choice of drugs for optimal management. For patients in the terminal phase, medication is often administered by the subcutaneous route (sc), either by injections given as required or by using a continuous subcutaneous infusion (CSCI).

Midazolam is a very effective, short acting anxiolytic that is well absorbed subcutaneously; in our experience small doses, e.g. 5–20mg/24h may be adequate to relieve fear and anxiety associated with breathlessness at the end of life in patients with advanced neurological disease. Where terminal agitation is contributing to symptom distress at the end of life, higher doses of midazolam are often required. Alternative drugs in this setting would include antipsychotics, such as levomepromazine (25–100mg/24h) or haloperidol (3–5mg/24h). Diamorphine is effective in relieving the sensation of breathlessness, again used in low dose, e.g. 5–10mg/24h. These drugs can be mixed together in a CSCI given via a syringe driver.

Neurodegenerative diseases

MND/ALS is the most common degenerative disorder of the motor-neuronal system occurring in adults. It is a progressive disease with no curative treatment, and the average prognosis is 3–4 years. The estimated incidence is 1.5–2 per 100,000 per year and increasing.[15] The clinical picture is characterized by fasiculations and progressive paresis of voluntary muscles, plus hyperreflexia and spasticity caused by concomitant involvement of upper and lower motor neurones.[16] Dyspnoea is a very common symptom, becoming a problem for up to 85 per cent of people with MND/ALS. Death usually occurs as a result of acute or acute on chronic ventilatory failure. Many people are frightened about this mode of death and express anxiety about 'choking'.[17]

Dyspnoea usually occurs as a direct result of respiratory muscle weakness, although other indirect symptoms such as thick mucous secretions and chronic hypoventilation also contribute. Any or all of the three muscle groups involved in normal breathing may be involved. As already described, it is this respiratory muscle weakness itself (and the subsequent afferent mismatch) that produces the sensation of dyspnoea. Infrequently, MND/ALS may present with respiratory failure, but for most patients, when the disease presents, there is usually reduced inspiratory, expiratory and upper airway muscle strength. Breathlessness is often the most severe symptom[18] and commonly presents as part of the complex of symptoms related to chronic nocturnal hypoventilation. This complex of symptoms includes daytime fatigue and sleepiness, poor concentration, difficulty sleeping and nightmares, morning headache, autonomic symptoms, depression and anxiety, reduced appetite and weight loss, recurrent or chronic respiratory infections, and diffuse neck and head pains.[19]

As already stated, respiratory failure is the principle cause of death in MND/ALS, and the rate of decline in respiratory function is the one of the few biological indicators shown to predict survival.[20] Since respiratory insufficiency is the most feared symptom of MND/ALS, patients often respond to the first episodes of dyspnoea with strong feelings of anxiety, and it is easy for them to enter an adverse cycle of dyspnoea-anxiety-worsening dyspnoea-worsening anxiety. Clear explanation of what is happening as described earlier in the chapter is essential. The use of anxiolytic medication as outlined in anxiety management also plays a vital role in management of breathlessness for people with MND/ALS.

Ventilation

A more specific treatment modality is ventilation. Mechanical ventilation is recognized to be effective in alleviating the symptoms of ventilatory failure in MND/ALS[21] but if this is achieved using a tracheostomy, it effectively leads to the patient becoming 'locked in'. It is rare for a fully informed patient to choose full mechanical ventilation via tracheostomy, although instances of patients with good quality of life over long periods of time have been reported.[22] Practices vary in different countries according to available resources, prevailing ethical considerations, and patient preferences. The option of non-invasive ventilation may be much more acceptable. Non-invasive positive pressure ventilation (NIPPV) has been shown to improve survival, and may slow rate of respiratory muscle decline for patients with MND/ALS.[23] Those who are able to use it successfully usually report improved dyspnoea and better sleep, although it is more difficult for people with predominantly bulbar symptoms to tolerate. To be effective it needs to be delivered for at least four hours each day, preferably at night.[23] Decisions about the use of non-invasive ventilation depend on the patient's informed choice of it as a management option, ability to use the facemask (which can feel claustrophobic) and the availability of a carer to set up the apparatus. Use of ventilatory support in this way may cause patients to live longer with more progressive disability[24-25], and this raises important ethical issues around decision-making for these patients and their carers. As the disease progresses, non-invasive ventilation may be increasingly required, until it is needed 24 hours a day. This can put a huge burden on the patient and their carers. It is particularly important with this treatment, therefore, to highlight to the patient and carer that it can be stopped whenever the patient wishes.

NIV can be withdrawn in a decremental way e.g. an hour at a time over days, or stopped in one go. It is impossible to predict the effect that stopping NIPPV will have on the patient's prognosis, but they and their carers need to know it may be precipitous. The relief of any acute symptoms of breathlessness and or anxiety can be managed either by sublingual lorazepam or buccal or subcutaneous midazolam. If the patient's condition does deteriorate very rapidly, a syringe driver administering continuous medication may be indicated. Again, it is obviously important that these eventualities are discussed fully prior to withdrawal of the NIPPV.

Movement disorders

Parkinson's disease is the most common movement disorder, and is addressed more fully below. The respiratory problems arising in Huntington's disease relate primarily to the dysphagia that is a common symptom of the motor component of Huntington's disease. Aspiration pneumonia is a common problem, and active measures to reduce risk of aspiration are therefore important.

Parkinson's disease

Breathlessness is frequent problem for patients with Parkinson's disease, occurring in 40 per cent of patients surveyed.[26] It commonly goes unrecognized, however, in the face of the more severe motor problems. Maximal static, inspiratory and expiratory pressures are reduced, as well as maximal inspiratory and expiratory flows. Patients with Parkinson's disease may also be unable to generate the necessary rise in peak expiratory flow required for effective cough. As a symptom, breathlessness can fluctuate with long-term levodopa treatment in a similar way to the well-described motor fluctuations. Although a survey of non-motor fluctuations in 50 patients with Parkinson's disease found dyspnoea less commonly than some other symptoms, dyspnoea was highly correlated with level of disability, and addressing it is therefore important for improving quality of life.[27] The cause of death in Parkinson's disease is commonly respiratory,[28,29] and active management of respiratory symptoms in the terminal phase needs careful attention.

Neuroinflammatory disorders

Neuroinflammatory diseases share the same pathological finding of foci of degeneration in the myelin sheath of nervous tissue. Multiple sclerosis (MS) is the commonest neuroinflammatory, demyelinating disease, which affects the central nervous system. It is also the commonest cause of chronic neurodisability in young adults, with a median age of onset of 31 years and prevalence in Britain of 80–100/100,000 population. It particularly affects the spinal cord, optic nerves and brainstem.

MS has a variable and unpredictable natural course which makes it particularly difficult to manage. Symptoms may appear and then disappear, only to reappear in a relapsing/remitting (RR) way for 85 per cent of people. These episodes occur at irregular intervals and, despite disease-modifying therapies, over time recovery is incomplete and a burden of disability and symptoms accumulates for the patient. Up to 90 per cent of people with RR disease progress to secondary progressive MS and suffer irreversible disability, which inexorably escalates.

Death from MS directly is very rare, and the most common cause of death is infection[30] Breathlessness is most commonly associated with respiratory infection, and as with Parkinson's disease, it correlates with the degree of disability. The later stages of MS are marked by severe fatigue and immobility. Weakness and dysphagia contribute to poor nutrition and cachexia, all of which in turn predispose to an enhanced risk of infection. MS also causes cognitive deficit in 40–60 per cent of people, with severe dysfunction in a third.[31] This makes involving the patient in the decision-making process about the appropriateness of active management of a respiratory infection and symptoms with antibiotics, oxygen therapy and possible ventilatory support all the more difficult.

Vascular disorders affecting the nervous system

In this group of neurological conditions, breathlessness is most commonly associated with respiratory infection. The prevalence of breathlessness as a symptom in this group of conditions is not known. Interventions are focused on treatment of the underlying infection, where appropriate, and general management strategies towards relief of breathlessness, as outlined above. Very careful consideration should be given to the appropriateness of treating the underlying infection, based on considerations of stage of illness, comorbidity, expected prognosis, patient preference, and balance of treatment benefits, as against illness/treatment burdens. Identifying patient preference is particularly challenging, since there may well be cognitive impairment and/or communication difficulties. Advance planning is especially valuable, if feasible.

Dementia

Although included here under vascular disorders, dementia may also be neurodegenerative. Pneumonia is markedly more common among those dying of advanced dementia that among those dying from cancer.[32] Despite this, the prevalence of breathlessness among those dying from dementia is low (8.2 per cent compared to 27.6 per cent in cancer patients in the same study). This may be because of the subjective nature of breathlessness as a symptom, and associated difficulties in detecting it in the presence of severe cognitive impairment.

Stroke

In the palliative day care setting, stroke is one of the three major diagnoses besides cancer.[33] Acute hemiplegia due to stroke is associated with an increased risk of death due to respiratory causes. Most of this increased risk is due to chest infections, but pulmonary embolus is reported in up to 9 per cent of those admitted with acute stroke.[34] The pathophysiology of breathlessness in stroke is unclear, but reduced diaphragmatic and intercostal muscle excursion on the hemiplegic side in voluntary breathing have been described.[35]

Ethical considerations

Ethical considerations in the management of breathlessness in neurological disease centre on informed consent. Competent patients are able to participate in the decision-making process and the planning of their care. It is for them to decide whether they wish to have treatment or not. In patients with neurodegenerative diseases such as Parkinson's disease or dementia, it is therefore appropriate to attend to end-of-life treatment decisions before a person becomes incompetent to express their preferences either because of communication difficulties or cognitive impairment. The slow nature of the progression of this degeneration should allow the patient, their family and the medical team time to discuss a disease-specific advance plan; for example, whether or not to have antibiotics to treat an infection, which is the underlying cause of their breathlessness. This can be formalised as an Advance Directive if the patient wishes. Similarly, patients with MND/ALS, where the most feared symptom is breathlessness caused by respiratory insufficiency, can discuss the use of NIPPV as soon as breathlessness develops, and before progressive dysarthria makes communicating very difficult. Refusal of medical treatment by competent patients, including that for breathlessness, is an implicit part of the doctrine of informed consent and must be respected.

Role of terminal sedation

Sedation of a patient who is imminently dying is considered when a symptom is refractory to management in any other way. The clinical management of breathlessness in the terminal phase has been covered earlier in the chapter. Should these measures fail to control a patient's breathlessness and they remain imminently dying and with an unacceptable level of distress, then terminal sedation may be indicated. This is defined as 'the intention of inducing and maintaining deep sleep but not deliberately causing death, in a very special circumstance'.[36] The drug of choice is empirically that which is also effective for the prevalent symptom with or without the use of a second agent such as a benzodiazepine. Ethically, the clinical decision to sedate a patient with the possibility in so doing of shortening a patient's life expectancy is distinct from euthanasia. This is because the intention is different. The validity of this derives from the doctrine of double effect, which distinguishes between the primary therapeutic intent (that of relief of the suffering caused by the breathlessness) and the possible second unintended consequence of an accelerated death (arising from the unavoidable, untoward consequence of decreased consciousness).

Conclusion

This chapter has considered the general mechanisms of the symptom and management of breathlessness in neurological disease. The causes of breathlessness in specific conditions have been described and the particular implications of these discussed. The majority of these conditions are degenerative in nature. They share the common feature that they all will at some point inexorably progress and will likely become resistant to curative interventions. The degree to which this is so varies between the diseases, but for all of them the goals of treatment, the methods used, and the decision-making under-taken must be openly discussed and shared with the patient and their families. The focus should always be the best quality of life for the particular individual and their family, and, when the time comes, the most appropriate death[37] with the least possible suffering.

References

1. Simon PM, Schwartzstein RM, Weiss JW, Lahive K, Fencl V, Teghtsoonian M *et al.* Distinguishable sensations of breathlessness induced in normal volunteers [see comment]. *American Review of Respiratory Disease* 1989; **140**(4): 1021–7.

2. Simon PM, Schwartzstein RM, Weiss JW, Fencl V, Teghtsoonian M, Weinberger SE. Distinguishable types of dyspnea in patients with shortness of breath [see comment]. *American Review of Respiratory Disease* 1990; **142**(5): 1009–14.

3. Manning HL, Schwartzstein RM. Dyspnoea and the control of breathing. In: Altose MT, Kamakami T, eds. *Control of Breathing in Health and Disease.* New York: Marcel Dekker, 1999, 105–135.

4. Spinelli A, Marconi G, Gorini M, Pizzi A, Scano G. Control of breathing in patients with myasthenia gravis. *American Review of Respiratory Disease* 1992; **145**(6): 1359–66.

5. Manning HL, Schwartzstein RM. Dyspnoea and the control of breathing. In: Altose MT, Kamakami T, eds. *Control of Breathing in Health and Disease.* New York: Marcel Dekker, 2004, 105–135.

6. Nishimura Y, Tsutsumi M, Nakata H, Tsunenari T, Maeda H, Yokoyama M. Relationship between respiratory muscle strength and lean body mass in men with COPD. *Chest* 1995; **107**(5): 1232–6.

7. Polkey MI, Lyall RA, Moxham J, Leigh PN. Respiratory aspects of neurological disease. *J Neurol Neurosurg Psychiatry* 1999; **66**(1): 5–15.

8. Lyall RA, Donaldson N, Polkey MI, Leigh PN, Moxham J. Respiratory muscle strength and ventilatory failure in amyotrophic lateral sclerosis. *Brain* 2001; **124**(Pt 10): 2000–13.

9. Bredin M, Corner J, Krishnasamy M, Plant H, Bailey C, A'Hern R. Multicentre randomised controlled trial of nursing intervention for breathlessness in patients with lung cancer. *BMJ* 1999; **318**(7188): 901–4.

10. Ahmedzai S. Palliation of respiratory symptoms. In: Doyle D, Hanks GWC, MacDonald N, eds. *Oxford Textbook of Palliative Medicine.* Oxford: Oxford University Press, 1998.

11. Ahmedzai S, Carter R, Mills RJ, Moran F. Effects of nabilone of pulmonary function. In: *Proceedings of the Oxford Symposium on Cannabis.* Oxford: IRL Press, 1984, 371–377.

12. Ripamonti C. Management of dyspnea in advanced cancer patients. *Supportive Care in Cancer* 1999; **7**(4): 233–43.

13. Gay PC, Edmonds LC. Severe hypercapnia after low-flow oxygen therapy in patients with neuromuscular disease and diaphragmatic dysfunction. *Mayo Clin Proc* 1995; **70**(4): 327–30.

14. Jennings AL, Davies AN, Higgins JP, Gibbs JS, Broadley KE. A systematic review of the use of opioids in the management of dyspnoea. *Thorax* 2002; **57**(11): 939–44.

15. Lilienfeld DE, Chan E, Ehland J, Godbold J, Landrigan PJ, Marsh G *et al.* Rising mortality from motoneuron disease in the USA, 1962–84. *Lancet* 1989; **1**(8640): 710–13.

16. Borasio GD, Appel SH, Buttner U. Upper and lower motor neuron disorders. In: Brant T, Caplan LR, Dichgans J, eds *Neurological Disorders: Course and Treatment.* San Diego, CA: Academic Press, 1996, 811–17.

17. O'Brien T, Kelly M, Saunders C. Motor neurone disease: a hospice perspective. *BMJ* 1992; **304**(6825): 471–3.
18. Borasio GD, Miller RG. Clinical characteristics and management of ALS. *Semin Neurol* 2001; **21**(2): 155–66.
19. Voltz R, Borasio GD. Palliative therapy in the terminal stage of neurological disease. *J Neurol* 1997; **244**(Suppl 4): S2–S10.
20. Haverkamp LJ, Appel V, Appel SH. Natural history of amyotrophic lateral sclerosis in a database population. Validation of a scoring system and a model for survival prediction. *Brain* 1995; **118**(Pt 3): 707–19.
21. Howard RS, Wiles CM, Loh L. Respiratory complications and their management in motor neuron disease. *Brain* 1989; **112**(Pt 5): 1155–70.
22. Smith RA, Gillie E, Licht J. Palliative treatment of motor neurone disease. In: de Jong JMBV, ed. *Handbook of Clinical Neurology*, pp. 459–73 volume **15**: Diseases of the motor system. New York: Elsevier, 1998.
23. Kleopa KA, Sherman M, Neal B, Romano GJ, Heiman-Patterson T. Bipap improves survival and rate of pulmonary function decline in patients with ALS. *J Neurol Sci* 1999; **164**(1): 82–8.
24. Pinto AC, Evangelista T, Carvalho M, Alves MA, Sales Luis ML. Respiratory assistance with a non-invasive ventilator (Bipap) in MND/ALS patients: survival rates in a controlled trial. *J Neurol Sci* 1995; **129**(Suppl): 19–26.
25. Aboussouan LS, Khan SU, Meeker DP, Stelmach K, Mitsumoto H. Effect of noninvasive positive-pressure ventilation on survival in amyotrophic lateral sclerosis. *Ann Intern Med* 1997; **127**(6): 450–3.
26. Witjas T, Kaphan E, Azulay JP, Blin O, Ceccaldi M, Pouget J et al. Nonmotor fluctuations in Parkinson's disease: frequent and disabling. *Neurology* 2002; **59**(3): 408–13.
27. Witjas T, Kaphan E, Azulay JP, Blin O, Ceccaldi M, Pouget J et al. Nonmotor fluctuations in Parkinson's disease: frequent and disabling. *Neurology* 2002; **59**(3): 408–13.
28. Lees AJ. Comparison of therapeutic effects and mortality data of levodopa and levodopa combined with selegiline in patients with early, mild Parkinson's disease. Parkinson's Disease Research Group of the United Kingdom. *BMJ* 1995; **311**(7020): 1602–7.
29. Wermuth L, Stenager EN, Stenager E, Boldsen J. Mortality in patients with Parkinson's disease. *Acta Neurol Scand* 1995; **92**(1): 55–8.
30. Sadovnick AD, Ebers GC, Wilson RW, Paty DW. Life expectancy in patients attending multiple sclerosis clinics. *Neurology* 1992; **42**(5): 991–4.
31. McDonald WI, Ron MA. Multiple sclerosis: the disease and its manifestations. *Philos Trans R Soc Lond B Biol Sci* 1999; **354**(1390): 1615–22.
32. Mitchell SL, Kiely DK, Hamel MB. Dying with advanced dementia in the nursing home. *Arch Intern Med* 2004; **164**(3): 321–6.
33. Higginson IJ, Hearn J, Myers K, Naysmith A. Palliative day care: what do services do? Palliative Day Care Project Group. *Palliat Med* 2000; **14**(4): 277–86.
34. Oppenheimer S, Hachinski V. Complications of acute stroke. *Lancet* 1992; **339**(8795): 721–4.
35. Fluck DC. Chest movements in hemiplegia. *Clin Sci* 1966; **31**(3): 383–8.
36. Poulain F, Pourchet S. Palliative Sededation – report of the working group of the EAPC. In: Abstracts of the 2nd Congress of the EAPC Research Network. *European Association for Palliative Care*; 2002, 240.
37. Cherny NI, Coyle N, Foley KM. Guidelines in the care of the dying cancer patient. *Hematol Oncol Clin North Am* 1996; **10**(1): 261–86.

7

Breathlessness in children

Stephen Liben

Definition of terms

In this chapter the terms dyspnea, breathlessness, air hunger, chest pain, and shortness of breath will be used interchangeably to describe the sensation experienced when breathing feels difficult, painful, laboured, or uncomfortable. A consensus statement on dyspnea[1] gives the following definition:

> Dyspnea is a term used to characterize a subjective experience of breathing discomfort that consists of qualitatively distinct sensations that vary in intensity. The experience derives from interactions among multiple physiological, psychological, social and environmental factors, and may induce secondary physiological and behavioural responses.

It is important to stress that the feeling/perception of unpleasantness is central to the diagnosis of dyspnea. Similar to the definition of pain, which emphasizes subjective experience even in the absence of actual tissue damage, dyspnea occurs whenever the patient says it occurs. Like pain again, dyspnea, as a felt sensation, is influenced by an individual's psychological state, personality and previous experience.

The importance of using an accurate definition of dyspnea cannot be overstated since misunderstandings between dyspnea and other forms of respiratory signs/symptoms may lead to inappropriate treatments. In this author's experience with paediatric palliative care the three signs most commonly confused with dyspnea are tachypnea, noisy (rattly, mucousy), and shallow breathing. These three signs *may or may not* be associated with a sensation of shortness of breath (dyspnea or breathlessness).

Tachypnea

Tachypnea means breathing with a respiratory rate that is greater than normal for age. Tachypnea may be an adaptive physiological sign in response to normal physical exertion or exercise and is not necessarily associated with the sensation of dyspnea. Tachypnea may occur without dyspnea when it is in response to increased central drive from, for example, a brain tumour. Alternatively tachypnea may occur concomitantly with dyspnea in the presence of meta-static pulmonary lesions.

Noisy breathing

Noisy breathing without dyspnea may occur due to movement of air through an altered airway, such as in a child with a tracheostomy. Noisy breathing sometimes called the 'death rattle' may also occur during the dying process and in unconscious children it may not be associated with dyspnea. In such situations it is often the onlookers (parents and professional caregivers) who are distressed by the 'noisy breathing' in the presence of a calm and relaxed child whose noisy breathing does not appear to be causing them any discomfort.

Shallow breathing

Shallow breathing means breathing with a decreased tidal volume and may occur at the end of life in the absence of any signs of dyspnea. Alternatively in a child with a pleural tumour shallow breathing may occur due to 'splinting' as deeper breaths may cause more pain. Such shallow breathing is the result of pain and distress and occurs together with dyspnea.

Case example

John was born with generalized weakness and recurrent bouts of respiratory failure resulting in multiple intubations and prolonged periods of time on mechanical ventilation. At age 1 year he was tracheostomized and was fully dependent on mechanical ventilation. When John was comfortable and doing well he was a happy baby able to smile and follow faces with his eyes. His repertoire of facial expressions was limited, but those who knew him best agreed that John certainly looked very different when he was relaxed and happy versus when he was upset or in pain. When John was taken off the ventilator for brief periods of time his face would register panic and placing him back on the respirator would quickly return him to what appeared to be a comfortable state. During periods of respiratory infections John's ventilator settings were adjusted (with an increased respiratory rate and tidal volume) both to normalize his oxygen saturation/carbon dioxide level as well as to decrease his caregiver's perception of his level of distress. During these episodes opioids (morphine via the gastrostomy tube) were used intermittently in addition to adjusting the ventilator settings. On the whole these adjustments were successful in maintaining a reasonable level of comfort for John. He had generalized hypotonia, poor suck and swallow and received feeds via a gastrostomy tube.

At age 2 years he was diagnosed with a rare form of myopathy. By age 4 years his weakness had progressed to the point where he was essentially paralysed and he began to have very frequent and severe episodes of pneumonia. He also developed chronic lung disease with increasing requirements for oxygen and appeared to be in respiratory distress much of the time, requiring frequent suctioning for secretions from his tracheostomy tube. He was placed on inhaled steroids as well as oral glycopyrrolate to help decrease the quantity of his airway secretions. His parents and other caregivers agreed that John's quality of life had become very low and that he was spending much of his life in discomfort and pain. During an episode of severe pneumonia his oxygen saturations stayed in the low 70s in spite of the administration of 100 per cent oxygen. He was placed on continuous morphine that was titrated to an assessment of his level of comfort from his facial expressions. After 5 days his respiratory function deteriorated and the decision was made to take him off the ventilator and allow him to die. His mother was helped in finding the words to explain to John what was happening and why in a way that was appropriate to a 4-year-old's developmental understanding of death and congruent with that family's communication style and spiritual beliefs (John was told that he was very sick and that it was time for him to go to a place where he would feel good and where his grandmother who had predeceased him would be waiting to help take care of him). When he was taken off the ventilator his baseline dose of morphine was maintained and he was given as needed boluses equal to one hour's worth of his morphine infusion every 10 minutes, titrated to his facial expressions. He died one hour later in the arms of his mother.

Epidemiology of breathlessness in paediatric palliative care

Although the exact prevalence is not known, given the current literature on symptoms at the end of life in children, it is reasonable to state that dyspnea is a commonly encountered symptom in dying children. Most of what we know about dyspnea and related respiratory symptoms at the end-of-life comes from studies looking at signs and/or symptoms of children with cancer. In one institution, a chart review spanning 11 years of children receiving palliative care for cancer found that 40 per cent of children had respiratory symptoms during the last three months of life.[2] A study examining the records of 28 children enrolled in a palliative home care program over a four-year period found severe respiratory problems in 39 per cent. The causes attributed to dyspnea were aspiration pneumonia, lung metastasis, brain tumours and heart failure. The authors commented that end-stage dyspnea was found to be particularly worrisome to parents.[3] A retrospective analysis of how children die in one Canadian hospital found that most died while in intensive care and that opioids were prescribed for dyspnoea/and or respiratory distress in 25 per cent of children.[4] Eighty per cent of parents responding to a telephone interview, a mean of three years after the death of their child from cancer, reported their child suffered from dyspnea in the last month of life with about 40 per cent stating that their child had suffered 'a great deal' or 'a lot' as a result. In this same study parents reported that dyspnea was treated 65 per cent of the time but was successfully treated in only 16 per cent of those surveyed. Of concern was a related finding that dyspnea was reported by parents but not by the physician 20 per cent of the time, while conversely reported by the physician but not by the parent only 11 per cent of the time.[5] Collins and colleagues[6] reported on the symptoms of children aged 10–18 years old in 159 children with cancer. Both cough and dyspnea were prevalent and were associated with significant distress. The location of death was significant in that the last week of life of children in an intensive care unit had half the prevalence of cough and dyspnea when compared to death on the wards. A more recent study out of Japan[7] examined the medical records of 28 children who died of cancer over a seven-year period. Although there were small numbers of children described in this study, a significant finding was the greater percentage of dyspnea in children with leukemia/lymphoma versus those with brain tumours.

A chart review of the end-of-life care of children with cystic fibrosis showed that almost half were reported to have both dyspnea and chest pain and most received opioids from between one hour to more than one month before death.[8] There remains a dearth of literature on the prevalence and severity of dyspnea in children dying from illnesses other than cancer. From the data that exists to date it appears that dyspnea is both a common and very significant symptom for both the affected children as well as for their caregivers.

Assessing breathlessness in children

Given the subjective nature of breathlessness, the best measurement remains that of self-report. Measurement scales, such as the modified Borg scale, originally developed for adults, have been modified for the self-report of breathlessness but they have not been applied to end of life care in children.[9] For younger children in whom self-report is more problematic, Kendrich has refined a self-rating scale that attempts to standardize language.[10] In addition to self-report and visual analogue scales, attempts at more objective measurements of dyspnea have included having children with cystic fibrosis take a deep breath and then count out loud to 15 wherein the number of breaths taken to complete the count is the score[11] For children who are able to verbalize how they feel, creating a scale that is simple for the child to use and that incorporates their own language is more likely to be clinically relevant in day to day practice. Children may describe the sensation of dyspnea/ breathlessness in many different ways. For example one study looked at the different terms 39 school age children with asthma used to describe their breathing on a 'bad breathing day'.[12] These children most frequently described their breathing as 'It is hard to breathe'. Words chosen most often were 'wheezy', 'short of breath', and 'tight'. Importantly this group of children with chronic asthma coped with their dyspnea by the use of medications, change in position, decreased activity, and fluids: in short, many of the same coping mechanisms used by adults.

For the many children in paediatric palliative care who are not able to talk either by virtue of their young age or advanced illness, self-report of dyspnea is impossible. For these children the frequency and intensity of their breathlessness will need to be assessed by others, most often their parents and the professional caregivers who know them best. Although this dependence on the subjective judgement of someone other than the patient to define dyspnea makes research into dyspnea at the end-of-life fraught with difficulty, these limitations are thankfully less important in day-to-day practice. It may be difficult to standardize, but the subjective assessment of breathlessness made by looking at the non-verbal language of the child (facial expression and posture) often is a sensitive measure of the respiratory distress of children. By their nature parents are always and continually responding to the non-verbal needs of their children and the facial expression of someone with obvious air hunger may be difficult to describe but is not hard to recognize. Responding to a child's perceived non-verbal distress is at present the best way of rating and responding to perceived signs of breathlessness. Such assessments work best when a clinician listens carefully to what those who know the child best have to say both about his or her breathlessness as well as to overall comfort. When in doubt it may be worthwhile to assume that breathlessness may be a factor in a child's non-verbal expression of distress and a trial of medication or non-drug therapy may be attempted to assess whether distress is relieved. For example should a non-verbal child show, through their facial expression, signs of respiratory distress, it might be prudent to assess their airway and breathing and if compromised attempt measures at alleviating the respiratory symptom to see if overall distress is alleviated.

Causes of dyspnea in advanced disease in children

There are myriad causes of dyspnea in a child which involve many of the branches of general paediatric medicine and paediatric respiratory medicine in particular. It is not within the scope of this chapter to address the aetiology and management of all causes of dyspnea with which a child with advanced disease might present. For example a child may have asthma in addition to the diagnosis of a brain tumour. At the end of life for this child it is possible that his asthma may be a significant cause of dyspnea and its treatment, based on current asthma guidelines, is well described in standard paediatric textbooks. In addition, given the paucity of data on dyspnea in paediatric palliative care there is little data correlating specific disease entities with dyspnea in paediatric palliative care. Classification systems for dyspnea may be based on the time course: acute, subacute, chronic, or recurrent. Alternatively dyspnea can be classified according to the type of sign or symptom it presents as: wheezing, stridor, rales, cough, haemoptysis, and pleural/chest pain. An even more detailed classification might be based on pathology: primary and secondary lung disease, causes of congestive failure, upper and lower airway pathologies and so on. In paediatric palliative care a classification based on the most commonly encountered causes of dyspnea might include dividing aetiologies into cancer (solid tumour versus the leukemias) and non-cancer-related causes (see Table 7.1).

Whichever classification schema is utilized it must be recognized that an individual patient may have dyspnea from different causes at different phases of their illness trajectory. In addition, despite the wide range of initial diagnoses that may be found in paediatric palliative care the final common pathway that most often leads to dyspnea is shared by many disorders. For example, fatal inborn errors of metabolism often lead to convulsions and coma. Dyspnea in this setting is often a result of the combined effects of acidemia along with aspiration pneumonia. In children with central nervous system injury from a wide variety of disorders (e.g. cerebral palsy, neonatal hypoxia and severe seizure disorders) dyspnea may present as a result of chronic aspiration of food or saliva. In cardiac failure due to many different congenital heart defects the final common pathway to dyspnea is often fluid overload syndromes with congestive heart failure. Clinically dyspnea may result from one of three perturbations of the respiratory system due to an *increase* in:

1 Respiratory drive driven by an increased respiratory load which occurs, for example, in obstructive and restrictive lung disease or pleural disease.
2 The amount of respiratory work needed in order to breathe such as in the presence of hyperinflated lungs or neuromuscular weakness.

Table 7.1 Cancer-related causes of dyspnea in advanced disease

Direct tumour effects	Indirect tumour effects	Cancer treatment effects
Invasion/replacement of lung parenchyma	Hypercoaguability – pulmonary emboli	Immunosuppression-infection/pneumonias
Large or small airway obstruction	Immunosuppression – infection	Radiotherapy – pneumonitis
Pleural effusion	Wasting/cachexia	Chemotherapy – pulmonary fibrosis
Ascites/abdominal distension	Paraneoplastic/endocrine-bronchospasm	Chemotherapy – congestive heart failure
Superior vena cava syndrome	Anaemia	Effects of surgical interventions on lung parenchyma/airways

Table 7.2 Non-cancer-related causes of dyspnea in advanced disease

Pulmonary	Cystic fibrosis	Hypoplastic lungs	Bronchopulmonary dysplasia	Primary pulmonary hypertension	Severe kyphoscoliosis
Cardiac	Congestive heart failure	Hypoplastic left heart syndrome	Complex-uncorrectable congenital heart disease	Myocarditis	Severe pericardial disease
Neurological–neuromuscular	Anoxic encephalopathy	Spinal Muscular atrophy	Muscular dystrophy	Myopathies	Spinal cord injuries
Metabolic/ systemic disorders	Inborn errors with acidosis	Renal failure	Anaemia	Abdominal distension/ obesity	Mitochondrial disorders

3 Ventilatory demands such as occurs with an increased metabolic rate, anaemia, hypoxemia, or pulmonary vascular disease.[13]

With each presentation of breathlessness a thorough re-evaluation of possible causes based on the approach that would be taken for a child at any stage of illness needs to be undertaken. Perhaps the greatest obstacle to successfully treating dyspnea in paediatric-advanced disease is the myth that dying is inevitably a painful process associated with breathlessness and gasping. A careful reassessment coupled to pathophysiologically-based therapeutic trials will often lead to relief of dyspnea at all stages of illness, including during the dying process.

Management of breathlessness in children

In the management of breathlessness in children with advanced disease it is first and foremost necessary to clearly identify the goals of treatment. The goal of the treatment of dyspnea is to reduce the child's perceived unpleasant or painful sensation of breathlessness or air hunger. Treatment may not diminish the outward manifestations of respiratory distress (i.e.: tachypnea may persist) but aims instead to eliminate the child's inner feeling/sensation of dyspnea. This may be important to articulate to both parents and professional caregivers who may not be aware that a child who appears relaxed but tachypneic is not necessarily experiencing breathlessness as a perceived sensation. In fact, the effects of drugs in the benzodiazepine and opioid class are often to decrease the sensation of dyspnea without necessarily altering the respiratory pattern.

First principles of treatment of dyspnea are to treat the underlying cause when and if possible. For example if a local tumour is impinging upon large airways or causing superior vena-caval obstruction then consideration may be given to a trial of steroids and local radiotherapy, and in some instances chemotherapy, particularly in the case of chemotherapy-sensitive lymphomas. If dyspnea is due to anaemia then a transfusion or the use of erythropoetin should be considered. Although more commonly utilized in adult palliative care there may be times when a pleural tap to relieve pleural effusions may be useful. More often, however, and depending on the cause, pleural fluid may rapidly reaccumulate and recurrent pleural taps may cause more discomfort than good.[14]

Drug treatments

Opioids are the mainstay of the drug management of dyspnoea in children with advanced disease. The mechanisms of action of opioids remain not fully elucidated but likely relate to opioid effects that serve to decrease the sensitivity of central PCO_2 receptors and by acting as a sedative. Thus opioids alleviate dyspnoea by decreasing the perception of breathlessness. Commonly held false beliefs that opioids cause apnoea unnecessarily keep some children from receiving the relief of dyspnea that is possible when opioids are used appropriately. Although there is little data comparing the doses of opioids required to relieve pain versus those required for the relief of dyspnoea, clinical practice appears to favour the use of opioids with the same dosage guidelines as those used for pain control in children.[15] Nebulized morphine has been used as a treatment for dyspnoea in the management of symptoms arising from cystic fibrosis with some success, but there is a need for further study before clear recommendations can be made on its regular use.[16]

The specific opioids used, route, and frequency of administration will be based on patient-dependent factors similar to those guiding the use of opioids to control pain. Dyspnoea of short duration can be treated on an as needed (prn) basis with short-acting opioids such as morphine (start dose in the opioid naïve child of 0.3 mg/kg/dose orally) or intravenous fentanyl (0.5 micrograms/kg/dose i.v.). Should dyspnoea persist for days to weeks then the initial prn doses of short-acting opioids can be used to calculate the equivalent in longer acting preparations. For patients with predictable long-term dyspnoea, such as those with cystic fibrosis, it may be advisable to use a long-acting opioid such as transdermal fentanyl with the addition of a short-acting opioid such as morphine administered orally on an as needed basis. Careful titration of opioids may have a tremendous effect on improving quality of life for children with dyspnoea of advanced disease. For severe or sudden dyspnoea, such as may occur with pulmonary embolus or pneumothorax, the use of intravenous (in an environment with the appropriate equipment and support) or subcutaneous opioids may be necessary. For children cared for in the home it may be helpful to have pre-prepared doses of morphine suppositories available in the event of dyspnoea that often occurs at the same time as difficulty swallowing. As with the use of any opioid the clinician needs to prevent the predictable and treatable side-effects of opioids, such as constipation.[15] A significant obstacle to the appropriate use of opioids to manage dyspnoea is often the pervasive myths that parents may hold with regard to opioid use. Parents may mistakenly believe that their children will become 'addicts' and may be reluctant to articulate their beliefs. The clinician will need to address these myths about opioids (such as addiction) and educate parents about the appropriate use of opioids to control dyspnoea.

Benzodiazepines are the other major class of drugs used to treat dyspnoea in children. Benzodiazepines act by decreasing the anxiety associated with breathlessness and may be used together with opioids as first line drug treatment of dyspnoea. Benzodiazepines have the advantage of ease of administration (sublingual or per rectum) and rapidity of onset in children who are unable to swallow. In situations where dyspnoea is associated with panic, benzodiazpeines can be especially useful. A typical start dose is 0.05 mg/kg/dose for oral lorazepam and 0.2–0.3 mg/kg/dose for oral diazepam. These dosages are generally the same as those used to treat anxiety.

Cannabinoids may also be used in the treatment of dyspnoea, although there may be significant problems with dysphoria. Cannabinoids may act via their bronchodilator effect together with altering the sensitivity to PCO_2 in addition to their likely role in altering the central perception of breathlessness. Synthetic cannabinoids such as dronabinol have been used mostly for their antiemtic effects but may play a role in selected patients with chronic dyspnoea.

Steroids may be used to manage dyspnoea in children in specific instances, either for their direct effects on the tumour or for their anti-inflammatory effects in reactive airways disease. Diuretics have a role in the management of dyspnoea resulting from congestive heart failure and occasionally in partial renal failure when the kidneys remain responsive to a forced diuresis.

Inhaled oxygen's potential effects on dyspnoea remain controversial (see Chapter 12 of this textbook). It appears that 'blow by' oxygen may be no more efficacious than 'blow by' room air (for example as delivered by a standard desktop or hand-held fan). In some patients oxygen appears to have a role in decreasing dyspnoea and when available it may be a useful therapy to initiate as a trial. For children dying in the home oxygen may be complicated and/or expensive to organize and the use of a free-flow of room air may be just as beneficial. It is *not* useful to have a continuous oxygen saturation monitor attached to a child in the terminal/dying stage of illness. Should this happen the monitor inevitably becomes the focus of attention rather than the child themself. If a trial of oxygen is initiated all involved should understand the goal of therapy: that is that oxygen will be given and titrated to comfort and not to a predetermined oxygen saturation.

Non-drug treatments

Educating caregivers as to what to expect, together with offering an initial treatment plan for managing dyspnoea, can do much to alleviate the often high degree of caregiver anxiety about the possibility of their child suddenly developing breathlessness. It is particularly important in home care to plan in advance for the possibility that dyspnoea may occur in the middle of night. A care plan that includes having a professional available for immediate consultation by phone together with the availability of 'start' doses of opioids and benzodiazpeines in the home can do much to alleviate caregiver distress. In addition to pharmacological treatments for breathlessness in children it may also help to avoid an overly high room temperature and maintain humidity. There is evidence that cold facial stimulation by providing a free flow of air by the face (via a fan or open window) may reduce breathlessness in adults and may help with some children.[17] This kind of non-invasive treatment has the added value in that is a helpful therapy that can be initiated and adapted by the child or parents without special training. Positioning may also alleviate distress and trials should be made with the child sitting up or alternatively changing from lying on one side to another. Gentle chest physiotherapy may be helpful in instances of increased sputum production, particularly in cystic fibrosis. In younger children and infants who swallow sputum rather than expectorate the risks of aspiration must be weighed against the potential benefits of chest physiotherapy.

In older children who are able to cooperate, the use of relaxation therapy, distraction, and guided imagery (hypnosis) may be helpful in reducing anxiety associated with chronic dyspnoea.[18] Another aspect to adjusting to chronic breathlessness in children involves educating the child and parents about the role of activity pacing in response to changes in the child's ability to play and be active. Activity pacing may involve encouraging children to learn to schedule activities when they are less breathless, when medications are at their peak effectiveness, or to take a prn dose for activities known to cause breathlessness. Such activity pacing requires taking a thorough history and adapting the child's daily schedule accordingly (Personal communication, D. Drouin 2004).

Ventilatory support

Ventilation may be supported by mechanical means and is a common feature in children who die in paediatric and neonatal intensive care units: it may be invasive or non-invasive.

Mechanical ventilation

Invasive mechanical ventilation is the use of positive pressure ventilation administered to the child via an endotracheal or tracheostomy tube. Children with progressive degenerative neuromuscular disease, such as spinal muscular atrophy, may have been placed on chronic long-term mechanical ventilation via a tracheostomy. Such ventilator-dependent children may become dyspnoeic due to specific problems related to their particular ventilator, airway, or lungs. The management of dyspnoea in these chronically ventilated children requires specialist paediatric respiratory care as well as specialized training of parents should the child be cared for at home. In advanced stages of illness when dying begins and routine ventilator management provides neither adequate ventilation nor relief from dyspnoea any longer then the management of dyspnoea becomes similar to that for the non-ventilated child with the use of opioids and anxiolytics coupled with non-pharmacological treatments.

Non-invasive ventilation

Non-invasive ventilatory support in the form of a fitted facial or nasal mask is especially useful in neuromuscular disorders where respiratory failure and dyspnoea are associated with decreased muscular ability to breathe over long periods of time. In adolescents with Duchenne's muscular dystrophy, for example, many years of stable overall function and good quality of life may be possible with the addition of non-invasive mechanical ventilatory support. In these young men the use of a fitted nasal mask may begin with the application of continuous positive airway pressure (CPAP) for specific periods of time (often overnight). As respiratory failure progresses the mode of mechanical ventilation may be increased from CPAP to biphasic positive airway pressure (BiPAP) support. As such mechanisms of ventilatory support become easier to apply and more pervasive they will undoubtedly play an increasingly import-ant role in the management of dyspnoea in children with advanced disease. As with other methods of management of dyspnoea in children, mechanical ventilation is but one option and is almost always coupled with the other modes of dyspnoea treatment mentioned in this chapter.

Secretions

Excess airway secretions may become a chronic problem for children with neurodegenerative disease. The inability to coordinate swallowing may result in chronic aspiration of saliva into the airway. In addition, airway secretions may cause noisy breathing in children too weak to have a productive cough. For children with chronic problems handling their airway secretions, regular suctioning of the mouth may help alleviate distress. In some children suction-ing is well tolerated including aspiration of the nasal passages. In many other children suctioning is clearly a very unpleasant and noxious procedure and it may be preferable to passively allow secretions to appear in the mouth with careful positioning and then remove the mouth secretions with very gentle suctioning or wiping with a cloth. For chronic loose airway secretions a trial of a secretion-drying agent such as glycopyrrolate (50 micrograms/kg/dose) may be beneficial. Glycopyrrolate may sometimes succeed in decreasing the quan-tity of secretions but can make the existing secretions more viscous and thus more difficult to remove with coughing or suctioning.

In cystic fibrosis there is an exaggerated inflammatory response to infection and chronic infection with *pseudomonas aeruginosa*. Excess mucous can cause airway obstruction and predisposes to infection. Therapeutic modalities in cystic fibrosis include antibiotics, chest physiotherapy, anti-cholinergic agents and anti-inflammatory agents. Mucolytic agents such as N-acetylcysteine and human recombinant DNASE have recently been added to treatment regimens in some centres.

Terminal care for respiratory symptoms

For late onset secretions in the terminal phase of illness the sounds made by the child (so-called 'death rattle') may be more disturbing for onlookers and care-givers rather than for the child themself. In this case carefully explaining that the child is not bothered by the sounds may help to alleviate caregiver distress. At times scopolamine may be also be used to help dry excessive secretions.

Terminal breathing patterns may include gasping, rapid shallow or agonal/ataxic breathing, or Cheyne–Stokes respiration. At these times careful reassurance and explanation of what the dying process involves is often helpful in alleviating caregiver distress. Listening to caregivers' concerns, carefully reassessing for possible dyspnoea, and selectively adding both drug and non-drug treatments that seek to improve comfort at the end of life together make up one of the cornerstones of the practice of paediatric palliative care.

References

1. **American Thoracic Society:** Dyspnoea, Mechanisms, Assessment, and Management: A Consensus Statement. *Am J Resp Crit Care* 1999; **159**: 321–40.
2. **Hain R, Patel N, Crabtree S, Pinkerton R.** Respiratory symptoms in children dying from malignant disease. *Palliative Medicine* 1995; **9**: 201–6.
3. **St Laurent-Gagnon** Paediatr Child Health 1998; Pediatric Palliative Care in the Home 3(3): 165–8.
4. **McCallum D, Byrne P, Bruera E.** How children die in hospital. *J Pain and Symptom Management* 2000; **20**(6): 417–23.
5. **Wolfe J, Grier HE, Klar N, Levin SB, Ellenbogen JM, Salem-Schatz S, Emanuel EJ, Weeks JC.** Symptoms and suffering at the end-of-life in children with cancer. *NEJM* 2000; **342** (5): 326–33.
6. **Collins JJ, Byrnes ME, Dunkel IJ, et al.** (2000) The measurement of symptoms in children with cancer. *J ofPain and Symptom Management* 2000; **19**(5): 363–77.
7. **Hongo T, Watanabe C, Okada S, Inoue N et al.** Analysis of the circumstances at the end-of-life in children with cancer: symptoms, suffering, and acceptance. *Paediatrics International* 2003; **45**, 60–4.
8. **Robinson WM, Ravilly S, Berde C, Wohl ME.** End-of-life care in cystic fibrosis. *Pediatrics* 1997; **100**(2): 205–9.
9. **Borg G.** *Borg's Perceived Exertion and Pain Scales* . Stockholm: Human Kinetics, 1999.
10. **Kendrick KR.** Can a self-rating 0–10 scale for dyspnea yield a common language that is understood by ED nurses, patients, and their families? *J Emerg Nursing* 2000; **26**(3): 233–4.
11. **Prasad SA, Randall Sd, and Balfour-Lynn IM.** Fifteen count breathlessness score: an objective measure for children. *Ped Pulmonology* 2000; **30**(1): 56–62.
12. **Carrieri VK, Kieckhefer G, Janson-Bjerklie S and Souza J.** The sensation of pulmonary dyspnea in school-age children. *Nursing Research* 1991; **40**(2): 81–5.
13. **Tobin MJ.** Dyspnea: pathophysiologic basis, clinical presentation, and management. *Arch Intern Med* 1990; **150**: 1604–13.
14. **Hain R, Patel N, Crabtree S, Pinkerton R.** Respiratory symptoms in children dying from malignant disease. *Palliative Medicine* 1995; **9**: 201–6.
15. **World Health Organization.** *Cancer Pain Reliefand Palliative Care in Children.* World Health Organization, Geneva, 1998.
16. **Cohen SP and Dawson TC.** Nebulized morphine as a treatment for dyspnoea in a child with cystic fibrosis. *Pediatrics* 2002; **110**(3): e 38.

17. **Schwartzstein RM, Lahive K, Pope A, Weinberger SE, Weiss JW.** (1987) Cold facial stimulation reduces breathlessness induced in normal subjects. *Am Rev Respir Dis* 1987; **136**: 58–61.
18. **Anbar RD.** Self-hypnosis for management of chronic dyspnoea in pediatric patients. *Pediatrics* 2001; **107**(2): e 21.

8

Respiratory muscle function in breathlessness

Michael I. Polkey

Introduction

Dyspnoea is a complex phenomenon but, in relation to the respiratory muscles, dyspnoea is most likely to occur when the load on the respiratory muscle pump exceeds its capacity (Figure 8.1). In this chapter the function of the respiratory muscle and its interaction with the respiratory system is discussed in health and disease. Although it should be noted that dyspnoea frequently occurs in the absence of respiratory muscle weakness, the concept that imbalance of load and capacity of the respiratory muscles may contribute to dyspnoea is supported by the clinical value of unloading the respiratory muscle pump using non-invasive mechanical ventilation.

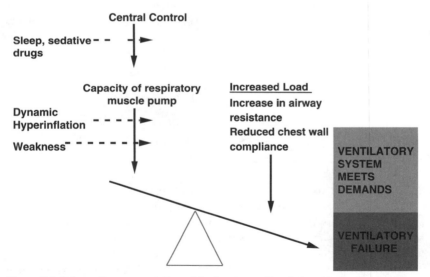

Figure 8.1 Schematic representation of the load capacity relationship for the respiratory muscle pump.

Respiratory muscles in health

In health, inspiration is an active process whereas expiration at rest is a passive process driven by lung and chest wall recoil. However expiration can, in the absence of flow limitation, be augmented by expiratory muscle activity and this is observed during exercise[1] and postural change.[2] Of the inspiratory muscles the most important is the diaphragm accounting for 70 per cent of ventilation in man[3] but additional contributions are made by the scalenes and intercostals.[4] Histologically the respiratory muscles are striated skeletal muscles and subject to the same physiological and disease processes that effect, for example limb muscle. The diaphragm has bilateral cortical innervation[5] but, except where cortical control is necessary (for example during speech or eating), respiration is normally automatic. Abnormalities of respiratory muscle control occasionally give rise to respiratory symptoms. Peripheral nerve may of course lose function as a result of disease processes but there are no known physiologic processes which impair function. Similarly neuro-muscular junction abnormalities, in the form of myasthenic syndromes and paraneoplastic syndromes, are a recognised cause of respiratory muscle weakness but physiologic processes affecting the neuromuscular junction are not known to limit performance.

Of the physiological processes affecting peripheral muscle the most import-ant in relation to the diaphragm are length and fatigue. All skeletal muscle has an optimal length, L_o, where contraction yields a maximum tension. In man L_o lies below residual volume so that hyperinflation results in diminished tension generation (Figure 8.2). This is particularly of relevance to patients

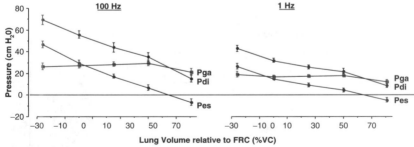

Figure 8.2 Data showing the tension generated by single (right panel) and paired stimuli with a 10ms interstimulus interval (left panel) in normal humans. Pdi is transdiaphragmatic pressure while Poes and Pga are the intrathoracic pressure and intra-abdominal pressure respectively. Note that as lung volume approaches total lung capacity (TLC) the tension generated by the diaphragm is markedly reduced mainly as a result of reduced intrathoracic pressure generation. Data adapted from (56).

with chronic obstructive lung disease who are hyperinflated at rest[6] and develop acute hyperinflation, termed dynamic hyperinflation, during exercise[7] or bronchoconstriction.

Fatigue is defined as a reversible loss in tension generation (i.e. weakness) which results from activity under load and which is reversible by rest.[8] Based on the nature of the stimulus applied, peripheral muscle fatigue may be 'high' (e.g. 50Hz or greater) or low-frequency fatigue. Since phrenic nerve discharge frequencies in man are in the region 10 to 20 Hz[9] the form of fatigue thought to be of most clinical relevance is low-frequency fatigue. Low-frequency diaphragm fatigue is most conveniently identified by the demonstration of a reduction in the transdiaphragmatic pressure elicited by a single bilateral phrenic nerve stimulation. Although diaphragm fatigue can be produced in highly committed healthy volunteers during maximal voluntary exercise[10] or during maximal voluntary hyperventilation[11] it has proved impossible to identify diaphragm fatigue in patients with COPD[12–14] and other medical conditions,[15,16] suggesting that it is not common in clinical practice. In addition even when produced in healthy volunteers, performance of the respiratory muscle pump is only minimally affected,[10,17] suggesting that fatigue is not a major contributor to dyspnea.

Some laboratory evidence exists to support the concept that respiratory muscle weakness may increase the sensation of respiratory effort. In a classic experiment, using the technique of partial neuromuscular blockade, Campbell et al.[18] showed that estimation of the size of an added respiratory load depended on the magnitude of the motor command which was inversely related to strength. In a later experiment the same group[19] asked subjects to maintain a fixed negative pressure against a closed airway in order to generate respiratory muscle fatigue. Once the muscles were fatigued an added inspiratory load appeared greater when presented at the end of a sustained contraction than after a comparable period of breath-holding. A clinical model which is amenable to study in this regard is of patients with advanced emphysema performing exhaustive treadmill walking. Physiologic changes indicating excessive inspiratory muscle loading occur at peak exercise in the absence of low frequency fatigue. If non-invasive ventilation is applied during exercise this both reverses these changes but also reduces dyspnoea.

Interestingly, isolated diaphragm paralysis in otherwise healthy patients causes symptoms only at high levels of exercise.[20] It also used to be considered that such patients were at high risk of nocturnal respiratory failure[21] which is of course a concern in patients with generalized neuromuscular disease (see below). Recent data, however, indicates that isolated diaphragm paralysis is not associated with respiratory failure,[22] most likely because central nervous system (CNS) plasticity permits the recruitment of extradiaphragmatic inspiratory muscles during rapid eye movement sleep.[23]

Respiratory muscle contributions to breathlessness in disease

Disease of nerve and muscle

Respiratory muscle weakness is a feature of a number of neuromuscular conditions. Acute respiratory muscle weakness occurs in a range of conditions including Guillain-Barré Syndrome,[24] envenomation[25] and organophsophate poisoning[26] and was of course a common feature in poliomyelitis. In these conditions management of respiratory failure using endotracheal ventilation is of critical importance. For more slowly progressive conditions respiratory muscle weakness may significantly precede the need for mechanical ventilation, even for those conditions where it is considered appropriate. The most commonly encountered conditions in the western world are motor neurone disease (amyotrophic lateral sclerosis) and muscular dystrophies. In such patients significant respiratory muscle weakness may precede the development of symptoms (Table 8.1) because more general neuromuscular weakness

Table 8.1 Inspiratory muscle strength in 10 patients with MND free of respiratory symptoms

Patient No	Cough Pga	MEP	Tw Pga	Sn Pdi	Sn Poes	Tw Pdi
17	110	31	14.8	78	66	28.1
18	96	56	27.8	49	50	5.5
19	77	71	37.6	67	52	23.5
20	53	24	22.0	70	50	21.2
21	89	18	42.0	97	47	31.5
22	74	71	7.9	42	55	7.0
23	170	95	23.0	181	90	33.0
24	129	91	21.5	144	91	39.4
25	50	62	11.6	86	75	23.4
26	213	10	24.0	95	68	23.7
Mean SD	52	30	10.7	45	21	10.7

Data from (57). These data (in CM H_2O) are from MND patients who were asymptomatic and serving as a control group for patients with respiratory symptoms. A sniff Poes less than 60 cm H_2O indicates inspiratory muscle weakness which is present in 5 of 10 controls.

prevents the patient exercising to a level where the diaphragm weakness would cause symptoms. Thus breathlessness during wakefulness and while erect is an unusual presenting feature of respiratory muscle involvement in these conditions. More usually the patient presents with features suggestive of nocturnal hypoventilation – these being morning headache or a sensation of fuzziness or being 'hungover' coupled with unwanted daytime somnolence. However the patient may complain of orthopnea or, more rarely, dyspnoea on immersion in water. In both these cases the mechanism is a reduction in vital capacity[27,28] consequent on the diaphragm's inability to defend itself against the weight of the abdominal organs and hydrostatic pressure respectively. Patients are often offered non-invasive ventilation (NIV) at this point and available data confirm the clinical impression that this therapy improves symptoms and quality of life.[29] NIV is not a treatment for the underlying condition and so inevitably the weakness of the respiratory muscles progresses. Such patients may develop increasing or total ventilator dependence and these patients may then experience breathlessness during spontaneous breathing efforts.

Movement disorder

Dyspnoea is not a primary feature of movement disorders; however, unwanted respiratory movements may cause distress. The best known example is hiccups[30] but rarely patients present with more profound respiratory dystonias.[31] Patients with Parkinson's disease and other related syndromes, may present with symptoms attributable to vocal cord closure. L-Dopa responsive patients occasionally experience respiratory discomfort associated with the drug but usually prefer to accept this discomfort if the drug is beneficial overall.

Chronic obstructive pulmonary disease (COPD)

Dyspnoea, particularly on exercise, is a characteristic feature of COPD. At rest the inspiratory muscles are at a disadvantage due to hyperinflation which leads to the universally accepted finding that such patients generate reduced inspiratory pressures,[32–34] although this reduction is appropriate[35] when the degree of hyperinflation is considered. Earlier studies considered that diaphragm fatigue accompanied exercise in COPD[36] but as noted this has proved impossible to replicate using phrenic nerve stimulation techniques. In fact available data suggest the diaphragm in COPD is fatigue-resistant both because of changes in fibre type[37] and also because shortened muscle is less susceptible to fatigue.[13,38] Patients with COPD do demonstrate excessive inspiratory muscle loading, manifest by slowing of the maximal relaxation rate, both during weaning from mechanical ventilation[39] and during exercise.[40,41] Therefore it is plausible that perception of this loading contributes to dyspnea;

certainly in the exercise model non-invasive ventilation unloads the inspiratory muscles[42] and extends walking distance.[43] Other interventions which unload the inspiratory muscles also reduce dyspnoea.[44]

Chronic heart failure

Dyspnea is a feature of chronic heart failure (CHF); interestingly symptoms correlate poorly with indices of left ventricular function.[45,46] Most early reports suggested that inspiratory muscle strength was reduced in CHF[47] but a study from our laboratory using more detailed measurement has shown that this is not so as shown in Figure 8.3.[48] The inspiratory muscles are excessively loaded during exercise in heart failure[49] but the magnitude

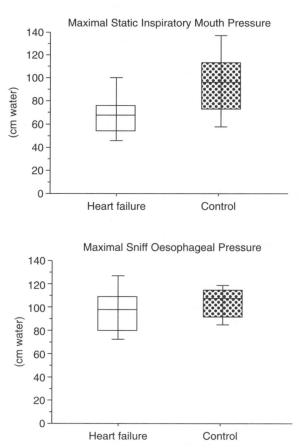

Figure 8.3 Using a traditional test of inspiratory muscle strength, the maximal static pressure, patients with CHF appear weak. Using the more recently developed test of maximal sniff oesophageal pressure the differences are more modest. Data from (48).

is less than observed in patients with COPD. In addition recent data has established that low frequency diaphragm fatigue does not follow cycle exercise in CHF[15] which is consistent with the known fibre type change towards more Type I fibres in CHF.[50] Although some investigators consider that inspiratory muscle endurance is reduced in CHF[51] our own studies suggest that this is due to a maladaptive change in breathing strategy rather than an intrinsic muscular problem.[52]

Cancer

Cachexia is a feature of advanced malignancy and respiratory muscle strength is known to be reduced in conditions characterized by weight loss such as anorexia nervosa.[53] Surprisingly few data are available concerning inspiratory muscle strength in malignancy but it seems that maximal static pressures are reduced in cancer patients and that this has a bearing on symptoms[54] Respiratory muscle weakness can complicate small cell lung cancer by virtue of the Lambert Eaton syndrome.[55]

Summary

Leaving rarities aside, the respiratory muscles are thought to contribute to dyspnoea because of an imbalance between the load placed on the respiratory muscles and their capacity. The most recent data suggests that fatigue, as opposed to weakness, does not contribute to symptoms in health or disease.

References

1. **Ewig JM, Griscom NT, Wohl MEB.** The effect of the absence of abdominal muscles on pulmonary function and exercise. *Am J Respir Crit Care Med* 1996; **153**: 1314–21.
2. **De Troyer A.** Mechanical role of the abdominal muscles in relation to posture. *Respir Physiol* 1983; **53**(3): 341–53.
3. **Mead J, Loring SH.** Analysis of volume displacement and length changes of the diaphragm during breathing. *J Appl Physiol* 1982; **53**: 750–5.
4. **Raper AJ, Taliaferro W, Thompson J, Shapiro W, Patterson JL.** Scalene and sternomastoid muscle function. *J Appl Physiol* 1966; **21**: 497–502.
5. **Similowski T, Straus C, Coic L, Derenne JP.** Facilitation-independent response of the diaphragm to cortical magnetic stimulation. *Am J Respir Crit Care Med* 1996; **154**: 1771–7.
6. **Sharp JT, Van Lith P, Nuchprayoo CV, Briney R, Johnson FN.** The thorax in chronic obstructive lung disease. *Am J Med* 1968; **44**: 39–46.
7. **Dodd D, Brancatisano T, Engel L.** Chest wall mechanics during exercise in patients with severe chronic airflow obstruction. *Am Rev Respir Dis* 1984; **129**: 33–8.
8. **NHLBI Workshop summary.** Respiratory muscle fatigue. Report of the Respiratory Muscle Fatigue Workshop Group. *Am Rev Respir Dis* 1990; **142**: 474–80.

9. De Troyer A, Leeper JB, McKenzie DK, Gandevia SC. Neural drive to the diaphragm in patients with severe COPD. *Am J Respir Crit Care Med* 1997; **155**: 1335–40.

10. Johnson BD, Babcock MA, Suman OE, Dempsey JA. Exercise-induced diaphragmatic fatigue in healthy humans. *J Physiol (Lond)* 1993; **460**: 385–405.

11. Polkey MI, Kyroussis D, Hamnegard C-H, Hughes PD, Rafferty GF, Moxham J, *et al.* Paired phrenic nerve stimuli for the detection of diaphragm fatigue. *Eur Resp J* 1997; **10**: 1859–64.

12. Polkey MI, Kyroussis D, Keilty SEJ, Hamnegard CH, Mills GH, Green M, *et al.* Exhaustive treadmill exercise does not reduce twitch transdiaphragmatic pressure in patients with COPD. *Am J Respir Crit Care Med* 1995; **152**: 959–64.

13. Polkey MI, Kyroussis D, Hamnegard C-H, Mills GH, Hughes PD, Green M, *et al.* Diaphragm performance during maximal voluntary ventilation in chronic obstructive pulmonary disease. *Am J Respir Crit Care Med* 1997; **155**: 642–8.

14. Laghi F, Cattapan SE, Jubran A, Parthasarathy S, Warshawsky P, Choi YS, *et al.* Is weaning failure caused by low-frequency fatigue of the diaphragm? *Am J Respir Crit Care Med* 2003; **167**(2): 120–7.

15. Kufel TJ, Pineda LA, Junega RG, Hathwar R, Mador MJ. Diaphragmatic function after intense exercise in congestive heart failure patients. *Eur Respir J* 2002; **20**(6): 1399–405.

16. El-Kabir DR, Polkey MI, Lyall RA, Williams AJ, Moxham J. The effect of treatment on diaphragm contractility in obstructive sleep apnea syndrome. *Respir Med* 2003; **97**(9): 1021–6.

17. Luo YM, Hart N, Mustfa N, Lyall RA, Polkey MI, Moxham J. Effect of diaphragm fatigue on neural respiratory drive. *J Appl Physiol* 2001; **90**(5): 1691–9.

18. Campbell EJ, Gandevia SC, Killian KJ, Mahutte CK, Rigg JR. Changes in the perception of inspiratory resistive loads during partial curarization. *J Physiol* 1980; **309**: 93–100.

19. Gandevia S, Killian K, Campbell E. The effect of respiratory muscle fatigue on respiratory sensations. *Clin Sci* 1981; **60**: 463–6.

20. Hart N, Nickol AH, Cramer D, Ward SP, Lofaso F, Pride NB, *et al.* Effect of severe isolated unilateral and bilateral diaphragm weakness on exercise performance. *Am J Respir Crit Care Med* 2002; **165**(9): 1265–70.

21. Newsom-Davis J, Goldman M, Loh L, Casson M. Diaphragm function and alveolar hypoventilation. *Q J Med* 1976; **177**: 87–100.

22. Laroche CM, Carroll N, Moxham J, Green M. Clinical significance of severe isolated diaphragm weakness. *Am Rev Resp Dis* 1988; **138**(4): 862–6.

23. Bennett JR, Dunroy HM, Corfield DR, Hart N, Simonds AK, Polkey MI, *et al.* Respiratory muscle activity during REM sleep in patients with diaphragm paralysis. *Neurology* 2004; **62**(1): 134–7.

24. Chevrolet JC, Delamont P. Repeated vital capacity measurements as predictive parameters for mechanical ventilation need and weaning success in Guillain Barre syndrome. *Am Rev Respir Dis* 1991; **144**: 814–18.

25. Singh G, Pannu HS, Chawla PS, Malhotra S. Neuromuscular transmission failure due to common krait (*Bungarus caeruleus*) envenomation. *Muscle Nerve* 1999; **22**: 1637–43.

26. Goswamy R, Chaudhuri A, Mahashur AA. Study of respiratory failure in organophosphate and carbamate poisoning. *Heart Lung* 1994; **23**: 466–72.

27. Schoenhofer B, Koehler D, Polkey MI. Influence of immersion in water on muscle function and breathing pattern in patients with severe diaphragm weakness. *Chest* 2004; **125**(6): 2069–74.

28. Allen SM, Hunt B, Green M. Fall in vital capacity with posture. *Br J Dis Chest* 1985; **79**: 267–71.

29. Lyall RA, Donaldson N, Fleming T, Wood C, Newsom-Davis I, Polkey MI, *et al.* A prospective study of quality of life in ALS patients treated with noninvasive ventilation. *Neurology* 2001; 57(1): 153–6.

30. Launois S, Bizec JL, Whitelaw WA, Cabane J, Derenne JP. Hiccup in adults: an overview. *Eur Respir J* 1993; 6(4): 563–75.

31. Braun N, Abd A, Baer J, Blitzer A, Stewart C, Brin M. Dyspnea in dystonia. A functional evaluation. *Chest* 1995; 107: 1309–16.

32. Byrd RB, Hyatt RE. Maximal respiratory pressures in chronic obstructive lung disease. *Am Rev Respir Dis* 1968; 98: 848–56.

33. Gibson G, Pride N, Clark E. Function of the diaphragm in patients with severe hyperinflation. *Am Rev Respir Dis* 1979; 119: 175–7.

34. Similowski T, Yan S, Gauthier AP, Macklem PT, Bellemare F. Contractile properties of the human diaphragm during chronic hyperinflation. *N Engl J Med* 1991; 325: 917–23.

35. Polkey MI, Kyroussis D, Hamnegard C-H, Mills GH, Green M, Moxham J. Diaphragm strength in chronic obstructive pulmonary disease. *Am J Respir Crit Care Med* 1996; 154: 1310–7.

36. Roussos C, Fixley M, Gross D, Macklem PT. Fatigue of the inspiratory muscles and their synergic behaviour. *J Appl Physiol* 1979; 46: 897–904.

37. Levine S, Kaiser L, Leferovich J, Tikunov B. Cellular adaptations in the diaphragm in chronic obstructive pulmonary disease. *N Engl J Med* 1997; 337: 1799–806.

38. Sacco P, McIntyre DB, Jones DA. Effects of length and stimulation frequency on fatigue of the human tibialis anterior muscle. *J Appl Physiol* 1994; 77: 1148–54.

39. Goldstone JC, Green M, Moxham J. Maximum relaxation rate of the diaphragm during weaning from mechanical ventilation. *Thorax* 1994; 49: 54–60.

40. Kyroussis D, Polkey MI, Keilty SEJ, Mills GH, Hamnegard C-H, Moxham J, *et al.* Exhaustive exercise slows inspiratory muscle relaxation rate in chronic obstructive pulmonary disease. *Am J Respir Crit Care Med* 1996; 153: 787–93.

41. Kyroussis D, Johnson LC, Hamnegard CH, Polkey MI, Moxham J. Inspiratory muscle maximum relaxation rate measured from submaximal sniff nasal pressure in patients with severe COPD. *Thorax* 2002; 57(3): 254–7.

42. Polkey MI, Kyroussis D, Mills GH, Hamnegard C-H, Keilty SEJ, Green M, *et al.* Inspiratory pressure support reduces slowing of inspiratory muscle relaxation rate during exhaustive treadmill walking in severe COPD. *Am J Respir Crit Care Med* 1996; 154: 1146–50.

43. Keilty SEJ, Ponte J, Flemming TA, Moxham J. Effect of inspiratory pressure support on exercise tolerance and breathlessness in patients with severe stable chronic obstructive pulmonary disease. *Thorax* 1994; 49: 990–4.

44. Man WD, Mustfa N, Nikoletou D, Kaul S, Hart N, Rafferty GF, *et al.* Effect of salmeterol on respiratory muscle activity during exercise in poorly reversible COPD. *Thorax* 2004; 59(6): 471–6.

45. Fink LI, Wilson JR, Ferraro N. Exercise ventilation and pulmonary artery pressure in chronic stable congestive heart failure. *Am J Cardiol* 1986; 57: 249–53.

46. Wilson JR, Rayos G, Yeoh TK, Gothard P, Bak K. Dissociation between exertional symptoms and circulatory function in patients with heart failure. *Circulation* 1995; 92: 47–53.

47. Chua TP, Anker SD, Harrington D, Coats AJ. Inspiratory muscle strength is a determinant of maximum oxygen consumption in chronic heart failure. *Br Heart J* 1995; 74(4): 381–5.

48. Hughes PD, Polkey MI, Harris ML, Coats A, Moxham J, Green M. Diaphragm strength in chronic heart failure. *Am J Respir Crit Care Med* 1999; **160**: 529–34.

49. Hughes PD, Hart N, Hamnegard CH, Green M, Coats AJ, Moxham J, *et al.* Inspiratory muscle relaxation rate slows during exhaustive treadmill walking in patients with chronic heart failure. *Am J Respir Crit Care Med* 2001; **163**(6): 1400–3.

50. Tikunov B, Levine S, Mancini D. Chronic congestive heart failure elicits adaptations of endurance exercise in diaphragmatic muscle. *Circulation* 1997; **95**: 910–16.

51. Walsh JT, Andrews R, Johnson P, Phillips L, Cowley AJ, Kinnear WJ. Inspiratory muscle endurance in patients with chronic heart failure. *Heart* 1996; **76**(4): 332–6.

52. Hart N, Kearney MT, Pride NB, Green M, Lofaso F, Shah AM, *et al.* Inspiratory muscle load and capacity in chronic heart failure. *Thorax* 2004; **59**(6): 477–82.

53. Murciano D, D. R, Pingleton S, Armengaud MH, Melchior JC, Aubier M. Diaphragmatic function in severely malnourished patients with anorexia nervosa. *Am J Respir Crit Care Med* 1994; **150**: 1569–74.

54. Dudgeon DJ, Lertzman M, Askew GR. Physiological changes and clinical correlations of dyspnea in cancer outpatients. *J Pain Symptom Manage* 2001; **21**(5): 373–9.

55. Laroche CM, Mier AK, Spiro SG, Newsom-Davis J, Moxham J, Green M. Respiratory muscle weakness in the Lambert-Eaton myasthenic syndrome. *Thorax* 1989; **44**(11): 913–18.

56. Polkey MI, Hamnegard C-H, Hughes PD, Rafferty GF, Green M, Moxham J. Influence of acute lung volume change on contractile properties of the human diaphragm. *J Appl Physiol* 1998; **85**: 1322–8.

57. Polkey MI, Lyall RA, Green M, Leigh PN, Moxham J. Expiratory muscle function in amyotrophic lateral sclerosis. *Am J Respir Crit Care Med* 1998; **158**: 734–41.

9

Pulmonary rehabilitation

Nha Voduc, Katherine Webb and Denis E. O'Donnell

Pulmonary rehabilitation is defined by the American Thoracic Society (ATS) as 'a multidisciplinary program of care for patients with chronic respiratory impairment that is individually tailored and designed to optimize physical and social performance and autonomy'.[1] Although the potential benefits of pulmonary rehabilitation were initially questioned, an abundance of clinical research performed over the past two decades has clearly established the importance of rehabilitation in the care of patients with chronic respiratory disease. This chapter will introduce and describe the contents of a pulmonary rehabilitation program, review the benefits of rehabilitation, and discuss specifically the effects of rehabilitation on dyspnea.

Components of pulmonary rehabilitation

The exact content of a rehabilitation program should be tailored to meet the specific needs of the patient and will also vary between programs. Nevertheless, most programs contain four major components: exercise training, education, psychosocial/behavioral intervention and outcome assessment. These interventions are provided by a multidisciplinary team of health professionals. This team would typically include physiotherapists, respiratory therapists, occupational therapists, nutritionists, pharmacists, psychologists, nurses and social workers. In many programs, physicians serve as medical directors. Physicians are required to assess patients prior to enrolment into the program, to confirm eligibility and ensure optimization of all medical conditions prior to commencement of training. Physicians may also be involved in follow-up after completion of the program and in the communication of outcomes to other physicians.

Exercise training

Among the four major components of pulmonary rehabilitation, only exercise training has been clearly demonstrated to improve clinical outcomes in controlled studies. Exertional dyspnea is the most common symptom of COPD and progresses inexorably as the disease advances. To avoid dyspnea, patients will often abstain from various dyspnea-provoking activities. Reduced activity levels over time result in skeletal muscle deconditioning and unfitness. Eventually, minor activities become associated with severe dyspnea and the patient becomes virtually immobile and housebound (Figure 9.1). Fortunately, this devastating dyspnea–disability spiral can successfully be broken by a structured exercise reconditioning program.

Exercise training can improve both maximal exercise capacity and exercise endurance in normal individuals. However, there was skepticism regarding the ability of patients with advanced respiratory disease to reach the exercise intensity necessary to produce a training effect. Recent evidence, however, has demonstrated that a clear training effect is still possible, even in patients with significant respiratory impairment. Casaburi and colleagues observed reductions in lactic acidosis during submaximal exercise, in patients with COPD who received exercise training.[2] These findings implied that despite ventilatory impairment, these patients were able to perform exercise of sufficient intensity to produce changes in muscle metabolism. This conclusion was subsequently confirmed by Maltais and associates, who demonstrated these improvements in peripheral muscle oxidative capacity using percutaneous muscle biopsy.[3]

The predominant training modality in most rehabilitation programs is endurance training: 20–30 minute sessions are recommended, at a frequency

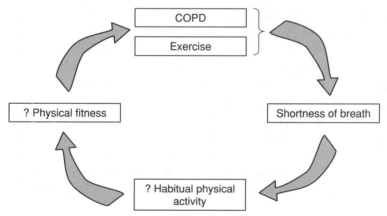

Figure 9.1 The dyspnea–disability spiral. Patients with COPD will often avoid dyspnea-provoking activities which results in skeletal muscle deconditioning and unfitness. Over time, even minor activities will become associated with severe dyspnea and the patient becomes virtually immobile and housebound in a vicious cycle.

of 2–5 sessions per week. The frequency of the sessions will be determined, in part, by the resources available to the rehabilitation program. The exact exercise prescription will vary between programs. Training at intensities above anaerobic threshold[4] or at 60–75 per cent of maximum work rate are advocated, although Ries and colleagues showed that patients with very severe disease (and thus a relatively low maximum work rate) can benefit from training at an even higher percentage of their maximum work rate.[5] Practically speaking, many rehabilitation programs will adjust the exercise prescription to patient symptoms and exercise tolerance; the intensity will be gradually increased as patient performance improves.

Decreased mobility is frequently reported by patients with respiratory disease and thus, lower extremity training is emphasized during pulmonary rehabilitation. The majority of studies examining exercise training in patients with chronic lung disease have focused on the benefits of lower extremity training. However, the performance of many activities of daily living involves upper extremity muscles and these muscles may even serve an accessory role in ventilation. This reasoning would suggest a role for upper extremity training although the utility of this modality remains uncertain. Upper extremity training clearly improves performance of tests involving the upper extremities but has not been shown to consistently improve either ventilation or quality of life.[6]

Strength training is not included in all rehab programs, but recent work suggests that strength training does offer complementary benefits to endurance training. In separate studies, both Ortega and Panton noted that strength training not only improved peripheral muscle strength but walking distance as well, when compared with endurance training alone.[7,8] As with upper extremity training, it remains to be proven whether the addition of strength training to endurance training is associated with any improvement in quality of life.

Respiratory muscle training has also been studied in patients with chronic lung disease. Chronic obstructive lung disease is frequently associated with increased ventilatory demands due to poor ventilation–perfusion mismatching, as well as impaired muscle function from hyperinflation. Both these factors contribute to an increased load on the muscles of respiration. It has been hypothesized that respiratory muscle training may contribute to dyspnea relief. Subsequently, several studies have shown that respiratory muscle strength can be increased by inspiratory muscle training using resistive loads[9] and that this may produce improvements in dyspnea and exercise capacity.[10] However, it remains unclear whether the addition of inspiratory muscle training to general exercise training results in any additive benefit with regards to either dyspnea relief or quality of life. General exercise training alone can significantly improve ventilatory muscle strength in patients with chronic obstructive lung disease.[11]

Education

The success of any rehabilitation program is contingent on patient motivation and compliance. It is not unreasonable to presume that education of patients and their families will not only increase patient understanding but also improve self-management skills and, potentially, long-term compliance with therapeutic interventions, such as medications and exercise. In reality, the true benefit of patient education in the setting of a rehabilitation program is very difficult to assess. Education is often incorporated with exercise training, and it is virtually impossible to have exercise training without some component of education. In one rehabilitation study conducted by Ries and associates, where education alone was used as a control, the combination of exercise and education was clearly superior.[12] In that study, the patients who only received education did not experience any significant improvement in either symptoms or exercise endurance compared to their baseline. In contrast, Bourbeau and colleagues demonstrated that an outpatient self-management program significantly reduced hospital admissions and improved quality of life in patients with COPD.[13] Strictly speaking, the program studied by Bourbeau was not a rehabilitation program but it did feature a comprehensive education component, suggesting that education is of benefit to patients, even in the absence of exercise training.

Education can be provided in small groups but may also be individualized. Topics of discussion may include basic pathophysiology of lung disease, proper use of medications, smoking cessation, self-management strategies, nutrition and end-of-life issues. Behavioral interventions such as energy conservation and breathing strategies (discussed below) are also commonly incorporated into educational sessions.

Psychological support and behavioral interventions

Dyspnea may have a significant affective component and thus it is not surprising that patients suffering from chronic lung disease may experience anxiety and reactive depression.[14,15] These symptoms can improve as patients participate in exercise training in a supportive and secure environment.[16] Although some patients with major psychological problems may require specific intervention by a psychologist or psychiatrist, this is usually not necessary for the majority of patients. Indeed, the usefulness of psychological therapy alone in patients with chronic lung disease remains uncertain. Lustig and colleagues observed that 15–20 rehabilitation sessions, which involved exercise, education and relaxation techniques, produced either comparable or superior effects on psychological outcomes, as an equivalent number of psychotherapy sessions.[17] However, it is possible that a subset of respiratory patients may benefit from psychotherapy. Eiser and associates evaluated the effects of psychotherapy on COPD patients who also experienced above-normal levels of anxiety (as assessed by Hospital Anxiety and Depression Scale), in a non-randomized pilot study. They found that these patients had a 24 per cent (72 m) improvement in their walking capacity, after six sessions of cognitive and behavioral psychotherapy.[18]

Behavioral interventions typically include education regarding energy conservation and breathing training. Energy conservation comprises a group of strategies aimed at minimizing energy expenditure during daily activities. The goal of energy conservation is to maximize functional capacity in an individual with very limited physiologic reserves. Breathing training techniques attempt to reduce dyspnea by altering breathing patterns. Pursed-lip breathing is one such technique that involves expiration against partially closed lips. Pursed-lip breathing reduces respiratory rate and minute ventilation,[19,20] but it has not been consistently shown to reduce dyspnea.

Although the evidence supporting the use of psychotherapy in pulmonary rehabilitation remains equivocal, many programs do incorporate some form of relaxation training and behavioral counseling into their curriculum.

Outcome assessment

Assessment of patient outcomes is an important component of any medical program. For the individual patient, this will serve to underscore the results of their efforts and potentially encourage them to continue training following completion of the program. For the rehabilitation team, a review of patient outcomes provides essential feedback on the effectiveness of the program. This information can be used to identify areas in need of improvement, modify components of the program or possibly even change patient enrolment criteria.

Ideally, the instrument or variable used for measuring outcomes would be simple and yet comprehensive; reproducible but also responsive to therapy. It should reflect changes in both patient quality of life and physiology. Unfortunately, this ideal instrument does not exist. Consequently, many rehabilitation programs use a combination of different tests. These tests can be arbitrarily divided into three categories: exercise tests, walking tests and symptom questionnaires.

Exercise tests measure patient performance against an adjustable workload. Exercise tests are typically performed on either a treadmill or cycle ergometer, although arm ergometers are occasionally used for patients unable to perform leg exercise. Exercise testing can be performed using an incremental protocol (gradually increasing workload) or a constant load (submaximal) protocol. Exercise tests are reproducible[21] and provide the most physiologic information of the three types of tests. Oxygen uptake, heart rate and ventilation are among the many variables that can be measured. Incremental exercise testing is frequently employed prior to commencement of exercise training. It can screen for important comorbidities (e.g., heart disease) and can be used to individualize the intensity of the future exercise regimen to the individual patients. Constant load exercise testing usually measures exercise duration at a constant load, which is usually set at a proportion of the patient's maximum workload (e.g., 75 per cent). This methodology is remarkably responsive to a wide variety of interventions.

Walking tests measure ambulatory capacity, either over a fixed duration of time (6- or 12-minute walk tests) or at predetermined speeds (shuttle walk). Walking tests have been shown to correlate with both measures of dyspnea and exercise capacity.[22] Unfortunately, the results of walking tests are also less reproducible, and can be influenced by learning effect and supervisor encouragement.[23] Nevertheless, their relative simplicity and minimal resource requirements (a long corridor or large room) have led to widespread use as outcome measures in pulmonary rehabilitation.

Exercise testing and walking tests provide insight into physiology and functional capacity but these tests do not directly measure the more subjective but equally important endpoints, such as symptoms or quality of life. Improvements in these parameters are clinically relevant and may not necessary correlate with measures of exercise capacity.[24] A number of scales are validated for the measurement of dyspnea. These range in complexity from the simple five-point Medical Research Council scale to the more comprehensive Baseline and Transition Dyspnea Indexes (BDI/TDI), developed by Mahler.[25] Quality of life can also be measured via disease-specific questionnaires: Chronic Respiratory Disease Questionnaire (CRDQ) and St. George's Respiratory Questionnaire (SGRQ). These questionnaires provide insight into the impact of rehabilitation on patient functioning that cannot be obtained from physiologic tests alone.

Practicality and availability of resources generally limit the number and type of tests employed by pulmonary rehabilitation programs for assessment of outcomes. Generally speaking, it is recommended that the outcome assessment include measures of symptoms, functional capacity and quality of life or health status. This is achieved by selecting a combination of 1–2 tests from each of the three main categories. This practice does not require excessive resources but provides a relatively comprehensive and objective assessment of patient outcomes.

Location

Pulmonary rehabilitation is provided in a variety of settings. A number of studies have proven the effectiveness of inpatient, outpatient and home-based pulmonary rehabilitation programs, although there is very little research comparing the different locations. Strijbos and colleagues[26] found that rehabilitation administered at home produced similar early improvements in exercise capacity and dyspnea to an outpatient hospital-based program. Additionally, these benefits were better maintained at 18 months follow-up in patients who underwent home-based exercise training. In contrast, Wedzicha and assoicates[27] found that home-based training did not benefit COPD patients suffering from severe breathlessness.

As with many other aspects of pulmonary rehabilitation, the choice of location should be individualized and influenced by available resources. Outpatient programs can usually accommodate a greater number of patients than inpatient programs. Inpatient programs are the most cost-intensive and should be reserved for the sickest patients, or for patients who lack access to transportation or who live a great distance from the rehabilitation center. These latter patients may find the difficulties associated with traveling back and forth several times per week to an outpatient program to be prohibitive. Home programs are most convenient for the patient but do require more resources from the rehab team's perspective than a centralized outpatient program. Furthermore, as alluded to above, home programs may not be appropriate for the most severely symptomatic patients.

Patient selection

The eligibility of an individual patient is determined by a pre-rehabilitation assessment. A physician is usually involved for this process. The physician will not only assess for the presence of contraindications to rehabilitation but also ensures that the patient's respiratory disease and any relevant comorbidities have been fully evaluated and that all medical therapy has been optimized prior to entry into the program.

Referral to a pulmonary rehabilitation program should be considered for *any* patient with chronic respiratory disease who continues to experience significant dyspnea or functional limitation, despite optimal medical management. Some clinicians refer only their most severely disabled patients for pulmonary rehabilitation. This practice may be a reflection of the enrollment patterns of the earlier rehabilitation studies (which tended to study patients with physiologically severe disease) but it is not necessary. If sufficient rehab resources are available, any patient with significant disability arising from their respiratory disease can be eligible for enrollment. Pulmonary rehabilitation has been shown to benefit patients with a wide range of physiologic impairment, although the relative benefit is less in patients with milder disease.[28,29]

Contraindications to enrollment would include: 1 conditions that might prevent the patient from benefiting from the rehabilitation process, or 2 conditions that place the patient at increased risk during exercise training (ATS guidelines).[1] Chief among the possibilities in the first category are poor motivation and disruptive behavior. Rehabilitation is a demanding process and a relatively high level of patient motivation is essential. Musculoskeletal conditions, such as arthritis, may impair ability to perform exercise but are not necessarily prohibitive. Exercise training can be tailored to circumvent musculoskeletal limitations, if these are not extensive. Conditions that are associated with increased risk to the patient would include severe pulmonary hypertension or unstable coronary artery disease.

The majority of pulmonary rehabilitation studies have focused on patients with COPD. This is not surprising as COPD is common and responds only partially to current pharmacological therapy. However, the benefits of re-habilitation are not limited solely to patients with this condition. There is evidence demonstrating benefit in patients with asthma,[30,31] cystic fibrosis[32] and even restrictive lung disease.[33]

The eligibility of (current) smokers for rehabilitation remains a controversial issue. It could be argued that patients who continue to smoke are directly contributing to the process which requires pulmonary rehabilitation in the first place and that these patients lack the motivation to benefit maximally from a rehabilitation program. Given that the availability of pulmonary rehabilitation may be limited, these resources should not be expended on smokers. This reasoning is similar to that used by lung transplant teams who routinely exclude current smokers. There is some limited evidence suggesting that smokers may still benefit from rehabilitation,[34] although retrospective analysis does suggest that smoking is associated with an increased likelihood of non-adherence with rehabilitation.[35] Obviously, the final decision will rest with individual rehabilitation programs; however, it should be noted that a smoking cessation program could easily be integrated into the education and supportive psychotherapy components of pulmonary rehabilitation.[36]

Benefits from pulmonary rehabilitation

The benefits of pulmonary rehabilitation have been demonstrated in several studies, although the magnitude of benefit is not consistent. Lacasse and associates published the earliest meta-analysis of pulmonary rehabilitation.[37]

When the results of 11 randomized, controlled studies were combined, rehabilitation was found to provide 55.7 m improvement in 6-minute walk distance (Figure 9.2). A post-hoc analysis suggested that the benefits were greater (93.8 m) in programs of longer duration (6 months). Pulmonary rehabilitation was also associated with an improvement in dyspnea and disease mastery (ability to cope with disease and its manifestations).

A more recent review of the pulmonary rehabilitation literature is found in the Cochrane Library.[38] The reviewers limited their analysis to randomized controlled trials of pulmonary rehabilitation in COPD. All eligible studies compared exercise training of at least four weeks in duration to conventional community care. A total of 23 studies were identified. A meta-analysis of these studies demonstrated clear improvements in quality of life. Eight of the 23 studies identified assessed quality of life via the chronic respiratory disease questionnaire (CRDQ). This is a validated tool that measures effect of respiratory disease on quality of life, in four separate domains: fatigue, emotional function, disease mastery and dyspnea. Rehabilitation produced improvements in all four domains. These improvements were not only statistically significant but exceeded the minimally clinically important difference (MCID) of the questionnaire (greater than 0.5 on a seven-point scale).

With regards to exercise capacity, statistically significant benefits were demonstrated by the meta-analysis but the magnitude of change was small. Fourteen of the 23 selected trials assessed maximal exercise capacity via incremental exercising test with cycle ergometry (exercise bike). The weighted mean difference with rehab was only 5.46 watts. Ten of 23 trials assessed functional exercise capacity with 6-minute walk testing. The weighted mean difference as

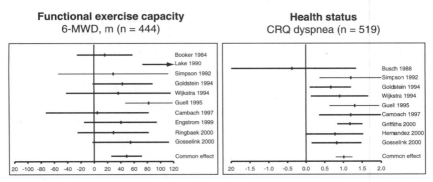

Figure 9.2 Effects of pulmonary rehabilitation on functional exercise capacity as measured by 6-minute walking distance (6-MWD m) and on health status as measured by the dyspnea dimension of the Chronic Respiratory Disease Questionnaire (CRQ). Results of a meta-analysis by LaCasse *et al.* (37, 38).

49 m. Although this improvement was statistically significant, it was below the estimated MCID for 6-minute walk testing.[39] These findings would suggest that pulmonary rehab produces only minimal improvements in exercise capacity: however, it should be noted that despite relatively stringent inclusion criteria, there was some heterogeneity in the nature of the rehab programs evaluated. Among the studies included in the analysis, there were differences in the severity of disease in the study population, content of the rehab program (with or without education, psychological support) and duration of training. These differences would likely influence the effectiveness of rehabilitation. For example, Guell and associates[40] evaluated the effectiveness of a 6 month rehabilitation program, for patients with severe COPD (FEV_1 35 per cent predicted). They found that rehabilitation produced a relatively large improvement in 6 minute walk distance (81 m). In comparison, Cambach and colleagues[30] evaluated a three-month program for patients with more moderate disease (FEV_1 59 per cent predicted). Although improvements in quality of life were still identified, rehabilitation did not produce any significant difference in functional exercise capacity for the COPD patients in this study. These two examples illustrate the heterogeneity present in the rehabilitation and highlight the inherent limitations of combining disparate studies.

The benefits of rehabilitation are also illustrated in a study conducted by Ries and colleagues.[12] This study was one of the largest randomized trials in rehabilitation but was not included in the Cochrane meta-analysis discussed above because patients in the control arm underwent an education program. A total of 119 outpatients with COPD were randomized into either an eight-week rehabilitation program or an eight-week education program. The authors selected different measures for assessment of exercise capacity and psychosocial outcomes. Compared to education alone, rehabilitation was associated with dramatic improvements in exercise endurance, as measured by constant load treadmill exercise (85 per cent vs 11 per cent increase in constant load exercise time). Significant improvements in dyspnea (assessed by University of California, San Diego Shortness of Breath Questionnaire) were also noted. Interestingly, this study did not demonstrate any significant effect of rehabilitation on quality of life. However, it was suggested by the investigators that the quality of life tool used (Quality of Well-Being scale) may not be sufficiently responsive to the benefits of rehabilitation.

The effect of pulmonary rehabilitation on healthcare utilization remains unclear. Older studies compared hospitalization rates before and after pulmonary rehabilitation and demonstrated impressive reductions in hospitalization.[41] However, the results from randomized controlled studies are conflicting. The study by Ries, mentioned above, found that rehabilitation was associated with only small and non-significant reductions in hospitalization and mortality. Another large study by Griffiths and associates also did not find any differences in frequency of hospitalization in the year following participation in a rehab program, however, the investigators did observe a 50 per cent reduction in duration of hospitalization (10.4 vs 21.0 days).[42] In contrast, a much smaller study (n = 26) by Behnke found that an 18-month home-based exercise program significantly reduced hospital admissions.[43] At this time, more research is required before definitive conclusions can be made regarding the effects of rehabilitation on hospitalization rates.

Mechanisms of dyspnea reduction

Dyspnea in COPD is multifactorial, but our knowledge of the source and mechanism of this common symptom continues to grow. During exercise, increased respiratory discomfort reflects the increased disparity between the central drive to breathe, which is increased in COPD, and the ventilatory response of the respiratory system, which is diminished because of the abnormal mechanics (i.e., neuromechanical dissociation). Central drive is increased because of increased chemical stimulation of the respiratory centre, resulting from: 1 increased CO_2 production at a given work rate; 2 reduced CO_2 elimination because of ventilation–perfusion abnormalities (fixed high physiological deadspace); and 3 early metabolic acidosis secondary to skeletal muscle deconditioning. On the other hand, the ventilatory response of the respiratory system for a given central drive is blunted because of functional weakness and overloading (elastic and resistive) of the muscles of breathing. In COPD, acute-on-chronic pulmonary overinflation, as a result of air trapping, reduces the ability of patients to increase ventilation during exercise because of the constraints it causes on tidal volume expansion. Neuromechanical dissociation may form the basis for the most prominent qualitative dimension of dyspnea in COPD, namely 'unsatisfied inspiration' (i.e., 'can't get enough air in').

Although there is an abundance of evidence demonstrating that dyspnea is improved following completion of pulmonary rehabilitation, the mechanisms for this improvement are still being investigated. It is likely that the dyspnea reduction produced by rehabilitation is multifactorial in etiology, a result of both physiologic and non-physiologic changes. In the past, particular emphasis was placed on the latter category, as early studies failed to demonstrate changes in physiology following rehabilitation. For example, it is suggested that rehabilitation serves to desensitize patients to dyspnea. In the course of exercise training, patients routinely experience some degree of dyspnea, however, the affective component of the dyspnea is gradually diminished by the supportive and secure environment of a rehab program. It would not be unreasonable to assume that patients would become acclimated to sensations of exertional dyspnea over time and that their improved exercise capacity is in part a reflection of increased tolerance for exertional dyspnea.[44] Research by Reardon and colleagues does provide some indirect support for the role of non-physiologic factors.[24] The authors assessed the effects of rehabilitation on 44 patients with chronic lung disease. They found that rehabilitation produced significant improvements in both functional exercise capacity and quality of life, however, these improvements were not linked. In this study, improvements in 12-minute walk distance did not correlate with either improvements in total CRDQ scores or even with only the dyspnea domain of the CDRQ questionnaire alone. Carreri-Kohlman and associates assessed the effects of coached and un-coached exercise training on 51 patients with COPD. They found that, with or without coaching, exercise training not only reduced ventilation but it also reduced dyspnea relative to ventilation. Thus, for a given minute ventilation, patients reported less dyspnea after exercise training. This observation would lend further support to the role of desensitization.

Over the last decade, evidence demonstrating physiologic changes following rehabilitation has become available (Table 9.1). O'Donnell and colleagues specifically studied the effects of exercise training on dyspnea in patients with severe obstructive lung disease.[45] In this controlled study, dyspnea was assessed by use of the Borg scale during exercise and the BDI/TDI questionnaire. Exercise responses before and after rehabilitation were rigorously measured with cycle exercise testing. The investigators found that group which underwent exercise training achieved much higher peak work rates on the cycle ergometer. Furthermore, comparisons of physiologic response at a standardized work rate demonstrated significant reductions in ventilation in

Table 9.1 Physiological effects of exercise training

1. Reduced ventilatory demand:
   – Increased efficiency
   – Reduced metabolic acidosis, increased oxidative capacity

2. More efficient breathing pattern (i.e., ↑ tidal volume, ↓ breathing frequency)
   – Reduced dynamic hyperinflation

3. Improved ventilatory muscle strength and endurance

4. Improved peripheral muscle strength

5. Improved cardiovascular function

patients who completed exercise training. This reduction in ventilation correlated best with reductions in exertional dyspnea. Incidentally, chronic dyspnea, as measured by BDI/TDI, also decreased significantly by 2.8 units. This improvement was well above the minimum clinically meaningful difference of 1 unit for the TDI and was considerably greater in magnitude than the changes obtainable by individual bronchodilators.

Given that pulmonary function is not changed, the most likely cause of reduced ventilation (and consequently, reduced dyspnea) following exercise training is a reduction in metabolic demand (Figure 9.3). This may have two sources: improved mechanical efficiency and reduction in lactic acid production. Improvement in mechanical efficiency (skill of performance) was demonstrated by the O'Donnell study mentioned above, which found a reduction in the slope of the oxygen uptake (VO_2) and work rate relationship. This hypothesis is supported indirectly by the Ries study, which also found that improvements in peak work rate were several times greater than improvements in peak VO_2.

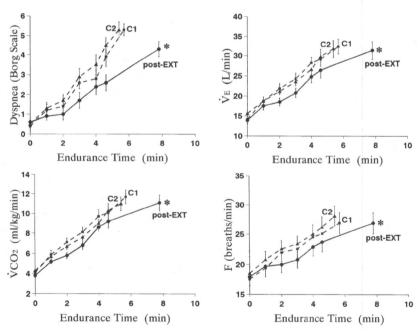

Figure 9.3 Ventilatory responses to constant-load cycle exercise after exercise training (EXT). Slopes of dyspnea (measured by the modified Borg scale), ventilation (V_E), carbon dioxide output (VCO_2) and breathing frequency (F) over time fell significantly (*p <0.05) after EXT (circles, solid lines) compared with a control period (dashed lines). C1 = pre-control (squares), C2 = post-control/pre-EXT (triangles).

Reductions in lactic acid production during exercise may be another important contributor to the reduced ventilatory demands seen following exercise training. Lactic acid is a by-product of anaerobic metabolism. As lactic acid is metabolized, carbon dioxide is produced, which in turn drives ventilation. Previous work has demonstrated alterations in skeletal muscle composition and oxidative capacity in patients with COPD.[46,47] These impairments likely contribute to the functional disability experienced by these patients. Exercise training can potentially reverse these changes and reduce lactic acidosis by increasing the oxidative capacity of the peripheral muscles. In a previously mentioned study, Casaburi and colleagues found reductions in lactic acidosis during exercise testing in patients who completed a high-intensity exercise program.[2] A relatively small alteration in blood lactate levels was shown to be associated with large changes in ventilation (2.5 L/min ventilation for each 1 mEq/L lactate).

Recently, the additional insights into the mechanism of dyspnea reduction were provided by Gigliotti and associates.[48] The investigators assessed the exercise responses of 20 patients with COPD before and after a pulmonary rehabilitation program. As with previous studies, ventilation was decreased at a given workload. A change in ventilatory pattern was also observed, with significant reductions in respiratory rate and an increase in tidal volume. Inspiratory capacity (IC) during a standardized work rate was also significantly increased, suggesting that the changes in ventilatory pattern permitted improved lung emptying (reduced hyperinflation). It has been previously demonstrated that IC, as a surrogate measure for hyperinflation, is an important determinant of dyspnea.[49] Hyperinflation during exercise places constraints on the expansion of tidal volume and increases work of breathing, both of which contribute to the dyspnea experienced by patients with COPD. By reducing ventilatory demand, pulmonary rehabilitation appears to reduce hyperinflation and, consequently, exertional dyspnea. Interestingly, this study also provided evidence of non-physiologic effects on dyspnea. The authors noted that at a standardized minute ventilation, the sensation of exertional dyspnea was decreased following rehabilitation. Given that IC, respiratory rate and tidal volume at standardized ventilation remained constant, this would suggest that patients do develop some desensitization to dyspnea following rehabilitation.

In summary, the mechanisms underlying the salutary effects of exercise training on dyspnea remain incompletely understood and likely involve a myriad of small physiological changes that culminate in a net positive sensory effect (Table 9.2). These include reduced ventilatory demand secondary to improved efficiency and reduced metabolic acidosis that follows peripheral

Table 9.2 Putative mechanisms of dyspnea relief in response to exercise training

↓ Ventilatory drive:	↓ metabolic acidosis
	↓ sympathetic system activation
	↓ ventilatory muscle weakness
+	
↑ Dynamic mechanical output:	↓ dynamic hyperinflation
	↑ muscle pump performance
= Enhanced neuromechanical coupling of the respiratory system	

muscle training. The favorably altered metabolic milieu at the peripheral muscle level may also reduce ergo-receptor stimulation of ventilation. Reduced ventilation at any given work rate during exercise will result in less air trapping in flow-limited patients. Combining these effects, reduced central drive together with increased ventilatory capacity (secondary to reduced dynamic lung hyperinflation) will result in enhanced neuromechanical coupling. Moreover, improved strength of the ventilatory muscles means that less electrical activation (neural drive) is required for a given force-generating capacity, which in itself is likely to result in a decreased sense of inspiratory effort. Exercise training also addresses the affective dimension of dyspnea. Thus, desensitization to respiratory discomfort over the period of exercise training in a supportive environment is undoubtedly important.

Duration of benefits

The majority of studies described thus far have examined and established the short-term benefits of pulmonary rehabilitation. As with many other therapies in medicine, less information is available regarding long-term outcomes. Ries and colleagues followed patients enrolled in an eight-week outpatient pulmonary rehabilitation program for a duration of six years. Despite monthly reinforcement sessions for one year, it was noted that the improvements from pulmonary rehabilitation tended to diminish over time. After one year, there was a significant diminution in exercise performance and an increase in symptoms. After two years, there was no significant difference between the rehab group and the control group, which received only education.[12]

It is possible that the design and duration of the rehabilitation program may influence long-term outcomes. In a previously mentioned study, Strijbos and associates compared the effects of a 12 week hospital based outpatient rehab program to a 12 week home-care program.[26] After completion of training, both groups received instructions to continue exercising, but without any supervision. The follow-up of this study was relatively complete, with data available for 41 of 45 patients at 18 months. Similar to the Ries study, the exercise performance and exertional dyspnea of patients receiving hospital-based training declined from the peak achieved at the completion of the program and was not significantly different from baseline measurements by 12 months. In contrast, the exercise performance and dyspnea of patients receiving the home-based program continued to improve and remained significantly greater than baseline at the end of the study.

Troosters and colleagues evaluated the effects of a longer duration rehabilitation program.[50] Patients received three 1.5 hour outpatient sessions per week for three months, followed by two sessions per week for three months. The validity of this study was diminished by a relatively high dropout rate (31 per cent at 6 months and 36 per cent at 18 months). Nevertheless, the authors did find that the benefits of rehabilitation appeared to be maintained at 18 months.

Most recently, Ries and associates[51] evaluated the effectiveness of maintenance program following completion of a pulmonary rehabilitation program. One hundred and seventy-two subjects were randomized into either a 12-month maintenance program or standard care, which commenced after the eight-week rehab program. The maintenance program consisted of weekly telephone calls and monthly reinforcement sessions, which included supervised exercise. Twenty-four month follow-up data was available for 129 of the original 172 patients. During this time, there was no change in pulmonary function. The 12-month maintenance program appeared successful in maintaining the physiological and subjective benefits of rehab, for the duration of the program. However, these benefits were gradually lost after the maintenance program was concluded. At 12 months after the maintenance program ended (two years after completion of rehabilitation) there was little difference between the two arms.

Based on available evidence, it would appear that setting, duration and follow-up all have important implications on the long term effects of rehabilitation. This conclusion is not surprising and, indeed, would appear intuitive. It is possible that the optimal rehabilitation program would be longer in duration and be home-based. However, such a program would be more demanding in terms of resources and may not be appropriate for all patients. For patients who undergo a more 'conventional' 6–8 week outpatient rehab program, periodic maintenance programs may be indicated, possibly for an indefinite period of time.

Conclusion

Pulmonary rehabilitation is a proven and effective therapy for patients with respiratory disease. Although not all pulmonary patients will be eligible, pulmonary rehabilitation has the potential for producing important improvements in both quality of life and exercise capacity. At this time, it is not known what constitutes an 'optimal' rehabilitation program, although this would likely be clarified with future research. Rehabilitation should be a consideration for all respiratory patients who continue to experience disability despite appropriate pharmacological therapy for their condition.

References

1. **American Thoracic Society.** Pulmonary rehabilitation – 1999. *Am J Respir Crit Care Med* 1999; **159**: 1666–82.
2. **Casaburi R, Patessio A, Ioli F, et al.** Reductions in exercise lactic acidosis and ventilation as a result of exercise training in patients with obstructive lung disease. *Am Rev Respir Dis* 1991; **143**: 9–18.
3. **Maltais F, Leblanc P, Simard C, Jobin J, Bérebé C, Bruneau J, et al.** Skeletal muscle adaptation to endurance training in patients with chronic obstructive pulmonary disease. *Am J Respir Crit Care Med* 1996; **154**: 442–7.
4. **Casaburi R, Wasserman K, Patessio A, et al.** A new perspective in pulmonary rehabilitation: anaerobic threshold as a discriminant in training. *Eur Respir J* 1989; **2**: 618s–623s.
5. **Ries AL, Archibald CJ.** Endurance exercise training at maximal targets in patients with chronic obstructive pulmonary disease. *J Cardiopulmonary Rehabil* 1987; **7**: 594–601.
6. **Lake FR, Henderson K, Briffa T, et al.** Upper limb and lower limb exercise training in patients with chronic airflow obstruction. *Chest* 1990; **97**: 1077–82.
7. **Ortega F, Toral J, Cejudo P, Villagomez R, Sanchez H, et al.** Comparison of effects of strength and endurance training in patients with chronic obstructive pulmonary disease. *Am J Respir Crit Care Med* 2002; **166**: 669–74.
8. **Panton LB, Golden J, Broeder CE, Browder KD, et al.** The effects of resistance training on functional outcomes in patients with chronic obstructive pulmonary disease. *Eur J Appl Physiol* 2003; **91**(4): 443–9.
9. **Belman MJ, Shadmehr R.** Targeted resistive ventilatory muscle training in chronic pulmonary disease. *J Appl Physiol* 1988; **65**: 2726–35.
10. **Lisboa C, Villafrance C, Leiva A, Cruz E, et al.** Inspiratory muscle training in chronic airflow limitation: effect on exercise performance. *Eur Respir J* 1997; **10**: 537–42.
11. **O'Donnell DE, McGuire M, Samis L, Webb KA.** General exercise training improves ventilatory and peripheral muscle strength and endurance in chronic airflow limitation. *Am J Respir Crit Care Med* 1998; **157**: 1489–97.
12. **Ries AL, Kaplan RM, Limberg TM, Prewitt LM.** Effects of pulmonary rehabilitation on physiologic and psychosocial outcomes in patients with chronic obstructive pulmonary disease. *Ann Intern Med* 1995; **122**: 823–32.
13. **Bourbeau J, Julien M, Maltais F, Rouleau M, Beaupré A, Begin R, et al.** Reduction of hospital utilization in patients with chronic obstructive pulmonary disease: a disease-specific self-management intervention. *Arch Intern Med* 2003; **163**: 585–91.

14. **Agle DP, Baum GL.** Psychosocial aspects of chronic obstructive pulmonary disease. *Med Clin North Am* 1977; **61**(4): 749–58.
15. **Light RW, Merrill EJ, Despars JA, Gordon GH, Mutalipassi LR.** Prevalence of depression and anxiety in patients with COPD: Relationship to functional capacity. *Chest* 1985; **87**: 35–8.
16. **Emery C, Leatherman NE, Burker EJ, MacIntyre NR.** Psychological outcomes of a pulmonary rehabilitation program. *Chest* 1991; **100**: 613–17.
17. **Lustig FM, Hass A, Castillo R.** Clinical and rehabilitation regimen in patients with COPD. *Arch Phys Med Rehabil* 1972; **53**: 315–22.
18. **Eiser N, West C., Evans S, et al.** Effects of psychotherapy in moderately severe COPD: A pilot study. *Eur Respir J* 1997; **10**: 1581–4.
19. **Breslin EH.** The pattern of respiratory muscle recruitment during pursed-lip breathing. *Chest* 1992; **101**(1): 75–8.
20. **Mueller RE, Petty TL, Filley GF.** Ventilation and arterial blood gas changes induced by pursued lips breathing. *J Appl Physiol* 1970; **28**: 254–8.
21. **Noseda A, Carpiaux JP, Prigogine T, Schmeber J.** Lung function, maximum and submaximum exercise testing in COPD patients: Reproducibility over a long interval. *Lung* 1989; **167**: 247–57.
22. **Mahler DA, Weinberg DH, Wells CK, Feinstein AR.** The measurement of dyspnea. Contents, interobserver agreement, and physiologic correlates of two new clinical indexes. *Chest* 1984; **85**: 751–8.
23. **Guyatt GH, Pugsley SQ, Sullivan MJ, et al.** Effect on encouragement on walking test performance. *Thorax* 1984; **39**: 818–22.
24. **Reardon J, Patel K, Zuwallack RL.** Improvement in quality of life is unrelated to improvement in exercise endurance after outpatient pulmonary rehabilitation. *Cardiopulm Rehabil* 1993; **13**: 51–4.
25. **Mahler DA, Wells CK.** Evaluation of clinical methods for rating dyspnea. *Chest* 1988; **93**: 580–6.
26. **Strijbos JH, Postma DS, van Altena R, Gimeno F, Koeter GH.** A comparison between an outpatient hospital-based pulmonary rehabilitation program and a home-care pulmonary rehabilition program in patients with COPD. A follow-up of 18 months. *Chest* 1996; **109**: 366–72.
27. **Wedzicha JA, Bestall JC, Garrod R, Garnham R, et al.** Randomized controlled trial of pulmonary rehabilitation in severe chronic obstructive pulmonary disease patients, stratified with the MRC dyspnoea scale. *Eur Respir J* 1998; **12**: 363–9.
28. **Zuwallack RL, Patel K, Reardon JZ, et al.** Predictors of improvement in the 12-minute walking distance following a six week outpatient pulmonary rehabilitation program. *Chest* 1991; **99**: 805–8.
29. **Cox NJM, Hendricks JC, Binkhorst RA, van Herwaarden CLA.** A pulmonary rehabilitation program for patients with asthma and mild chronic obstructive pulmonary diseases (COPD). *Lung* 1993; **171**: 235–44.
30. **Cambach W, Chadwick-Straver RVM, Wagenaar RC, et al.** The effects of a community-based pulmonary rehabilitation program on exercise tolerance and quality of life: A randomized controlled trial. *Eur Respir J* 1997; **10**: 104–13.
31. **Cochrane LM, Clark CJ.** Benefits and problems of a physical training programme for asthmatic patients. *Thorax* 1990; **43**: 345–51.
32. **de Jong W, Grevink RG, Roorda RJ, Kaptein AA, et al.** Effect of a home exercise training program in patients with cystic fibrosis. *Chest* 1994; **105**: 463–8.

33. **Foster S, Thomas H.** Pulmonary rehabilitation in lung disease other than chronic obstructive pulmonary disease. *Am Rev Respir Dis* 1990; **141**: 601–4.
34. **Singh SJ, Vora VA, Morgan MDL.** Does pulmonary rehabilitation benefit current and non-smokers? *Am J Respir Crit Care Med* 1999; **159**: A764.
35. **Young P, Dewse M, Fergussen W, Kolbe J.** Respiratory rehabilitation in chronic obstructive pulmonary disease: predictors of non-adherence. *Eur Respir J* 1999; **13**: 855–9.
36. **Lacasse Y, Maltais F, Goldstein RS.** Smoking cessation in pulmonary rehabilitation: goal or prerequisite? *J Cardiopulm Rehabil* 2002; **22**(3): 148–53.
37. **Lacasse Y, Wong E, Guyatt GH, King D, Cook DJ.** Meta-analysis of respiratory rehabilitation in chronic obstructive pulmonary disease. *Lancet* 1996; **348**: 1115–19.
38. **Lacasse Y, Brosseau L, Milne S, Martin S.** Pulmonary rehabilitation for chronic obstructive pulmonary disease. The Cochrane Library 2004; 1.
39. **Redelmeier DA, Bayoumi AM, Goldstein RS, *et al.*** Intrepreting small differences in functional status; the six minute walking test in chronic lung disease. *Am J Respir Crit Care Med* 1997; **155**: 1278–82.
40. **Guell R, Casan P, Belda J, Sangenis M, *et al.*** Long-term effects of outpatient rehabilitation of COPD. *Chest* 2000; **117**: 976–83.
41. **Hudson LD, Tyler ML, Petty T.** Hospitalization needs during an outpatient rehabilitation program for severe chronic airway obstruction. *Chest* 1976; **70**: 606–10.
42. **Griffiths TL, Burr ML, Campbell IA, Lewis-Jenkins V, Mullins J, Shiels K, *et al.*** Results at 1 year of outpatient multidisciplinary pulmonary rehabilitation: a randomized controlled trial. *Lancet* 2000; **355**: 362–8.
43. **Behnke M, Jorres RA, Kirsten D, Magnussen H.** Clinical benefits of a combined hospital and home-based exercise programme over 18 months in patients with severe COPD. *Monaldi Arch Chest Dis* 2003; **59**: 44–51.
44. **Belman MJ, Brooks SM, Ross DJ, *et al.*** Variability of breathlessness measurement in patients with chronic obstructive pulmonary disease. *Chest* 1991; **99**: 566–71.
45. **O'Donnell DE, McGuire M, Samis L, Webb KA.** The impact of exercise reconditioning on breathlessness in severe chronic airflow limitation. *Am J Respir Crit Care Med* 1995; **152**: 2005–13.
46. **Maltais F, Simard AA, Simard C, *et al.*** Oxidative capacity of skeletal muscle and lactic acid kinetics during exercise in normal subjects and in patients with COPD. *Am J Respir Crit Care Med* 2004; **153**: 288–93.
47. **American Thoracic Society, European Respiratory Society.** Skeletal muscle dysfunction in chronic obstructive pulmonary disease. *Am J Respir Crit Care Med* 1999; **159**: S1–S40.
48. **Gigliotti F, Coli C, Bianchi R, Romagnoli I, *et al.*** Exercise training improves exertional dyspnea in patients with COPD. *Chest* 2003; **123**: 1794–802.
49. **O'Donnell DE, Revill SM, Webb KA.** Dynamic hyperinflation and exercise intolerance in chronic obstructive pulmonary disease. *Am J Respir Crit Care Med* 2001; **164**: 770–7.
50. **Troosters T, Gosslink R, Decramer M.** Short and long-term effects of outpatient rehabilitation in patients with chronic obstructive pulmonary disease: A randomized trial. *Am J Med* 2000; **109**: 207–12.
51. **Ries AL, Kaplan RM, Myers R, Prewitt LM.** Maintenance after pulmonary rehabilitation in chronic lung disease. *Am J Respir Crit Care Med* 2003; **167**: 880–8.

10

Surgical interventions to improve dyspnoea

Andrew J. Drain and Francis C. Wells

Introduction

All surgical procedures are a careful balance of risk against benefit, yet surgery for advanced disease in the chest is often regarded as being too interventional for patients with incurable disease. This approach frequently leaves patients with distressing symptoms, of which dyspnoea is one of the most frightening. It is exactly these cases however, where aggressive palliative intervention yields gratifying results and in many cases can alleviate or even abolish the dyspnoea.

Advanced malignant disease gives rise to most cases of dyspnoea that may benefit from surgical intervention and as such will take up the bulk of this chapter.

Malignant disease within the thorax

Malignant disease that gives rise to chest complications includes primary lung cancer, metastatic lung cancer, primary pleural malignancy (mesothelioma) and other mediastinal tumours (see Box 10.1).

This is not an exhaustive list but includes the most common malignant disorders that present in a regional thoracic centre. Despite the plethora of potential tumours, they all manifest their chest complications in similar ways (see Box 10.2). Consequently, the resulting dyspnoea arising from thoracic malignancy may be managed using well-tested and commonly used surgical techniques.

Airway obstruction

Airway obstruction is a common occurrence in patients with advanced bronchial carcinoma, but other malignancy such as lymphoma and metastatic

Box 10.1 Common causes of thoracic malignancy

Primary malignancy	Metastatic malignancy
Lung	Breast
Mesolithioma	Lymphoma
Oesophagus	Gynaecological
Mediastinal	Other (renal, sarcoma, melanoma)

Box 10.2 Causes of dyspnoea due to intra-thoracic malignancy

Airway obstruction
Pulmonary sepsis (including empyema)
Haemoptysis
Pleural effusion
Pericardial effusion

disease can also give rise to this complication. Symptoms are usually caused by loss of functioning lung, often accompanied by significant shunting of blood through non-aerated lung. Abscess formation, empyema and haemoptysis can all occur as an end result of the obstruction, with potentially fatal consequences.

There are several ways of clearing the obstructed lung. The first essential element is bronchoscopy (flexible or rigid) to evaluate the extent of obstruction. CT with or without 3-D reconstruction will further enhance this information by visualizing the length of the airway involved (see Figure 10.1).

Provided there is a patent bronchus beyond the site of obstruction, a way through the narrowed areas can usually be found although if the whole length of the bronchus is occluded this may not be possible. Definable obstructed segments can be opened up by a variety of techniques including balloon-dilatation (+/− stent insertion), laser therapy, loop diathermy, cryoablation, and local radiotherapy (brachytherapy).

Previously most of these would have required a rigid bronchoscope but many can now be done using a flexible bronchoscope, obtaining excellent images that are recordable and reproducible. These procedures all have risks and although exsanguination can occur with tumour-directed therapy (e.g. laser) or with stenting alone, most bleeding can usually be controlled with

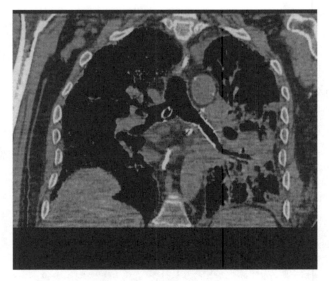

CT

Figure 10.1 Coronal CT showing left bronchial stent in place.

topical adrenaline. The most common surgical approach to airway obstruction is stenting and dilatation. There are now a large variety of stents available. Tracheal compression or collapse may be held open with a Montgomery T-tube – a silicone stent with a side arm that can be inserted through a tracheostomy incision. Variations on the Montgomery stent exist with a bifurcated distal limb to hold the carina and proximal bronchi open.

Cooper and colleagues reported an extensive experience over 15 years with bronchial stenting[2] demonstrating that excellent palliation is achievable with airway stents. While these stents are usually permanent, stent-exchange is feasible when required.[3] More recently, expandable metal stents are being placed via a flexible bronchoscope and then dilated to give maximal airway opening (see Figure 10.2).[2]

Local radiotherapy can also be used to help open obstructed airways and used in combination with the above techniques can relieve quite significant obstructions. The Cleveland Clinic showed how low-dose endobronchial radiation alone or combined with laser resection gave good to excellent symptom control.[4] Once airway patency has been achieved, close patient follow-up is required as there is a high likelihood of tumour growth causing further obstruction. These techniques can be repeated on several occasions allowing improved airway patency over a considerable timeframe.

Main indications for bronchial stent: Inoperable (patient) or unresectable (stage) lung cancer, following bronchial anastamosis (sleeve or transplant).

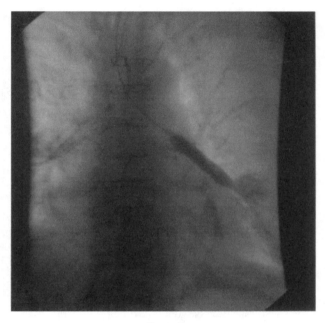

Stent 1

Figure 10.2 Screening image during bronchoscopic balloon dilatation (left). Note expandable stent on right.

Malignant pleural effusion

A pleural effusion is a common complication of primary pulmonary, primary pleural (mesothelioma) and metastatic thoracic disease. It is a major cause of dyspnoea in advanced malignancy, often with the primary site unidentified. The mechanism of the effusion may be due to either obstruction of the pleural drainage or overproduction of fluid from the pleura. In all cases it portends a poor prognosis with a reduced life expectancy, represents advanced malignant disease (e.g. stage IV lung cancer), and is not manageable by surgical resection.[5]

Mesothelioma, a pleural-based malignancy in which the most common presenting complaints are dyspnoea and chest pain, has a median survival from the time of diagnosis of seven to twelve months.[6] Malignant effusions associated with primary lung cancer also have a short survival time and together with breast cancer account for 50–65 per cent of all malignant effusions.[7] However, malignant pleural effusion is a complication for which there is usually good palliative surgical treatment available if the algorithm as set out in the BTS (British Thoracic Society) guidelines[8] is followed (see Figure 10.3).

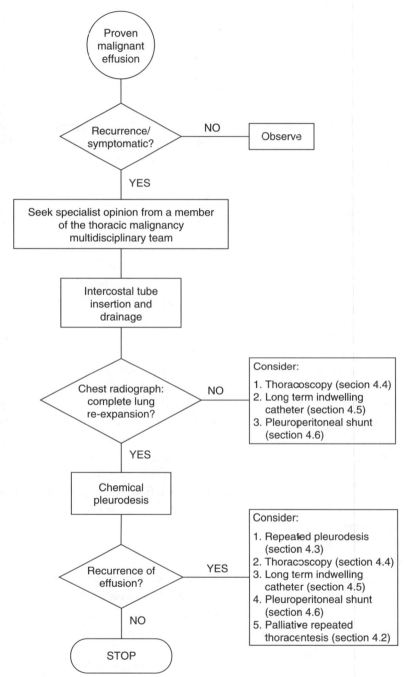

Figure 10.3 Options for management of malignant pleural effusion: BTS guidelines 2003.

While using this algorithm as an excellent guide, ultrasound or CT-guided chest drain insertion should be performed if there is uncertainty about the extent of the effusion, the proximity of underlying structures, or the degree of loculation of the collection. The danger of repeated chest drain insertion and the subsequent risk of empyema cannot be overstated.

Simple aspiration or even chest tube drainage is rarely enough and usually results in rapid re-accumulation of the fluid. The choice of management will depend upon whether the lung is capable of full expansion or not. If the lung will not re-expand, the space within the thorax will refill.

In considering first the situation where the lung will re-expand, a pleurodesis either by mechanical scarification of the parietal pleura or talc insufflation will, in the vast majority of cases, result in complete resolution of the problem with the lung adhering to the chest wall.[9]

If the lung will not re-expand because it is encased by advanced tumour, then the decision on what to do next will depend on the mobility of the mediastinum. If the mediastinum is fixed, then effusion will usually accumulate to a certain volume and then cease. Symptoms of dyspnoea in this circumstance are often due to fixation of the intra-thoracic structures by tumour, and the removal of a pleural collection may not radically alter the way a patient will feel.

If the mediastinum and the diaphragm are mobile, then the patient will become breathless as the fluid reaccumulates, due to increasing intra-thoracic pressure causing compression of the opposite lung. Under these circumstances a pleurectomy may be performed by either video-assisted thoracic surgery (VATS) or open thoracotomy. Both of these techniques are well described producing good symptom control and preventing recollection of effusion, associated lung collapse, infection and empyema.[10]

The use of a pleuro-peritoneal shunt is now infrequent but still has a role in some patients. These shunts are made of silicone and consist of three parts. First a central pumping chamber within which there is a simple flutter valve. When the chamber is compressed, fluid passes through the valve, which is similar to the finger of a surgical glove with the end cut off. The fluid cannot pass backwards. There is an inlet and outlet tube leading into and out of the chamber. Each of these tubes has multiple side holes to allow the fluid to enter or leave. The inlet tube is placed within the thorax via a small purse-string suture in the intercostal muscle while the outlet tube is placed in a similar fashion through the peritoneum. The pumping chamber is then placed subcutaneously to one side of the incision over the costal margin.

The chamber will contain up to 5 mls of fluid, hence repeated pumping is required throughout the day. This can be accomplished through clothing, however, once the patient has become accustomed to it. Pumping 40–50 times every 4–8 hours can keep the pleural space empty allowing most patients to be able to deal with this without significant difficulty.[11]

More modern devices, such as the pleuri-vac system, are a simpler 'patient-managed' chest drain systems. The pleuri-vac is inserted as a chest drain but then tunnelled through the skin before exiting. This allows the patient to empty the bag when required rather than the need for repeated and frequent pumping.

Talc pleurodesis is commonly performed on many patients in whom the lung does re-expand. The use of less aggressive agents such as tetracycline instilled into the pleural space via a chest tube is less effective. Some published information suggests they can be effective in up to 75 per cent of patients whereas talc pleurodesis is effective in about 90 per cent.[11]

It is important to remember that inserting a chest drain is a painful, frightening procedure. Always use adequate analgesia (local anaesthetic infiltration and systemic analgesics such as opioids) to keep the patient as comfortable as possible during the insertion. Once the drain is in the patient may have significant pain, particularly on movement, and need regular opioid analgesics for some days.

Pulmonary sepsis

The mainstay in the management of lung and pleural abscesses is, if possible, the removal of the pus together with appropriate antibiotic therapy in liaison with the microbiologist. For a lung abscess this can be done percutaneously using fine bore catheters placed under ultrasound or CT-guidance. If no fibrous rind or cortex has formed on the visceral surface then the lung should re-expand, collapsing the abscess. Once drainage ceases, the tube can be removed.

A pleural abscess (empyema) should always be carefully assessed with CT imaging to assess loculations and the degree of cortication on the visceral surface of the lung. There has been much debate surrounding medical versus surgical management of empyema and the use of intra-pleural thrombolytics. The evidence to date suggests that VATS is cost-effective if employed without delay as a primary treatment.[12] If, however, a trial of chest-tube drainage is to be attempted in the first two to three days, it should be augmented by a fibrinolytic agent such as urokinase. If the pleural sepsis does not resolve clinically and radiologically, more aggressive methods such as VATS should be employed without further delay.[13] If a fibrous cortex has formed then the lung is unlikely to re-expand and may necessitate a thoracotomy and decortication. One study has shown that an empirical treatment strategy combining intrapleural fibrinolysis with early surgical intervention resulted in shorter hospitalisations and lower mortality rates.[14]

Considering the comorbidity and prognosis of some patients with advanced malignancy, a simple rib resection may be all that is required to manage the empyema. This allows adequate drainage of the abscess with minimal surgical intervention

Haemoptysis

Haemoptysis is a common and disturbing accompaniment of airway involvement. It can often be well relieved with radiotherapy applied intraluminally (brachytherapy) or externally. Sadly in some cases, massive haemoptysis is a dreadful terminal event and nothing can (or should) be done other than to make the patient as comfortable as possible.

Palliative surgical resection

Surgical resection for chest malignancy with curative intent can be considered only if a good proximal clearance can be achieved. Palliative resection has no place in the management of lung cancer. However, even though excision of tumour with positive margins will not result in cure, it may bring about significant relief of symptoms including those from locally advanced disease. Inappropriate use of surgery can worsen the situation and even precipitate death. Bronchial stump breakdown, post-resection empyema and cardiac events leading to long-term hospitalisation make resection an option rarely appropriate in terminally ill patients.

Pericardial disease

The pericardium may be directly involved from pulmonary tumours and metastases. This commonly causes a pericardial effusion which may go on to cause tamponade and dyspnoea. Tamponade may be relieved by draining the fluid via the sub-xiphisternal approach (needle or fine-bore tube). As with pleural effusions however, recurrence of the fluid usually necessitates more definitive management.

A pericardial window may be carried out by VATS or through a direct anterior mini-thoracotomy. By either route a 2–4cm square of pericardium, usually anterior to the phrenic nerve is resected leaving direct drainage into the pleural space. A drain is left in the pleural space in patients without significant pleural disease. On removal of the drain, fluid from the pericardium is absorbed by the pleura or if a pleural effusion is present a shunt can be placed at the same time.

Laham et al. have described their experience with malignant pericardial effusions in 50 patients.[15] They describe a combination of methods and stress the importance of using the appropriate technique in an individual patient.

Oesophageal carcinoma

Oesophageal cancer is a formidable malignancy with the majority of patients incurable on presentation. The drawback of oesophagectomy is that it is a substantial operation with significant morbidity and mortality when in the wrong hands. In many cases oesophagectomy is a palliative procedure but with careful patient selection and an experienced team, cure is possible even with locally advanced disease. In those for whom cure is not achieved, resection reduces the likelihood of complications such as perforation, aspiration and local disease-related problems.

Oesophageal cancer most commonly gives rise to symptoms of dyspnoea through the processes mentioned in relation to thoracic malignancy in general and is therefore managed in a similar fashion. Two problems more related to oesophageal cancer than any other thoracic malignancy and therefore worthy of separate mention are tracheo-oesophageal fistula and aspiration secondary to luminal narrowing.

Stenting

If resection cannot be achieved or where distant metastases are present, oesophageal patency may be maintained in a variety of ways (Box 10.3).

Oesophageal stenting has become the most common technique for maintaining luminal patency in the face of inoperable disease. Prior to the availability of expandable stents, endo-luminal stents were frequently used. Examples of these include the Mousseau Barbin, Nottingham and Celestin tubes. None of these was entirely satisfactory due to the problems of dislodgement, regurgitation or distal displacement. The Mousseau-Barbin needed an open gastrostomy for placement and was generally used when unexpected

---

Box 10.3 Techniques for treatment of oesophageal obstruction

Dilatation
Stenting
Laser therapy
Radiotherapy
Chemotherapy
Surgical bypass

findings at laparotomy rendered the oesophagus unresectable. The Celestin tube had a high incidence of distal migration into the gastrointestinal tract, with an increased tendency to break up often causing perforation and mediastinitis or peritonitis.

The current forms of expandable metal stents (some covered by a plastic coating) have the advantage that they can be placed endoscopically over a guide wire and dilated to the appropriate size.[16] This also allows the insertion of further stents within the first. Covered stents are ideal for management of tracheo-oesophageal fistulae.[17] Although these endoscopically placed stents are an improvement compared to their predecessors, expandable stents can still migrate, erode (leading to life-threatening haemorrhage) and be complicated by perforation during their insertion.[18]

Main indications: Inoperable or unresectable carcinoma, recurrent disease, perforation

Surgical bypass

Extra-anatomical bypass is much less frequently used today, but still has a place in some cases of tracheo-oesophageal fistula. Stomach or colon are detached from their anatomical position and brought up to bypass the oesophagus which is left in its normal position and stapled off above and below the tumour. There is a high mortality from this procedure and it should be reserved for highly selected cases.

Non-malignant disease

Chronic breathlessness in advanced disease is of course not always secondary to malignancy. Some of the benign conditions that give rise to this can be ameliorated by surgical intervention (see Box 10.4).

Empyema management has been dealt with in the context of malignancy. Surgical management of emphysema (either by VATS or median sternotomy) has been looked at extensively recently with the lung volume reduction trial.[19]

Box 10.4 Non-malignant causes of chronic dyspnoea

Empyema
Emphysema and severe bullous disease
Tracheal compression (e.g. thyroid)
Idiopathic tracheal stenosis
Thromboembloic pulmonary hypertension

Although there was no overall increase in survival this demonstrated an improved increase in exercise capacity compared with best medical therapy. There were also other improvements for specific groups depending on the distribution of the emphysema.

Main indications for LVRS: heterogenous, mainly upper lobe disease, with no improvement on maximal therapy and pulmonary rehabilitation.

Breathlessness in heart failure has already been discussed in Chapter 5. From drainage of large pleural effusions and pericardial window formation to the use of mechanical ventricular assist and ultimately transplantation, surgery has and will continue to have an important role to play in the management of end-stage heart failure.

Pulmonary hypertension may now be successfully treated surgically with pulmonary thrombo-endarterectomy if the cause has been demonstrated to be secondary to chronic thromboembolism.[20] While the risks of this procedure remain high, in experienced hands it can provide excellent relief of symptoms and increased life expectancy.

Finally the surgeon should also be used in the management of dyspnoea when diagnosis is unclear. With improved surgical (e.g. VATS) and anaesthetic techniques, lung, pleural, mediastinal and hilar masses are all amenable to surgical biopsy with minimal morbidity and can be imperative to direct patient-focused and medically optimal therapy or palliation.

Conclusions

In keeping with the ethos of this book and patient management in general, treating patients with dyspnoea from advanced disease is best achieved through a multidisciplinary approach. For example, the most common malignant tumour within the thorax is that of the lung, but with only 15–20 per cent of lung cancer 'resectable' on presentation, many patients continue to be seen outside a specialist centre.[21] Palliative interventions may benefit many, but cannot be applied if there is no access to specialist help and dedicated multidisciplinary teams.

Patients with malignant or non-malignant disease can be denied access to proper investigation on the grounds that it is not worth it or may put the patient through unnecessary suffering. This will at times be the case, but all patients should be allowed to benefit from the opinion of a group of experts in the field thereby identifying patients for well-targeted palliative care. Particularly in malignant disease, dyspnoea can be rapidly and often permanently alleviated by surgical intervention.

References

1. Cooper JD, Pearson FG, Patterson A, Todd TR, Ginsberge RJ, Godlberg M, Waters P. Use of silicone stents in the management of airway problems. *Ann Thor Surg* 1989; 47(3): 371–8.

2. Wassermann K, Eckel H, Michel O, Muller RP. Emergency stenting of malignant obstruction of the airways: Long-term follow-up with two types of silicone prosthesis. *Journal of Thorac Cardiovasc Surg 1996;* 112(4): 859–66.

3. Suh HH, Dass KK, Pagliaccio PA, Taylor ME, Saxton JP, Tan M, Mehta AC. Endobronchial radiation therapy with or without neodymium yttrium aluminium garnet laser resection for managing malignant airway obstruction. *Cancer* 1994; 73(10): 2583–8.

4. Chernow B, Sahn SA. Carcinomatous involvement of the pleura. *Am J Med* 1977; 63; 695–702.

5. Molengraft van de FJJM, Vooijs GP. Survival of patients with malignant-associated effusions. *Acta Cytol* 1989; 33: 911–16.

6. Rusch VW. Diffuse malignant mesothelioma. In: Shields TW ed. *General Thoracic Surgery*, 4th edn, pp. 731–47, 1994. Williams & Wilkins, Baltimore.

7. DiBonito L, Falconieri G, Colauti I, *et al.* The positive pleural effusion. A retrospective study of cytopathological diagnosis with autopsy confirmation. *Acta Cytol* 1992; 36; 329–32.

8. G Antunes, Neville E, Duffy J, Ali N. BTS guidelines for the management of malignant pleural effusions *Thorax* 2003; 58 suppl 2: ii29–38.

9. Yim APC, Chung SS, Lee TW, Lam CK, Ho JKS. Thoracoscopic management of malignant pleural effusions. *Chest* 1996; 109(5): 1234–8.

10. Grossebner MW, Arifi AA, Goddard M, Ritchie AJ. Mesothelioma–VATS biopsy and lung mobilization improves diagnosis and palliation. *Eur J Cardiothorac Surg 1999;* 16(6): 619–23.

11. Petrou M, Kaplan D, Goldstraw P. Management of recurrent malignant pleural effusions. The complementary role of talc pleurodesis and pleuroperitoneal shunting. *Cancer* 1995; 75(3): 800–15.

12. Lim TK. Management of pleural empyemas. *Chest* 1999; 116(3): 845–6.

13. Bouros D, Schiza S, Tzanakis N, *et al.* Intrapleural urokinase versus normal saline in the treatment of complicated para-pneumonic effusions and empyema: a randomized, double blind study. *Am J Respir Crit Care Med* 1999; 159: 37–42.

14. Lim TK, Chin NK. Empirical treatment with fibrinolysis and early surgery reduces the duration of hospitalisation in pleural sepsis. *Eur Respir J* 1999; 13: 514–18.

15. Laham RJ, Cohen KJ, Kuntz RE, Bain DS, Lorell BH, Simons M. Pericardial effusion in patients with cancer: outcome with contemporary management strategies. *Heart* 1996; 75: 67–71.

16. Winkelbauer FW, Schoft R, Niederle B, Wilding R, Thurnber S, Lammer J. Palliative treatment of obstructing oesophageal cancer with nitinal stents: value, safety and long-term results. *Am J Roentgenol* 1996; 166(1): 79–84.

17. Han YM *et al.* Esophago-respiratory fistulae due to esophageal carcinoma: palliation with a covered Gianturco stent. *Radiology* 1996; 199(1): 65–70.

18. Acuras B, Rozanes I, Akpinar S, Tunaci A, Tunaci M, Acuras G. Palliation of malignant oesophageal strictures with self-expanding nitinol stents: drawbacks and complications. *Radiology* 1996; 199(3): 648–52.

19. **National Emphysema Treatment Trial Research Group.** A randomised trial comparing lung volume reduction therapy with medical therapy for severe emphysema. *N Engl J Med* 2003; **348**: 2059–73.

20. **Cerveri I, D'Armini AM, Vigano M.** Pulmonary thromboendarterectomy almost 50 years after the first surgical attempts. *Heart* 2003; **89**(4): 369–70.

21. **British Thoracic Society and Society of Cardiothoracic Surgeons of Great Britain and Ireland Working Party** (2001). Guidelines on the selection of patients with lung cancer for surgery. *Thorax* **56**, 89–108.

11

Non-pharmacological approaches
Virginia Carrieri-Kohlman

Introduction

The most recent definition of the symptom of dyspnea or breathlessness was developed by a multidisciplinary committee and defines dyspnea as '...a subjective experience of breathing discomfort that consists of qualitatively distinct sensations that vary in intensity. This experience is derived from interactions among multiple physiological, psychological, social and environmental factors and may induce secondary physiological and behavioral responses'.[1] This description extends the more physiological perspective of the earlier definition of '...difficult or labored breathing rated by the patient himself...'[2] to that of a symptom that may be influenced by psychological and social factors resulting in physiological and behavioral responses. This new and more comprehensive definition reflects the generalized description that a symptom is the consciously appreciated sensation of a physiologic problem and is the result of an interaction of multiple physiological, sociological and psychological factors.[3,4] It also acknowledges and provides evidence that strategies to modulate the symptom of dyspnea can target other dimensions of the symptom experience beyond the physiological domain, including cognitive, emotional, sensory, and behavioral dimensions.

Symptom perception models

Models of symptom perception propose stages of *acknowledgement, interpretation* and *assignment of meaning* that are sequential and shaped by each other.[5] An initial perception of an internal 'disturbance' or somatic sensation is followed by the individual assigning meaning or attribution to that sensation. This interpretation is known to be mediated by the individual's affect, personality, individual beliefs, past experiences with the symptom, expectations, motivation, and perception of available coping and self-care resources. Non-pharmacological treatments can be targeted to any of these stages of symptom perception, interpretation, or final responses.

More specifically the perception of dyspnea has been shown to be affected by cognitive variables of personality,[6] fatigue,[7] and emotions, including anxiety,[8] and depression.[9,10] How a person appraises a stressful situation, such as symptoms, and the meaning they assign to a physical sensation, can have a profound effect on their definition of the symptom as well as the emotional responses, individual coping responses, and healthcare behaviors.[5,11,12] Attention to the symptom,[13] the individual's confidence that he/she can manage the symptom,[14,15] and feelings of loss of control[16, 17] influence the level of dyspnea. Symptoms occur in a social context: therefore, the person's responses are reinforced and shaped by others, while also influencing the behavior of others.[18] Previous experience with the symptom,[13,19] the social context in which it is experienced,[20] living situation, and family conflict[21] may also affect the intensity and frequency of dyspnea.

Affective dimension of dyspnea

The theoretical perspectives of symptom perception outlined above inform the non-pharmacological strategies for breathlessness discussed in this chapter. The prescription and use of non-pharmacological strategies also assumes that the dyspnea experience is similar to other symptoms, such as pain, and includes sensory and affective dimensions, both of which influence each other.[22–24] Evidence for an 'unpleasant' or 'distressing' dimension of dyspnea is derived from clinical and research observations including: patients' actual descriptions of affective emotions they feel during episodes of shortness of breath,[7, 21] the synergistic cycle of anxiety and shortness of breath observed in both acute or chronic clinical situations, the reported influence of anxiety on dyspnea in patients with acute dyspnea,[25] the ability of patients to differentiate the intensity of experienced dyspnea from the anxiety and distress they are feeling,[26] and the findings using PET scanning and fMRI that there is cortical activation of the anterior insular cortex, a limbic structure, when healthy volunteers experience 'air hunger' in the laboratory.[27,28]

Dyspnea perception and response may be similar to a hypothesized sequential model for the affective component of the pain experience that has long been acknowledged and studied.[22] This model hypothesizes that there is immediate appraisal and affective emotional feelings, such as unpleasantness and distress that are associated with the sensory features of pain in the immediate context. In the second stage, affect is associated with the long-term implications of having pain and is based on the patient's memories, reflection about the implications of having pain and concern for the future.[29]

The study of and measurement of the affective dimension of dyspnea is in the early phases. At present there is little consensus on either the type on anxiety that should be measured or the method used to measure anxiety or distress. Some investigators have measured 'state' anxiety, or anxiety that is defined as situational anxiety during times that patients are short of breath, in patients with chronic obstructive pulmonary disease (COPD).[25,30] Others have measured anxiety as a separate emotion in terminal cancer patients at rest by asking 'How anxious are you'?.[31] This author has measured anxiety associated with dyspnea during exercise by asking the question 'How anxious or nervous are you about your shortness of breath?'.[32]

The impact of affective feelings or emotions on the sensation or intensity of shortness of breath becomes extremely important in advanced disease when medical treatments may not reduce the sensory dimension of dyspnea. It is then, when physiological causes of dyspnea cannot be improved and strategies to target physiological mechanisms are limited, that improving the affective dimension (i.e., decreasing the 'unpleasantness' or the anxiety associated with the symptom) becomes essential.

Cognitive-behavioral perspective

For the most part the non-pharmacological strategies proposed in this chapter are cognitive-behavioral strategies targeted toward altering the patient's central perception of dyspnea. Cognitive-behavioral strategies for helping patients cope with symptoms in advanced disease are based on the belief that there is an interaction between mind and body and more importantly that individuals can be taught new patterns of thinking, feeling and behaving to cope with symptoms. Cognition is the mental process by which knowledge is acquired, manipulated, and changed and is made up of thoughts, knowledge and assigned meaning. Cognitive strategies are attempts to modify thought processes, including thinking, feeling, and knowledge in order to modulate an unpleasant symptom.[33] A major tenet of the cognitive-behavioral approach is that symptoms occur in a social context and that there is a reciprocal relationship between cognition, behaviors, and the environment.[34] Behavioral strategies are defined as performances, activities or responses and are believed to change the person's environmental conditions.[5] Both cognitive and behavioral strategies provide mastery experiences, increase confidence in skills to control the symptom, and subsequently affect the magnitude of physiological responses to the symptom.[35]

Other major concepts within the cognitive-behavioral perspective are that of self-efficacy and control. Self-efficacy, a cognitive factor, and a key component in social cognitive learning theory, refers to a person's self-perceived ability or confidence that he/she can complete a task or cope with a given situation.[36] This perception is strongly influenced by the individual's belief that he/she can gain the motivation, use the cognitive resources and take the action needed to meet the situational demands.[35] Increased self-efficacy has been found to be related to higher tolerance for other symptoms.[37]

Increasing perceived self-efficacy for coping with a symptom can reduce that symptom in several ways.[38] People who believe they can alleviate a symptom, such as dyspnea, try management strategies they have learned and persevere in their attempts to decrease the symptom. On the other hand, those patients who do not feel confident in their ability to decrease their shortness of breath by some means give up readily if they do not get quick results. If individuals have confidence that they can cope with an increasing symptom, they also may have less negative anticipatory emotions about the symptom, and therefore, the symptom may not be as intense or enhanced by anxiety and panic. For example, if a person believes they can cope with the amount of dyspnea they will experience while climbing the stairs, their anxiety about climbing stairs may be less, which may result in less dyspnea while climbing the stairs. People who believe they can control their symptoms are more likely to tolerate unpleasant bodily sensations than those who believe there is nothing they can do to alleviate the symptom.[38] The aim of the strategies discussed in this chapter is to increase the patients' self-efficacy or mastery in their ability to control their dyspnea which may result in an improved quality of life.

Cognitive-behavioral strategies are typically 'self-management' strategies. Most of these strategies do not require a pharmaceutical prescription, therefore, the strategies can be used by a person to manage his or her shortness of breath with varied frequency in any situation (Table 11.1). Managing symptoms for a chronic illness on a daily basis requires that the patients monitor their physical and emotional status and make appropriate management decisions, adhere to recommended treatment protocols, interact with healthcare providers, and manage the effects of their illness on emotions, relationships and ability to function.[39] This self-management of the illness and its effects requires family support and a collaborative relationship with one or more healthcare providers. As the degree of breathlessness advances these functions may have to be assumed by the family or healthcare providers.

Selected non-pharmacological strategies

Broad categories of theoretical mechanisms that can be altered in efforts to reduce dyspnea include:

1 reducing ventilatory demand
2 reducing ventilatory impedance
3 improving muscle function and/or
4 altering the central perception of dyspnea.[40]

Most coping strategies for the breathless patient can be categorized in one of these four mechanisms, however, most non-pharmacological strategies that reduce dyspnea are guided by a cognitive-behavioral perspective and focus on changing the central perception of dyspnea.[41] There are, however, non-pharmacological strategies that primarily address physiological mechanisms. These strategies that target physiological mechanisms with published research evidence of effectiveness will be presented, followed by a discussion of those cognitive-behavioral strategies that focus on changing the central perception of the symptom.

Table 11.1 Self-care strategies for managing dyspnea reported by patients in selected studies

	Brown 1986 Adults lung cancer (N = 30)	Carrieri 1986 Adults Obs, Res, Vas (N = 68)	Carrieri-Kohlman 1991 Children, asthma (N = 39)	Janson 1992 Adults, asthma (N = 95)	Kwiatkowski 1995 Adults, COPD (N = 52)
Physiological					
Breathing strategies	×	×	×	×	
Pursed-lips breathing	×	×			×
Diaphragmatic breathing		×			×
Drink fluids		×	×	×	
Exercise	×	×			×
Positioning/posture	×	×		×	
Sit down		×	×		
Sit up			×		
Lie down		×			
Keep still		×	×	×	
Environmental/social					
Activity modification/ energy conservation		×		×	

(continues)

Table 11.1 (continued) Self-care strategies for managing dyspnea reported by patients in selected studies

	Brown 1986 Adults lung cancer (N = 30)	Carrieri 1986 Adults Obs, Res, Vas (N = 68)	Carrieri-Kohlman 1991 Children, asthma (N = 39)	Janson 1992 Adults, asthma (N = 95)	Kwiatkowski 1995 Adults, COPD (N = 52)
Advanced planning	×	×		×	
Decrease in activities	×	×		×	
Move slower	×				
Transfer ADLs to others	×	×			
Change in living arrangement	×				
Distancing from triggers	×	×		×	×
Fresh air		×	×	×	×
Seeking social support	×	×	×	×	×
Seeking medical care		×	×	×	
Cognitive/behavioral					
Self-monitoring		×		×	×
Self-regulation of meds	×		×	×	
Stress reduction	×	×		×	×
Distraction – diversion	×		×	×	×
Imagery				×	
Meditation, prayer	×	×			
Music	×	×		×	
Relaxation	×	×	×	×	×
Self-isolation	×	×			
Self-talk	×	×		×	×

Physiological strategies

The non-pharmacological strategies discussed in this section target physiological mechanisms and typically are components of a comprehensive pulmonary rehabilitation program.

Energy conservation

Energy conservation, activity modification, and advanced planning of activities can decrease dyspnea by decreasing the respiratory effort and work of breathing and the related fatigue. Energy conservation techniques gain even greater importance for the patient and the family in advanced disease when family resources and other assistance may become essential.

Most of the information known about the relationship between energy conservation techniques and dyspnea is reported in studies that describe the patients' experiences with the strategies[21,42,43] as there are no randomized clinical studies examining this relationship. Patients have described energy conservation techniques that help them manage their shortness of breath. These strategies include: pacing activities; slowing down; using good posture and breathing techniques with performance of any task; replacing hobbies and activities with those that require less effort; and advanced planning of activities with estimation of 'breathing stations'.[42,44] It is important to instruct patients that there is a crucial balance between pacing or resting and appropriate exercise. Graduated exercise and activity to stay physically conditioned is emphasized, while at the same time stressing the need to accept a slower pace. Quality exercises should replace needless activities. Patients need help with advanced planning for almost any activity. Trips are organized early to allow time to anticipate the availability of oxygen, the altitude, the potential for triggers/irritants, the amount of energy needed, and the scheduling of rest periods. Daily walks, restaurant lunches, and activities need to be planned to balance demanding tasks with rest periods. Most clinicians suggest a 'daily outline', dividing the day into phases with exact activities and scheduled rests. Activities can be substituted that are pleasurable, but require less effort. For example, hobbies such as playing cards can be suggested for less strenuous activity to replace the weekly golf game.

It is important to provide patients with strategies for managing their shortness of breath during each of their daily activities so that daily tasks can be completed more efficiently with less energy expenditure. Specific guidelines for completing activities of daily living such as grooming, bathing, showering, and dressing are available to use as visual aids when teaching patients and family.[45] It is important to review steps in self-care with the patient so that energy conservation techniques can be individualized for the patient's ability, daily routine, support resources, and home environment. Patients can be taught to avoid unnecessary movements including: minimizing steps in any task, avoiding overreaching and bending by arranging equipment closely, sitting and using good posture and body mechanics, planning the hardest chores for 'best breathing' times, using controlled pursed-lips breathing in performing any task, using slow smooth movements, and sitting whenever possible. Setting up proper working conditions includes working at proper work height, avoiding clutter in the work area, breaking the job down into steps, and sliding and pushing items rather than lifting. Management strategies for certain activities are published and include strategies for reducing short-ness of breath with dressing and bathing, sexual activity, homemaking, and meal preparation and eating.[46] A variety of recommendations to help patients conserve energy and minimize shortness of breath with activities of daily living are published extensively elsewhere.[45,47]

Breathing strategies

Breathing strategies can decrease ventilatory impedance by improving elim-ination of CO_2 and minimizing the mechanical effects of hyperinflation. Many patients who are short of breath have a tendency to take shallow breaths at a rapid rate.[16,48] This type of breathing pattern can increase dyspnea, and more importantly, it may escalate the anxiety or panic associated with increasing shortness of breath.[24,49] Helping the patient practice and develop a breathing pattern of slow, deep breathing becomes even more significant with the recent evidence that dynamic hyperinflation, with resulting restriction of tidal vol-ume, is the primary contributor to dyspnea during exercise.[50–52] As discussed later in this chapter, investigators have shown that patients can change their rate and depth of breathing through biofeedback while exercising.[53] Others have suggested that the traditional yoga pranayama technique of 4–4–8 can be modified for COPD patients to a 4–2–7–0 pattern, i.e., a count of 4 during inhalation, a count of 2 while holding the breath, a count of 7 for exhalation.[54] The length of inhalation and exhalation can be modified to accommodate the patient's abilities and music or distraction might be added if the patient is unable to count or needs greater relaxation. It is the focus on the breathing and the instructions that may help the patient ultimately develop a new breathing rhythm. Continual practice of this new breathing pattern, which includes reducing the respiratory rate, prolonging the expiratory time and using a gentle forced expiration, may ultimately become unconscious and automatic for the patient. Specific step-by-step exercises to alter breathing rhythm are published elsewhere.[16,55]

Pursed-lips breathing (PLB) is a very effective strategy for managing short-ness of breath for some patients. PLB increases tidal volume and vital capacity, decreases respiratory rate, improves gas exchange, and reduces dyspnea.[56–59] A group of investigators recently measured lung volumes with non-invasive measures and found that PLB decreased end-expiratory volume by decreasing respiratory rate and lengthening expiratory time, therefore, improving dyspnea.[60] Patients need to practice the correct method of PLB, emphasizing a deeper slow breath and practicing a long exhalation with the activity.

Places where patients know they can rest when they are short of breath were previously labeled 'breathing stations'.[44] While planning a daily excursion or trip the patient should be encouraged to remember where these rest places are so they can be used if necessary. During an acute episode of dyspnea, adults and children with chronic lung disease have described positions such as standing still, being 'motionless', 'keeping still', 'staying quiet' or finding a 'place to sit or lean on'.[42] During acute episodes a position that is often helpful in reducing dyspnea for patients is the head down and leaning forward position with arms supported either standing or sitting. This postural relief is thought to be due to an improvement in the mechanical efficiency of the diaphragm and optimal functioning of the accessory muscles.[61] Patients should always be encouraged to assume the position that is most comfortable for them, even during acute dyspnea when nurses, physicians or family members may think they should assume a different 'more comfortable' position.

Cognitive-behavioral strategies

Cognitive-behavioral strategies have been theoretically categorized as distraction or attention strategies. Research has shown that if the symptom is relatively brief, acute distraction is more effective for alleviating distress and increasing tolerance than attention to the stressor. However, as in chronic illness when the stressor (or symptom) is long term, attention has been found to be more beneficial when the individual may be more able to actively and successfully confront the situation.[62] In general, using attention coping strategies, e.g., symptom monitoring and information-seeking to cope with chronic symptoms, is associated with better illness adjustment, while avoidant coping strategies or distraction, e.g., hoping, ignoring, and attention diversion, result in higher levels of physical and psychological disability and a poorer adjustment to illness.[18] The categories of attention and distraction are not mutually exclusive, attention strategies can also provide distraction and vice versa. For instance, planning an outing with a supportive group of people with COPD may be an attention strategy, but it also may provide distraction for the patient. The strategies in this chapter focus on both the sensory and affective dimensions of dyspnea. In research concerning other symptoms, such as pain, different types of coping strategies were more effective depending on whether they addressed the sensory or affective dimension. However, to date investigators have not measured these two dimensions as separate outcomes in the study of dyspnea, and therefore, it is difficult to determine which dimension is being modified.

Distraction strategies

Relaxation exercises

Anxiety increases when dyspnea increases. Previously this has been primarily a clinical observation with anxiety increasing with increasing shortness of breath in a synergistic spiral resulting in severe shortness of breath and panic. Recently anxiety has been associated with increasing or high dyspnea in a controlled trial of asthma patients in an emergency room,[63] in COPD patients during treadmill exercise[64] and in cancer patients.[8] Since they are related, strategies that decrease this anxiety or modulate the level of distress might be expected to reduce dyspnea. Relaxation may have a physiological effect by reducing respiratory rate and increasing tidal volume, thus improving breathing efficiency and dyspnea.[65] One investigator studied the effect of relaxation on dyspnea in 10 patients with COPD compared with a control group that was instructed to relax, but not given specific instructions. Although dyspnea was significantly reduced for the relaxation group during treatment sessions, the scores were similar after four weeks.[66] In another study relaxation techniques used by patients with COPD decreased 'state' anxiety as well as the perception of dyspnea at rest.[30] However, in these preliminary studies immediate decreases in dyspnea did not persist outside the experimental session. They do provide beginning evidence that teaching a patient a program of relaxation to use when dyspnea increases may prevent the anxiety and dyspnea from escalating at the time. Relaxation needs to be tailored for the individual patient. There are many published methods with most including: the use of a quiet environment, a comfortable position, loose clothing, some type of word or imagery repeated in a systematic fashion, slow abdominal breathing with deep breaths and slow expirations, systematic tensing or relaxing of all muscles and gentle massage if desired.[55] Individualized tape recordings with a therapist can be used to coach patients throughout a session in the home.[67]

Music

Patients with chronic shortness of breath have described using many distraction strategies, such as watching TV, reading, talking on the phone, using the internet. Those spontaneously reported by one male are listed in (Table 11.2). Music is one of these strategies that has been tested with small samples. One investigator studied the effect of listening to music on dyspnea and anxiety during a home walking program for 24 COPD patients. There was a significant decrease in dyspnea immediately following the use of music as reported in a music diary and a significant decrease in dyspnea and anxiety following the use of music in week two. However, there were no significant changes

Table 11.2 Strategies for SOB used by a 64-year-old male with COPD

Read	Go fishing
Pray	Get on the Internet
Meditate	Take meds
Talk to a friend	Write
Pursed lips breathing	Watch TV
Listen to music	Take vitamins
Exercise	Cook
Relax	Shop
Get cool	Walk in the zoo
Go driving	Sleep
Take a shower	

in anxiety or dyspnea over the total five-week period.[68] Other investigators used a cross-over design to measure the effect of music on dyspnea and anxiety experienced by 30 individuals with COPD while walking. Participants walked without music for 10 minutes and for 10 minutes while listening to selected music in random order. There were no differences in the change from before to after the six minute walk (MW) for dyspnea or anxiety when the patients walked with or without music.[69]

Guided imagery

Clinically people seem to walk longer and move through greater dyspnea levels when they use some type of guided imagery, such as asking the person to think about or pretend they are walking in a place they enjoy. However, guided imagery has only been tested in one observational study with 19 COPD patients who met weekly for four weeks for one hour of practice with guided imagery.[70] A standard guided imagery script was read and subjects were asked to visualize the scene described. Audiotapes of the script were provided for practice. In this observational study there was no significant change in dyspnea, depression, quality of life, anxiety or functional status after the sessions.

Acupuncture and acupressure

Acupuncture and acupressure have shown early positive findings for their use in the management of dyspnea. Jobst compared the effects of 'traditional' and 'placebo' acupuncture in 24 COPD patients with 'disabling breathlessness'.[71] During 13 treatment sessions administered over three weeks acupuncture needles were inserted according to 'traditional acupuncture points', while in the other group the placebo needles were inserted in non-acupuncture 'dead points'. Both groups did improve their dyspnea on two different measurement scales and at the end of the six MW, the acupuncture group had significantly greater improvement than the placebo. Acupuncture was tested in 20 patients with cancer-related breathlessness.[72] Initially the patients received needles for ten minutes, these were then left in place for 90 minutes. Seventy per cent of the patients reported significantly improved relief in breathlessness, anxiety and relaxation that peaked at 90 minutes and lasted up to six hours. A nurse was present during this time for observation, therefore, it is difficult to know whether this relief was due to the acupuncture or the presence and reassurance of the nurse.

Maa and colleagues added an acupressure treatment to a pulmonary re-habilitation program to determine if there was additional improvement in dyspnea.[73] Thirty-one COPD patients were taught to apply pressure to seven accupoints that are believed to give relief to patients with dyspnea. Patients applied pressure daily at home for six weeks alternating with a sham acupres-sure. Dyspnea on a Visual Analogue Scale (VAS) was significantly less during the acupressure than the 'sham', however, there were no significant differences between the treatments in dyspnea measured by the Borg Scale or after the six MW. These same investigators later compared the effect of 'standard care' plus acupressure or acupuncture to 'standard care' in asthma patients with 'chronic obstruction'.[74] The acupuncture group received 20 treatments using five points previously hypothesized to provide relief for dyspnea[75] and the other group self-administered their acupressure daily for eight weeks. Although slightly improved, there were no significant differences between the standard care, acupuncture, or the acupressure groups in dyspnea measured by the VAS and modified Borg Scale after eight weeks. Both treatment groups had clinic-ally significant improvements in quality of life with the acupuncture group having the greatest improvements. Another group of investigators randomly assigned 44 COPD patients to a program of 'true acupoint' acupressure or 'sham' pressure points.[76] The true acupoint acupressure group had signifi-cantly greater improvement than the sham group in dyspnea, measured by the Pulmonary Functional Status and Dyspnea Questionnaire-Modifed scale (PFSDQ-M),[77] six MW, state anxiety and oxygen saturation. These early studies with small samples and questionable controls provide conflicting results. These early positive results need to be confirmed in larger controlled trials.

Biofeedback

Today e-Health technological advances in monitoring body systems is a rapidly growing area of research with findings being translated into clinical practice.[78,79] Patients are monitoring physiological data, such as peak flow rates and heart rate, that are often rapidly transferred to the provider. Therefore, it is conceivable that in the near future it will be much easier for a patient to use his/her own respiratory pattern as feedback to change his/her breathing pattern. Over the last decades in sporadic studies biofeedback was shown to reduce respiratory rate and paradoxical breathing, increase tidal volume, increase airway diameter, and decrease weaning time.[80,81] With the recent identification of dynamic hyperinflation as one of the primary mechanisms of dyspnea[52] there is even more reason to focus on helping patients change their breathing pattern. Recently a group of investigators[53] compared the efficacy of a six week 18-session program of ventilation-feedback combined with cycle exercise (VF^{+EX}), ventilation-feedback only (VF^{ONLY}), or exercise only (EX^{ONLY}) on exercise endurance and breathlessness in 39 COPD patients. The purpose of the feedback was to train patients to prolong their expiratory time and maintain tidal volume during exercise. The visual and auditory ventilation-feedback was an indicator of inhalation and exhalation (moving horizontal bar) presented on a screen with an audible alert when the time of expiration was met. After six weeks there was a significantly greater change in the exercise (VF^{+EX}) duration in the group who received feedback during exercise than those who just received the ventilatory feedback. The VF^{+EX} group also had significant improvements in dyspnea and breathing pattern parameters, including minute ventilation, tidal volume, frequency, and expiratory time.

Other investigators[82] examined the feasibility and outcomes of a breathing training program designed to change breathing pattern using heart rate variability (HRV) biofeedback and walking with pulse oximetry feedback. The major outcomes germaine to this chapter were the intensity and distress accompanying breathlessness measured on a Borg Scale after the six MW and dyspnea with activities, measured by the Pulmonary Functional Status and Dyspnea Questionnaire (PFSDQ-M).[77] Twenty patients with COPD participated in five weekly sessions of HRV biofeedback, which consisted of a computer display of a pacing stimulus with which they were told to match their breathing. This feedback was then replaced by a signal showing heart rate variability, which the patient was instructed to maximize. This biofeedback and practice was followed by four weekly sessions of walking practice with oximetry and instructions to walk at home. In this observational study respiratory rate decreased and tidal volume increased and there were significant improvements in distance and dyspnea distress after the six MW and self-reported activity impairments measured by the PFSDQ-M.

Hypnosis

Hypnosis is a trance state that combines a heightened inner awareness with a diminished awareness of one's surroundings. It is suggested that hypnosis may modify the cortical centers and the perception of dyspnea, however, the available studies are primarily with asthma patients. Dyspnea decreased in one patient with severe COPD who received hypnotically-induced relaxation and biofeedback in an effort to decrease his dyspnea during periods of anxiety.[83] Another 16 patients with asthma had a decrease in their dyspnea from pre- to immediately post-hypnosis and the decrease was sustained 30 minutes after hypnosis.[84] Seventeen children and adolescents who had chronic dyspnea with normal lung function that was not responsive to medical therapy were taught self-hypnosis in one or two sessions. Thirteen of the children reported their dyspnea and associated symptoms had resolved within one month of their final hypnosis session. Eleven believed that resolution of their dyspnea was attributable to hypnosis, because their symptoms cleared immediately after they received hypnosis or with the regular use of self-hypnosis.[85]

Social support

There is little controlled research on social support and symptoms in people with chronic dyspnea. In one cross-sectional interview survey, social support and the number of persons in the social support network and frequency of contact with others related to the intensity of dyspnea.[7] It is important to remember that social support for a specific task is more effective than general support. For example, social support focused on initiation or maintenance of exercise impacts motivational readiness[86] and increases adherence to exercise[87,88] more than general social support.

In people with chronic disease the provision of social support buffers stress,[89] influences self-management and adaptation to the illness,[90] improves functioning,[91, 92] and may even decrease the number of exacerbations in patients with COPD through improved immune functioning.[93] It is important to remember that social support is only beneficial if it corresponds to the individual's preference for the type, amount, source, and timing of support sources.[94]

Some patients with dyspnea prefer and may actually benefit from isolating themselves and limiting their interactions with friends and family. Dudley found that failure of patients with COPD to adequately use withdrawal during acute episodes of shortness of breath was associated with an increase in symptoms and psychological deterioration.[95] People hospitalized with acute dyspnea have suggested that healthcare providers and family permit them to withdraw and isolate themselves when they are experiencing severe dyspnea.[96] Other people with chronic dyspnea need and develop extensive networks and resources that provide a high level of social support.[97] Vicarious learning from other people, who have experienced the same symptom and tested successful strategies to decrease the symptom, is a powerful self-efficacy enhancing experience that allows individuals to develop a shared sense of commonality, acceptance, and normalization.[98,99] In an early study with 64 patients with COPD, a group workshop increased self-help skills at home, perhaps by group approval, encouragement, and support that increased confidence and motivation.[100] It is impossible to study the group effect separately from the many components of pulmonary rehabilitation programs (PR), however, social support provided in group sessions may be one of the major contributors to symptom reduction and improvement in quality of life found after structured PR programs.

Exercise as a strategy for changing central perception of dyspnea

One of the most powerful strategies for improving dyspnea with activity is exercise. The major benefits of exercise are attributed to the physiological effects of 'conditioning' or other physiological factors, including improvement in respiratory and peripheral muscle strength and changes in the pattern of breathing resulting in less dynamic hyperinflation with exercise.[50,101] Others have found decreases in dyspnea despite little change in outcomes that reflect physiological effects.[102–104] Possible mechanisms for the reduction in dyspnea without predominant physiological changes include: adaptation to the sensation[105]; a change in the scaling behavior of patients[106]; a type of placebo effect labeled a 'response shift' that connotes a change in the individual's perception of the symptom or frame of reference[107,108]; and desensitization to the symptom.[109,110] In any one patient it is difficult to know which of the many mechanisms is operant, but for clinical purposes it may not be very important. It is important that after performance of low intensity exercise in a controlled setting, studies have shown that patients rate their dyspnea lower for activities of daily living.[32,111]

Clinically, one approach to decreasing a patient's perceived dyspnea for a certain activity level has been to encourage exercise to the point that moderate dyspnea occurs, while coaching the patient to use strategies such as pursed-lips breathing and relaxation. If this procedure is performed in a supportive, safe environment with someone the patient trusts, the patient's fear of dyspnea may decrease while confidence is gained in the ability to control the symptom.

This empirical observation was reported by investigators who observed that control subjects described less anxiety with activities at home after participating in pre- and post-exercise testing.[112] The investigator suggested that this decrease in the anxiety may be due to a type of 'systematic desensitization' to dyspnea that occurred as a result of exposure to a greater than usual level of exercise in a safe, monitored environment.

Based on these findings and those from social cognitive learning theory[35] this author tested a dyspnea self-management program that included exercise. We hypothesized that similar to phobias and other symptoms, repeated exposure to dyspnea in a safe, monitored environment would result in increased and more effective coping skills, a change in the appraisal of the symptom, an increased tolerance for the symptom and finally a reduction in anxiety and distress associated with the dyspnea.[110] The dyspnea self-management did increase patients' control or self-efficacy for walking and managing dyspnea and the dyspnea intensity was less for a given level of ventilation.[32, 113] The precise mechanism of the decrease in dyspnea relative to ventilation after exercise is still unknown. Desensitization or another cognitive mechanism for reducing dyspnea may be especially important in advanced disease as the reduction occurs regardless of the patient's ability to improve physical exercise performance.[32,114,115]

Treatment programs for other symptoms place emphasis on how the treatment affects an individual's confidence and ability to cope with specific threats or sense of control over that symptom. Components of these programs may include:

1 mastery of graduated small components;
2 short-term goals;
3 physical support;
4 modeling of activities and coping strategies;
5 varied performance of the task; and
6 gradual increase in time with the feared stimulus (symptom).[116]

These strategies can be used during pulmonary rehabilitation or in the home to increase patients' tolerance for increasing dyspnea. It is important to advise patients that it is ok to be short of breath while exercising.

Alternative types of exercise – yoga

'Eastern' exercises, such as yoga or Tai-chi, may be alternatives to aerobic or endurance training for people who are limited by severe shortness of breath. These exercises may bring about relaxation, calmness, balance, and may promote changes in the pattern of breathing, including slow and deep breathing. Two investigators have measured some aspects of dyspnea in their study of yoga exercise training. Tandon[117] studied 11 males with COPD who received training in yoga breathing exercises and postures. A yoga teacher taught breathing exercises, using both abdominal and thoracic muscles and 10 yoga postures. A matched group received physiotherapy, including exercises for respiratory muscles, diaphragmatic breathing, and lower extremity exercises. Treatments for both groups were one hour three times a week for four weeks with decreasing sessions over nine months. More yoga subjects compared to the physiotherapy group stated that they had 'easier control' of their dyspnea attacks. More recently, Behera[118] studied a group of 15 males with chronic bronchitis who practiced eight body postures and five breathing exercises in the laboratory 30 minutes daily for one week and then continued in the home for three weeks with weekly reinforcement. There were significant reductions in dyspnea measured with a VAS at week four, but not at week two. Although both studies included a small number of male subjects and used non-validated measures of dyspnea, these findings provide preliminary evidence that light yoga may be an alternative exercise to decease dyspnea, especially in advanced disease when impaired mobility prohibits walking or biking.

Attention strategies

Symptom monitoring

The monitoring of daily symptoms is an intervention in itself that may affect the patient's rating of symptoms, adherence to a regimen, and heighten the patient's awareness of bodily sensations. For people with asthma monitoring of peak expiratory flow rate and symptoms is one of the essential components of effective self-management programs.[3,122] A few studies have shown that if COPD patients monitor their symptoms and/or use an action plan, there is earlier initiation of medical therapy and reduced resource utilization (Table 11.3). Patients who were provided an education booklet, action plan and a supply of prednisone and antibiotics, initiated medical treatment for their exacerbations earlier than patients who received usual care.[119] Gallefoss and colleagues compared the effects of a self-treatment plan with peak expiratory flow and symptom monitoring to a usual care group with COPD. Treatment subjects used less short-acting beta agonists, had an 85 per cent reduction in number of visits to their primary care provider,[120] and less overall costs.[121] Daily symptom monitoring also provides more accurate reflection of symptoms than recall during a weekly or monthly visit. Examples of diaries are published and can be used to develop an ongoing symptom-monitoring program for patients.

Table 11.3 Action plan for shortness of breath

If I have the following symptoms:
◆ Increased shortness of breath
◆ Change in mucous colour or amount
◆ Symptoms of a cold
◆ Sore throat
◆ Other_____
Contact health care provider and:
◆ Increase inhaler frequency to ___puffs every ___hours
◆ Start antibiotics
◆ Start and/or increase Prednisone to___ mg
◆ Monitor peak flow rates if prescribed
◆ If your shortness of breath has not improved in __ hours, contact your health care provider

Education

Asthma There is content specific to the teaching of asthma management and symptoms for children and adults in *Guidelines for the Diagnosis and Management of Asthma.*[122] Optimal self-management components in an asthma education program include: information and facts about asthma including correct inhaler use; self-monitoring of peak flow and/or symptoms; written action plan allowing self-adjustment of medications (individual); and regular clinician review of asthma control and medications. Education about symptoms in asthma is typically integrated into a self-management program. A meta-analysis of 12 studies of asthma self-management programs found that those that included 'education only' significantly improved knowledge of facts and improved perceived symptoms.[123] However, these 'education only' programs had no effect on hospitalizations, ER visits, unscheduled MD visits, lung function, medication use or days lost from work. In contrast, a more recent meta-analysis found that self-management programs that included not just education, but also medical review, self-monitoring of PEFR and symptoms, and a written action plan allowing self-management of medications resulted in decreased resource utilization,[124] nocturnal asthma,[125] symptoms,[126] and improved quality of life[124] when compared to usual controls.

COPD There has been much less study of educational or self-management programs for COPD patients. At present most of the education for COPD patients occurs as one component in structured pulmonary rehabilitation programs. Therefore, the effect of that education component alone has not been sufficiently studied. The individual programs for COPD that included only education and limited skills training have not significantly improved dyspnea.[119,121,127–130] With programs that have included education about dyspnea self-management strategies coupled with some type of exercise and reinforcing phone calls, a decrease was found in dyspnea with laboratory exercise sessions, a decrease in dyspnea with ADL was found after additional supervised exercise, and a decrease in dyspnea with ADL was found with with a home walking prescription.[113] Recent programs for patients with COPD that have provided self-management education, action plans, and prescriptions for antibiotics and steroids coupled with home visits, a limited exercise program, and regularly scheduled follow-up phone calls[120,131–133] reported significant reductions in healthcare utilization compared to usual care groups. This decrease in healthcare utilization could be presumed to mirror a reduction in symptoms, however, which component of these multi-treatment programs had the primary effect on the outcomes is unknown.

Lung cancer One group of investigators has reported a successful nurse clinic for lung cancer patients who completed the 'first line of treatment'.[134,135] A nursing clinic intervention for breathlessness patients was compared to a supportive group that received standard treatment for breathlessness during a weekly clinic visit. The nursing clinic consisted of assessment of breathlessness, teaching effective ways of coping with dyspnea, exploration of the meaning of dyspnea, breathing control, activity pacing, relaxation techniques, and psychosocial support. The intervention group improved their dyspnea at rest, performance status, and physical and emotional status significantly more than the control group at eight weeks. It is noteworthy that this nursing intervention improved dyspnea without an exercise prescription which has not been true of several other education only programs as discussed above.

Fans and air

One strategy that could be labeled an attention or distraction strategy that has been identified by patients who have chronic dyspnea is 'fresh air' or the use of fans to provide a stream of cold air to the face.[42] This clinical observation is supported by a laboratory study that investigated the effect of altering afferent information by directing a flow of cold air against the cheek in normal subjects and found a decrease in dyspnea.[136] A fan that allows the patient to breathe circulating cold air may be one of the most effective non-pharmacological strategies available for chronic dyspnea or acute dyspnea at end of life. This treatment is inexpensive, free of side-effects, and can be applied almost anywhere.[137]

Non-pharmacological strategies across the illness trajectory

Advanced disease can be conceptualized as many phases in an illness that interrupt or decrease the patient's functional abilities. For the purposes of this chapter these phases are labeled: active and stable; homebound with supported outings; acute exacerbations with hospitalization; homebound; and end-of-life with death in the hospital, hospice or home. It is helpful to examine the different strategies that can be used in each phase.

Active and stable

In this phase symptom management begins with the measurement of dyspnea (Table 11.4). The important task is to establish a baseline of shortness of breath that the patient and family can use to determine efficacy of new treatments and changes in the patient's symptom status. A symptom history should include asking about sensations experienced, the meaning of the symptom to the patient and the family, aggravating and alleviating factors, and strategies the patient uses to manage his/her dyspnea. The patient should be asked to give a rating of his/her shortness of breath and distress with the symptom with the most important activities of daily living on unidimensional scales. One of the standardized multidimensional instruments can be used to measure other dimensions of the dyspnea experience.[77,138–141] After a baseline is established dyspnea should be measured before and after (or during) a treatment to help the healthcare provider and patient determine the effective-

Table 11.4 Active and stable phase

Measurement of baseline symptoms
Assess and monitor symptoms and disease
Reduce risk factors
Manage stable COPD
Facilitate exercise, activity and teach self-care action plan
Manage acute exacerbations

ness of alternative strategies for the symptom. This is the time to build a shared partnership with the patient and family. Focus should be on the individual and what strategies he/she is using to manage his/her dyspnea. Self-care strategies used by other patients to manage their shortness of breath should be shared with the patient. The plan can incorporate those strategies tailored to the individual's own self care strategies, environment, and life style. This is the time to emphasize pulmonary rehabilitation programs if available, physical activity with a gradual increase in an established exercise regimen, active strategies such as support groups, and to replace strenuous activities like golf with less demanding activities such as card games or reading. The symptom of dyspnea can be targeted in clinic programs as described above in education strategies.

Homebound with supported outings

During this phase it is important for the patient to continue all strategies used in the previous phase for as long as possible (Table 11.5). Guidelines for conserving energy with ADL and homemaking need to be reinforced, especially if outside resources or family help is not possible. More often than the previous phase patients may often complain of other symptoms, such as anxiety and fatigue. Several studies have shown these symptoms may be synergistic. Dyspnea was found to be more severe in patients with more severe pain.[31] Seriously ill patients who had dyspnea and nausea experienced more pain[142] and the presence of fatigue increases dyspnea.[143] Fatigue and dyspnea are related and more severe when associated with anxiety and depression.[144] Symptom measurement may have to include an attempt to help the patient separate these symptoms in order to determine the primary one or that which is triggering the other. If patients have difficulty separating the symptoms it is important to share with them that patients have described that many of the same cognitive-behavioral strategies used for dyspnea can be used to manage

Table 11.5 Home bound with supported outings

Separate and target symptoms
Continue to use patients' self-care strategies
Change exercise prescription
Attention and Distraction Strategies
Peer support
Add oxygen therapy

their fatigue. These similar strategies such as rest, distraction, nutrition, and social support are listed in Table 11.6. In this phase it is important to realize that people with chronic dyspnea have developed a repertoire of strategies that can be used at home or when going out for an excursion or to see their healthcare provider. There are a variety of strategies patients use as evidenced by one man with COPD who spontaneously wrote the strategies he used listed in Table 11.2 when asked 'What things do you do for your shortness of breath?' Patients who are experiencing a high level of dyspnea for the first time need to be taught and have time to practice the strategies that other patients have found beneficial for managing their shortness of breath.

In this phase attention and distraction strategies can be reinforced and practiced, so they will become a 'habit' before, but also as, shortness of breath increases. Attention strategies might include monitoring of the symptom, advanced planning of activities, energy conservation and appropriate rests, and the use of a fan. Distraction strategies might include music, TV, the Internet, walks, reading, relaxation, guided imagery, self-talk, acupressure, or massage. This phase may require a change or decrease in the exercise regimen, however, optional exercises can replace walking, such as, daily weights, breaking up the exercise to smaller intervals, or chair aerobics. Support groups either organized or within the community can also help patients to learn strategies to cope with increasing dyspnea. Vicarious learning from peers who have developed ways to manage dyspnea is a potent source of self-efficacy or confidence that will help them to control their dyspnea. In the hypoxic COPD patient oxygen therapy may be added at this time to supplement the regular medication regimen.

Table 11.6 Patients' self-care strategies for managing fatigue

Category	Example
Modify activity and rest	Rest/nap, walk, modify activities
Alter sleep-wake pattern	Go to bed early, sleep most of day
Psychological strategies	Music, read, relaxation tape, acupuncture, homeopathy
Social interventions	Engage in hobbies, conversation, have dinner
Preservation of normality	Go to work, go shopping, write letters
Nutritional interventions	Take soothing drinks
Comfort and symptom relief	Hot bath, taking anti-emetics

Hospitalization phase

Patients with a severe exacerbation of COPD may require hospitalization. In qualitative interviews patients with shortness of breath in the hospitalization phase have described emotions of fear, anxiety, panic, helplessness and a feeling of urgency as if 'each breath was the last'.[96,145] Mechanically-ventilated patients have rated their dyspnea from mild to very severe, depending on different types of procedures, ventilator support, weaning periods, and the time in their illness trajectory.[146–148] During hospitalization is an excellent time for teaching patients new strategies that may help their shortness of breath. This teaching needs to begin early in the hospital stay when the patient is comfortable or during rest periods on the medical unit.[149] Hospitalized patients often have had previous experience with strategies that they have learned from others or developed themselves. The patient can be asked to describe or write down the strategies they typically use at home. Often a family or significant other can provide a list of the patent's previous adaptations for dealing with dyspnea. These strategies can be practiced and reinforced so that when the patient is more short of breath, e.g., during a weaning trial, the patient will have strategies that they know can help them to control their dyspnea. During a weaning trial the nurse can coach and model for the patient by standing by them and helping them to maintain a slow, rhythmic and deep pattern of breathing. The presence of the nurse or family, support for relaxation, a quiet calming environment, and breathing techniques that required patients only to imitate the nurse were preferred and seen as the most effective by hospitalized patients. Demonstration and modeling and 'staying with the patient to help them breath slowly and deeply' may be the most important teaching the clinician can do while the patient is experiencing acute dyspnea.[96] Hospitalization is an excellent time to review with the patient and family an action plan for assessing the patient's symptoms and appropriate treatment alternatives that may increase the patient's feeling of control and ultimately decrease the distress of the symptom[137] (Table 11.7).

Homebound phase

Most activities will need to be transferred to the home when advancing disease decreases mobility. During this homebound phase patients may still come to the outpatient clinic or physician office for assessment and palliative care treatment. Alternative options for continuation of exercise at home should be discussed with emphasis on places to walk in the home or yard and times when upper arm exercises can be done. Physical activity tailored to the patient's functional level ought to be recommended throughout the illness

Table 11.7 Hospitalization phase

Quiet, calm environment
Fans
Rating of dyspnea for baseline
Coach and modeling of breathing pattern
'Staying with' the patient
Practice old and new breathing strategies
Practice arm and leg exercises
Teach family about strategies for SOB

trajectory. To continue mobility and still reduce necessary exertion some type of wheelchair can be prescribed.

One alternative method of care, an outpatient palliative medicine consultation team, improved outcomes in patients with COPD, cancer or congestive heart failure who had a prognosis ranging from 1–5 years.[150] This program of multiple consultations by a palliative medicine team, advanced care planning, psychosocial support, and family caregiver training over a year was compared with a control group who received usual care in general medicine clinics. The patients who received the intervention from the consultation team had significantly less dyspnea, anxiety, improved sleep and spiritual well-being than the usual care group.

End of life phase

Care of pulmonary patients in the end of life phase has received more needed attention in the last few years. Greater than 70 per cent of a sample of patients, recently bereaved family members, and health care providers stated that pain and symptom management was the most important factor at the end of life.[151] 'Having symptoms under control' was one of six conceptual domains identified from a sample of family, patients, and literature review for the development of an instrument to measure the quality of dying and death.[152] Despite the importance given to symptom control by patients and families, the frequency of severe dyspnea for patients with pulmonary disease who die in the hospital remains great. Ninety percent of patients with COPD, 70 per cent of lung cancer patients and 52 per cent of patients with acute respiratory failure complained of severe dyspnea three days before their death.[153] The patient and family need to be supported in their use of opioids and oxygen for dyspnea relief at this time (Table 11.8).[40] In this phase support for breathing strategies

Table 11.8 End of life phase

Confidence in control of symptoms
Support for caregivers in use of oxygen and opioides
Oxygen
Opioids
Positioning
Pursed lips breathing
Distraction strategies
Fan
TV
Music
Massage

and comfortable positioning and the use of cognitive strategies, such as electric fans for circulating air, distraction and relaxation with TV, listening to a loved one read, and/or music should be the focus of care.

References

1. **American Thoracic Society.** Dyspnea. Mechanisms, assessment, and management: a consensus statement. *American Journal of Respiratory and Critical Care Medicine* 1999; **159**(1): 321–40.
2. **Comroe JH.** Some theories of the mechanisms of dyspnea. In: Howell JBL, Campbell EJM, eds *Breathlessness*, pp. 1–7. Oxford: Blackwell Scientific, 1966.
3. **Pennebaker JW.** *The Psychology of Physical Symptoms.* New York: Springer-Verlag, 1982.
4. **Larson P, Carrieri-Kohlman V, Dodd MJ, Douglas M, Faucett J, Froelicher ES,** *et al.* A model of symptom management. *Image: Journal of Nursing Scholarship* 1994; **26**: 272–76.
5. **Cioffi D.** Beyond attentional strategies: A cognitive-perceptual model of somatic interpretation. *Psychological Bulletin* 1991; **109**(1): 25–41.
6. **Chetta A, Gerra G, Foresi A, Zaimovic A, Del Donno M, Chittolini B,** *et al.* Personality profiles and breathlessness perception in outpatients with different gradings of asthma. *Am J Respir Crit Care Med* 1998; **157**(1): 116–22.
7. **Janson-Bjerklie S, Kohlman-Carrieri V, Hudes M.** The sensations of pulmonary dyspnea. *Nurisng Research* 1986; **35**(3): 154–9.
8. **Dudgeon DJ, Kristjanson L, Sloan JA, Lertzman M, Clement K.** Dyspnea in cancer patients: prevalence and associated factors. *J Pain Symptom Manage* 2001; **21**(2): 95–102.
9. **van Manen JG, Bindels PJ, Dekker FW, CJ IJ, van der Zee JS, Schade E.** Risk of depression in patients with chronic obstructive pulmonary disease and its determinants. *Thorax* 2002; **57**(5): 412–16.

10. Jones P, Wilson R. Cognitive Aspects of Breathlessness. In: Adams L, Guz A, eds *Respiratory Sensation*, pp. 311–39. New York: Marcel Dekker, 1996.

11. Dodd M, Janson S, Facione N, Faucett L, Froelicher ES, Humphreys J, *et al.* Advancing the science of symptom management. *Journal of Advanced Nursing* 2001; **33**(5): 668–76.

12. van Wijk CM, Kolk AM. Sex differences in physical symptoms: the contribution of symptom perception theory. *Soc Sci Med* 1997; **45**(2): 231–46.

13. Meek PM. Influence of attention and judgement on on perception of breathlessness in healthy individuals and patients with chronic obstructive pulmonary disease. *Nursing Research* 2000; **49**(1): 11–19.

14. Janson-Bjerklie S, Ferketich S, Benner P, Becker G. Clinical markers of asthma severity and risk: importance of subjective as well as objective factors. *Heart and Lung* 1992; **21**(3): 265–72.

15. Tsang A. Effectiveness of three interventions to improve self-efficacy for managing dyspnea in patients with COPD. *American Journal of Respiratory and Critical Care Medicine* 2001; **163**(5): A968.

16. Gallo-Silver L, Pollack B. Behavioral interventions for lung cancer-related breathlessness. *Cancer Practice* 2000; **8**(6): 268–73.

17. Roberts DK, Thorne SE, Pearson C. The experience of dyspnea in late-stage cancer. Patients' and nurses' perspectives. *Cancer Nurs* 1993; **16**(4): 310–20.

18. Keefe FJ, Dunsmore J, Burnett R. Behavioral and cognitive-behavioral approaches to chronic pain: recent advances and future directions. *Journal of Consulting and Clinical Psychology* 1992; **60**(4): 528–36.

19. Janson BS, Ruma SS, Stulbarg M, Carrieri VK. Predictors of dyspnea intensity in asthma. *Nurs Res* 1987; **36**(3): 179–83.

20. Pennebaker JW. Psychological factors influencing the reporting of physical symptoms. In: Stone AA, Turkkan JS, Bachrach CA, Jobe JB, Kurtzman HS, Cain VS, eds *The Science of Self Report: Implications for Research and Practice*, pp. 299–316. Mahwah, NJ: Lawrence Erlbaum Associates, 2000.

21. Brown ML, Carrieri V, Janson B, Dodd MJ. Lung cancer and dyspnea: the patient's perception. *Oncology Nursing Forum* 1986; **13**(5): 19–24.

22. Price DD, Harkins SW. The affective-motivational dimension of pain: a two stage model. *American Pain Society Journal* 1992; **1**(4): 229–39.

23. Gracely R, McGrath P, Dubner R. Validity and sensitivity of ratio scales of sensory and affective verbal pain descriptors: manipulation of affect by diazepam. *Pain* 1978; **2**: 19–29.

24. Dudgeon DJ, Lertzman M, Askew GR. Physiological changes and clinical correlations of dyspnea in cancer outpatients. *J Pain Symptom Manage* 2001; **21**(5): 373–9.

25. Gift A, Plaut M, Jacox A. Psychologic and physiologic factors related to dyspnea in subjects with chornic obstructive pulmonary disease. *Heart and Lung* 1986; **15**: 595–601.

26. Carrieri-Kohlman V, Gormley JM, Douglas MK, Paul SM, Stulbarg MS. Differentiation between dyspnea and its affective components. *West J Nurs Res* 1996; **18**(6): 626–42.

27. Banzett RB, Mulnier HE, Murphy K, Rosen SD, Wise RJ, Adams L. Breathlessness in humans activates insular cortex. *Neuroreport* 2000; **11**(10): 2117–20.

28. Evans KC, Banzett RB, Adams L, McKay L, Frackowiak RS, Corfield DR. BOLD fMRI identifies limbic, paralimbic, and cerebellar activation during air hunger. *J Neurophysiol.* 2002 Sep; **88**(3):1500–11.

29. **Price DD.** The dimensions of pain experience. In: *Psychological Mechanisms of Pain and Analgesia. Progress in Pain Research and Management,* pp. 43–70. Seattle, WA: International Association for the Study of Pain; 1999.

30. **Gift AG, Moore T, Soeken K.** Relaxation to reduce dyspnea and anxiety in COPD patients. *Nurs Res* 1992; **41**(4): 242–6.

31. **Dudgeon DJ, Lertzman M.** Dyspnea in the advanced cancer patient. *Journal of Pain and Symptom Management* 1998; **16**(4): 212–19.

32. **Carrieri-Kohlman V, Gormley JM, Douglas MK, Paul SM, Stulbarg MS.** Exercise training decreases dyspnea and the distress and anxiety associated with it. Monitoring alone may be as effective as coaching. *Chest* 1996; **110**(6): 1526–35.

33. **Turk D, Meichenbaum D, Genest M.** *Pain and Behavioral Medicine: A Cognitive-Behavioral Perspective.* New York: Guilford Press, 1983.

34. **Bandura A.** *Social Foundations of Thought and Action. A Social Cognitive Theory.* Englewood Cliffs, NJ: Prentice Hall, 1986.

35. **Bandura A.** *Self Efficacy: The Exercise of Control.* New York: W.H. Freeman and Co., 1997.

36. **Bandura A.** Self-efficacy mechanism in human agency. *American Psychologist* 1982; **37**(2): 122–47.

37. **Bandura A, O'Leary A, Taylor C, Gaunthier J, Gossard D.** Perceived self-efficacy and pain control: opioid and non-opioid mechanisms. *J Person Soc Psychol* 1987; **35**: 563–71.

38. **Bandura A.** Self-efficacy for mechanism in physiological activation and health-promoting behavior. In: Madden IV J, Barchas J, eds *Neurobiology of Learning. Emotion and Affect.* New York: Raven Press, 1991.

39. **Von Korff M, Gruman J, Schaefer J, Curry SJ, Wagner EH.** Collaborative management of chronic illness. *Annals of Internal Medicine* 1997; **127**(12): 1097–102.

40. **American Thoracic Society.** Dyspnea. Mechanisms, assessment, and management: a consensus statement. American Thoracic Society. *American Journal of Respiratory and Critical Care Medicine* 1999; **159**(1): 321–40.

41. **Carrieri-Kohlman V.** Coping strategies for the breathless patient. *European Respiratory Review* 2002; **12**(86): 1–4.

42. **Carrieri VJ, Janson-Bjerklie S.** Strategies patients use to manage the sensation of dyspnea. *West J Nurs Res* 1986; **8**: 284–305.

43. **Janson S, Reed ML.** Patients' perceptions of asthma control and impact on attitudes and self-management. *J Asthma* 2000; **37**(7): 625–40.

44. **Fagerhaugh SY.** Getting around with emphysema. *American Journal of Nursing* 1973; **73**(1): 94–9.

45. **Carrieri-Kohlman V, Stulbarg MS.** Dyspnea: assessment and management. In: Hodgkin JE, Celli BR, Connors GL, eds *Pulmonary Rehabilitation,* 3rd edn. New York: Lippincott Wiliams and Wilkins; 2000, 57–90.

46. **Carrieri-Kohlman V, Stulbarg M. Dyspnea.** In: Carrieri-Kohlman V, Lindsey A, West C, eds *Pathophysiological Phenomena in Nursing: Human Responses to Illness,* pp. 175–208, 3rd edn. St. Louis, Missouri: Saunders, 2003.

47. **AACVPR.** *Guidelines for Pulmonary Rehabilitation Programs,* 2nd edn. Champaign, IL: Human Kinetics, 1998.

48. **Kawut SM, Mandel M, Arcasoy SM.** Two faces of progressive dyspnea. *Chest* 2000; **117**(5): 1500–4.

49. Gift AG, Cahill CA. Psychophysiologic aspects of dyspnea in chronic obstructive pulmonary disease: a pilot study. *Heart Lung* 1990; **19**(3): 252–7.
50. O'Donnell DE, McGuire M, Samis L, Webb KA. The impact of exercise reconditioning on breathlessness in severe chronic airflow limitation. *Am J Respir Crit Care Med* 1995; **152**(6PH), 2005–13.
51. Belman MJ, Botnick WC, Shin JW. Inhaled bronchdilators reduce dynamic hyperinflation during exercise in patients with chronic obstructive pulmonary disease. *American Journal of Respiratory Critical Care Medicine* 1996; **153**: 967–75.
52. O'Donnell DE, Revill SM, Webb KA. Dynamic hyperinflation and exercise intolerance in chronic obstructive pulmonary disease. *American Journal of Respiratory and Critical Care Medicine* 2001; **164**(5): 770–7.
53. Collins E, Fehr L, Bammert C, O'Connell S, Laghi F, Hanson K, *et al.* Effect of ventilation-feedback training on endurance and perceived breathlessness during constant work-rate leg-cycle exercise in patients with COPD. *Journal of Rehabilitation Research and Development* 2003; **40**(Suppl 2) (5): 35–44.
54. Sharma V. personal communication, 2004.
55. Hodgkin JE, Celli BR, Connors GL. *Pulmonary Rehabilitation*. New York: Lippincott Wiliams and Wilkins, 2000.
56. Thoman RL, Stoker GL, Ross JC. The efficacy of pursed-lips breathing in patients with chronic obstructive pulmonary disease. *Am Rev Respir Dis* 1966; **93**(1): 100–6.
57. Mueller RE, Petty TL, Filley GF. Ventilation and arterial blood gas changes induced by pursed lip breathing. *J Appl Physiol* 1970; **28**: 784–9.
58. Tiep BL, Burns M, Kao D, Madison R, Herrera J. Pursed lips breathing training using ear oximetry. *Chest* 1986; **90**(2): 218–21.
59. Breslin EH. The pattern of respiratory muscle recruitment during pursed-lip breathing. *Chest* 1992; **101**(1): 75–8.
60. Bianchi R, Gigliotti F, Romagnoli I, Lanini B, Castellani C, Grazzini M, *et al.* Chest wall kinematics and breathlessness during pursed-lip breathing in patients with COPD. *Chest* 2004; **125**(2): 459–65.
61. Sharp JT, Drutz WS, Moisan T, *et al.* Postural relief of dyspnea in severe chronic obstructive pulmonary disease. *Am Rev Respir Dis* 1980; **122**: 201–13.
62. Suls J, Fletcher B. The relative efficacy of avoidant and nonavoidant coping strategies: a meta-analysis. *Health Psychology* 1985; **4**(3): 249–88.
63. Gift AG. Psychologic and physiologic aspects of acute dyspnea in asthmatics. *Heart Lung* 1990; **19**(3): 252–7.
64. Carrieri-Kohlman V, Gormley J, Eiser S, Demir-Deviren S, Nguyen H, Paul S, *et al.* Dyspnea and the affective response during exercise training in obstructive pulmonary disease. *Nursing Research* 2001; **50**(3): 136–46.
65. Gosselink R. Controlled breathing and dyspnea in patients with chronic obstructive pulmonary disease (COPD). *Journal of Rehabilitation Research and Development* 2003; **40**(5, Suppl 2): 25–33
66. Renfroe KL. Effect of progressive relaxation on dyspnea and state anxiety in patients with chronic obstructive pulmonary disease. *Heart Lung* 1988; **17**(4): 408–13.
67. Horsman J. Using tape recordings to overcome panic during dyspnea. *Respir Care* 1978; **23**: 767–8.
68. Bauldoff GS, Hoffman LA, Zullo TG, Sciurba FC. Exercise maintenance following pulmonary rehabilitation: effect of distractive stimuli. *Chest* 2002; **122**(3): 948–54.

69. Brooks D, Sidani S, Graydon J, McBride S, Hall L, Weinacht K. Evaluating the effects of music on dyspnea during exercise in individuals with chronic obstructive pulmonary disease: a pilot study. *Rehabilitation Nursing* 2003; 28(6): 192–6.

70. Moody LE, Fraser M, Yarandi H. Effects of guided imagery in patients with chronic bronchitis and emphysema. *Clinical Nursing Research* 1993; 2(4): 478–86.

71. Jobst K, Chen J, McPherson K, Arrowsmith J, Brown V, Efthimiou J, *et al.* Controlled trial of acupuncture for disabling breathlessness. *Lancet* 1986; 2: 1416–19.

72. Filshie J, Penn K, Ashley S, Davis C. Acupuncture for the relief of cancer-related breathlessness. *Palliative Medicine* 1996; 10: 1447–52.

73. Maa SH, Gauthier D, Turner M. Acupressure as an adjunct to a pulmonary rehabilitation program. *J Cardiopulm Rehabil* 1997; 17(4): 268–76.

74. Maa SH, Sun M, Hsu KH, Hung TJ, Chen HC, Yu CT, *et al.* Effect of acupuncture or acupressure on quality of life of patients with chronic obstructive asthma: a pilot study. *The Journal of Alternative and Complementary Medicine* 2003; 9(5): 659–70.

75. Stux G, Pomeranz B. *Acupuncture: Textbook and Atlas*. New York: Springer-Verlag, 1987.

76. Wu HS, Wu SC, Lin JG, Lin LC. Effectiveness of acupressure in improving dyspnoea in chronic obstructive pulmonary disease. *J Adv Nurs* 2004; 45(3): 252–9.

77. Lareau SC, Meek PM, Roos PJ. Development and testing of the modified version of the pulmonary functional status and dyspnea questionnaire (PFSDQ-M). *Heart Lung* 1998; 27(3): 159–68.

78. Gustafson DH, Robinson TN, Ansley D, Adler L, Brennan PF. Consumers and evaluation of interactive health communication applications. The Science Panel on Interactive Communication and Health. *American Journal of Preventive Medicine* 1999; 16(1): 23–9.

79. Gustafson DH, Hawkins R, Pingree S, McTavish F, Arora NK, Mendenhall J, *et al.* Effect of computer support on younger women with breast cancer. *J Gen Intern Med* 2001; 16(7): 435–45.

80. Sitzman J, Kamiya J, Johnson J. Biofeedback training for reduced respiratory rate in chronic obstructive disease: A preliminary study. *Nurs Research* 1987; 32: 218–23.

81. Holliday JE, Hyers TM. The reduction of weaning time from mechanical ventilation using tidal volume and relaxation biofeedback. *American Review of Respiratory Disease* 1990; 141(5 Pt 1): 1214–20.

82. Giardino, ND, Chan L, & Borson, S. Combined heart rate variability and pulse oximetry biofeedback for chronic obstructive pulmonary disease: preliminary findings. *Appl Psychophysiol Biofeedback*. (2004) Jun; 29(2):121–33.

83. Acosta AF. Tolerance of chronic dyspnea using a hypnoeducational approach: a case report. *Am J Clin Hypn* 1991; 33(4): 272–7.

84. Aronoff GM, Aronoff S, Peck LW. Hypnotherapy in the treatment of bronchial asthma. *Annals of Allergy* 1975; 34(6): 356–62.

85. Anbar RD, Self-hypnosis for management of chronic dyspnea in pediatric patientss. *Pediatrics* 2001: 107(2): E21.

86. Courneya KS, Plotnikoff RC, Hotz SB, Birkett NJ. Social support and the theory of planned behavior in the exercise domain. *American Journal of Health Behavior* 2000; 24(4): 300–8.

87. Wilcox S, Castro C, King AC, Housemann R, Brownson RC. Determinants of leisure time physical activity in rural compared with urban older and ethnically diverse

women in the United States. *Journal of Epidemiology and Community Health* 2000; **54**(9): 667–72.

88. **Oka RK, King AC, Young DR.** Sources of social support as predictors of exercise adherence in women and men ages 50 to 65 years. *Womens Health* 19995; **1**(2): 161–75.

89. **Cohen S, Wills TA.** Stress, social support, and the buffering hypothesis. *Psychological Bulletin* 1985; **98**(2): 310–57.

90. **Duncan TE, Duncan SC, McAuley E.** The role of domain and gender-specific provisions of social relations in adherence to a prescribed exercise regimen. *Journal of Sport and Exercise Psychology* 1993; **15**(2): 220–31.

91. **Graydon JE, Ross E.** Influence of symptoms, lung function, mood, and social support on level of functioning of patients with COPD. *Research in Nursing and Health* 1995; **18**(6): 525–33.

92. **Lee RN, Graydon JE, Ross E.** Effects of psychological well-being, physical status, and social support on oxygen-dependent COPD patients' level of functioning. *Research in Nursing and Health* 1991; **14**(5): 323–8.

93. **Uchino BN, Cacioppo JT, Keicolt-Glaser JK.** The relationship between social support and physiological processes: A review with emphasis on underlying mechanisms and implications for health. *Psychological Bulletin* 1996; **119**(3): 488–531.

94. **Jacobson DE.** Types and timing of social support. *Journal of Health and Social Behavior* 1986; **27**: 250–64.

95. **Dudley DL, Glaser, Jorgenson BN, Logan DL.** Psychosocial concomitants to rehabilitation in chronic obstructive pulmonary disease. Part 1. Psychosocial and psychological considerations. *Chest* 1980; **77**: 413–20.

96. **DeVito AJ.** Dyspnea during hospitalizations for acute phase of illness as recalled by patients with chronic obstructive pulmonary disease. *Heart Lung* 1990; **19**(2): 186–91.

97. **Burkhardt CS.** Coping strategies of the chronically ill. *Nursing Clinics of North America* 1987; **22**: 543–50.

98. **Borkman TJ.** *Understanding Self-help/Mutual Aid.* Piscataway, New Jersey: Rutgers University Press, 1999.

99. **Spiegel D.** *Living Beyond Limits.* New York: Times Book, 1993.

100. **Ashikaga T, Vacek PM, Lewis SO.** Evaluation of a community-based education program for individuals with chronic obstructive pulmonary disease. *Journal of Rehabilitation* 1980; **46**(2): 23–7.

101. **O'Donnell DE, Lam M, Webb KA.** Measurement of symptoms, lung hyperinflation, and endurance during exercise in chronic obstructive pulmonary disease. *American Journal of Respiratory and Critical Care Medicine* 1998; **158**(5 Pt 1): 1557–65.

102. **Niederman MS, Clemente PH, Fein AM, Feinsilver SH, Robinson DA, Ilowite JS, *et al.*** Benefits of a multidisciplinary pulmonary rehabilitation program. Improvements are independent of lung function. *Chest* 1991; **99**(4): 798–804.

103. **Berry MJ, Rejeski WJ, Adair NE, Zaccaro D.** Exercise rehabilitation and chronic obstructive pulmonary disease stage. *American Journal of Respiratory and Critical Care Medicine* 1999; **160**(4): 1248–53.

104. **Maltais F, LeBlanc P, Jobin J, Berube C, Bruneau J, Carrier L, *et al.*** Intensity of training and physiologic adaptation in patients with chronic obstructive pulmonary disease. *American Journal of Respiratory and Critical Care Medicine* 1997; **155**(2): 555–61.

105. **Helson H.** *Adaptation-Level Theory: An Experimental and Systematic Approach to Behavior.* New York: Harper and Row, 1964.

106. **Hoogstaten J.** Influence of objective measures on self-reports in a retrospective pre-test post-test design. *Journal of Experimental Education* 1985; **53**: 207–10.

107. **Sprangers MAG, Schwartz CE.** Integrating response shift into health-related quality-of-life research: a theoretical model. *Social Science and Medicine* 1999; **48**: 1507–15.

108. **Gibbons FX.** Social comparison as a mediator of response shift. *Social Science and Medicine* 1999; **48**: 1517–30.

109. **Haas F, Salazar-Schicchi J, Axen K.** Desensitization to dyspnea in chronic obstructive pulmonary disease. In: Casaburi R, Petty T, eds *Principles and Practice of Pulmonary Rehabilitation,* pp. 241–51. Philadelphia: W B Saunders, 1993.

110. **Carrieri-Kohlman V, Douglas MK, Gormley JM, Stulbarg MS.** Desensitization and guided mastery: treatment approaches for the management of dyspnea. *Heart Lung* 1993; **22**(3): 226–34.

111. **Normandin EA, McCusker C, Connors M, Vale F, Gerardi D, ZuWallack RL.** An evaluation of two approaches to exercise conditioning in pulmonary rehabilitation. *Chest* 2002; **121**(4): 1085–91.

112. **Levine S, Weiser P, Gillen J.** Evaluation of a ventilatory muscle endurance training program in the rehabilitation of patients with chronic obstructive pulmonary disease. *Am Rev Respir Dis* 1986; **133**: 400–6.

113. **Stulbarg MS, Carrieri-Kohlman V, Demir-Deviren S, Nguyen HQ, Adams L, Tsang AH, *et al.*** Exercise training improves outcomes of a dyspnea self-management program. *J Cardiopulm Rehabil* 2002; **22**(2): 109–21.

114. **Ramirez-Venegas A, Ward JL, Olmstead EM, Tosteson AN, Mahler DA.** Effect of exercise training on dyspnea measures in patients with chronic obstructive pulmonary disease. *J Cardpulm Rehabil* 1997; **17**(2): 103–9.

115. **Belman MJ, Brooks LR, Ross DJ, Mohsenifar Z.** Variability of breathlessness measurement in patients with chronic obstructive pulmonary disease. *Chest* 1991; **99**(3): 566–71.

116. **Williams SL.** Guided mastery treatment of agoraphobia: Beyond stimulus exposure. *Prog Behav Modif* 1990; **26**: 89–121.

117. **Tandon MK.** Adjunct treatment with yoga in chronic severe airways obstruction. *Thorax* 1978; **33**(4): 514–17.

118. **Behera D.** Yoga therapy in chronic bronchitis. *Journal of the Association of Physicians of India* 1998; **46**(2): 207–8.

119. **Watson P, Town G, Holbrook N, Dwan C, Toop L, Drennan C.** Evaluation of a self-management plan for chronic obstructive pulmonary disease. *Eur Resp J* 1997; **10**: 1267–71.

120. **Gallefoss F, Bakke PS.** Impact of patient education and self-management on morbidity in asthmatics and patients with chronic obstructive pulmonary disease. *Respir Med* 2000; **94**(3): 279–87.

121. **Gallefoss F, Bakke PS.** Cost-benefit and cost-effectiveness analysis of self-management in patients with COPD–a 1-year follow-up randomized, controlled trial. *Respir Med* 2002; **96**(6): 424–31.

122. National Heart, Lung and Blood Institute. National Asthma Education and Prevention Program. Expert Panel Report II: Guidelines for the Diagnosis and Management of Asthma. National Institutes of Health Publication No. 97–4051. Bethesda, MD. 1997

123. Gibson P, Powell H, Couglan J, Wilson A, Abramson M, Haywood P, *et al.* Self-management education and regular practitioner review for adults with asthma (Cochrane Review). In: *The Cochrane Library.* Oxford: Update Software; 2003.

124. Lahdensuo A, Haahtela T, Herrala J, Kava T, Kiviranta K, Kuusisto P, *et al.* Randomised comparison of guided self management and traditional treatment of asthma over one year. *BMJ* 1996; 312(7033): 748–52.

125. Allen RM, Jones MP, Oldenburg B. Randomised trial of an asthma self-management programme for adults. *Thorax* 1995; 50(7): 731–8.

126. Wilson SR, Starr-Schneidkraut N. State of the art in asthma education: the US experience. *Chest* 1994; 106(4 Suppl): 197S–205S.

127. Howland J, Nelson EC, Barlow PB, McHugo G, Meier FA, Brent P, *et al.* Chronic obstructive airway disease. Impact of health education. *Chest* 1986; 90(2): 233–8.

128. Sassi-Dambron DE, Eakin EG, Ries AL, Kaplan RM. Treatment of dyspnea in COPD. A controlled clinical trial of dyspnea management strategies [see comments]. *Chest* 1995; 107(3): 724–9.

129. Zimmerman BW, Brown ST, Bowman JM, Garcia-Rio F, Pino JM, Gomez L, *et al.* A self-management program for chronic obstructive pulmonary disease: relationship to dyspnea and self-efficacy. *Rehabil Nurs* 1996; 21(5): 253–7.

130. Lorig KR, Sobel DS, Stewart AL, Brown BW, Jr., Bandura A, Ritter P, *et al.* Evidence suggesting that a chronic disease self-management program can improve health status while reducing hospitalization: a randomized trial. *Medical Care* 1999; 37(1): 5–14.

131. Bourbeau J, Julien M, Maltais F, Rouleau M, Beaupre A, Begin R, *et al.* Reduction of hospital utilization in patients with chronic obstructive pulmonary disease: a disease-specific self-management intervention. *Arch Intern Med* 2003; 163(5): 585–91.

132. Monninkhof E, van der Valk P, van der Palen J, van Herwaarden C, Zielhuis G. Effects of a comprehensive self-management programme in patients with chronic obstructive pulmonary disease. *Eur Respir J* 2003; 22(5): 815–20.

133. Gravil J, Al-Rawas O, Cotton MM, Irwin A, Stevenson R. Home treatment of exacerbations of chronic obstructive pulmonary disease by an acute respiratory assessment service. *Lancet* 1998; 351: 1853–5.

134. Corner J, Plant H, A'Hern R, Bailey C. Non-pharmacological intervention for breathlessness in lung cancer. *Palliat Med* 1996; 10(4): 299–305.

135. Bredin M, Corner J, Krishnasamy M, Plant H, Bailey C, A'Hern R. Multicentre randomised controlled trial of nursing intervention for breathlessness in patients with lung cancer. *BMJ* 1999; 318: 901–4.

136. Schwartzstein RM, Lahive K, Pope A, Weinberger SE, Weiss JW. Cold facial stimulation reduces breathlessness induced in normal subjects. *Am Rev Respir Dis* 1987; 136(1): 58–61.

137. Hansen-Flaschen J. Advanced lung disease: palliation and terminal care. *Clnics in Chest Medicine* 1997; 18(3): 645–55.

138. Hyland ME, Singh SJ, Sodergren SC, Morgan MP. Development of a shortened version of the Breathing Problems Questionnaire for use in a pulmonary rehabilitation clinic: a purpose-specific, disease specific questionnaire. *Qual Life Res* 1998; 7(3): 227–233.

139. Jones PW, Quirk FH, Baveystock CM, Littlejohns P. A self-complete measure of health status for chronic airflow limitation. The St. George's Respiratory Questionnaire. *American Review of Respiratory Disease* 1992; 145(6): 1321–7.

140. Guyatt GH, Berman LB, Townsend M, Pugsley SO, Chambers LW. A measure of quality of life for clinical trials in chronic lung disease. *Thorax* 1987; 42(10): 773–8.

141. **Eakin EG, Resnikoff PM, Prewitt LM, Ries AL, Kaplan RM.** Validation of a new dyspnea measure: the UCSD Shortness of Breath Questionnaire. University of California, San Diego. *Chest* 1998; 113(3): 619–24.
142. **Desbiens NA, Mueller RN, Connors AF, Wenger NS.** The relationship of nausea and dyspnea to pain in seriously ill patients. *Pain* 1997; 71(2): 149–56.
143. **Stone P, Richards M, A'Hern R, Hardy J.** A study to investigate the prevalence, severity and correlates of fatigue among patients with cancer in comparison with a control group of volunteers without cancer. *Ann Oncol* 2000; 11(5): 561–7.
144. **Smith EL, Hann DM, Ahles TA, Furstenberg CT, Mitchell TA, Meyer L, Maurer LH, Rigas J, Hammond S.** (2001) Dyspnea, anxiety, body consciousness, and quality of life in patients with lung cancer. *J Pain Symptom Manage.* Apr; 21 (4):323–9.
145. **Heinzer MM, Bish C, Detwiler R.** Acute dyspnea as perceived by patients with chronic obstructive pulmonary disease. *Clin Nurs Res* 2003; 12(1): 85–101.
146. **Lush MT, Janson BS, Carrieri VK, Lovejoy N.** Dyspnea in the ventilator-assisted patient. *Heart Lung* 1988; 17(5): 528–35.
147. **Connelly B, Gunzerath, L., Knebel, A.** A pilot study exploring mood state and dyspnea in mechanically ventilated patients. *Heart Lung* 2000; 29: 173–9.
148. **Knebel AR, Janson-Bjerklie SL, Malley JD, Wilson AG, Marini JJ.** Comparison of breathing comfort during weaning with two ventilatory modes. *Am J Respir Crit Care Med* 1994; 149(1): 14–18.
149. **Carrieri KV.** Dyspnea in the weaning patient: assessment and intervention. *AACN Clin Issues Crit Care Nurs* 1991; 2(3): 462–73.
150. **Rabow MW, Dibble SL, Pantilat SZ, McPhee SJ.** The comprehensive care team: a controlled trial of outpatient palliative medicine consultation. *Arch Intern Med* 2004; 164(1): 83–91.
151. **Steinhauser KE, Christakis NA, Clipp EC, McNeilly M, McIntyre L, Tulsky JA.** Factors considered important at the end of life by patients, family, physicians, and other care providers. *JAMA* 2000; 284(19): 2476–82.
152. **Patrick DL, Engelberg RA, & Curtis R.** (2001) Evaluating the Quality of Dying and Death. *J Pain and Symptom Manage.* 22:717–726
153. **Lynn J, Teno JM, Phillips RS, Wu AW, Desbiens N, Harrold J, et al.** Perceptions by family members of the dying experience of older and seriously ill patients. SUPPORT Investigators. Study to Understand Prognoses and Preferences for Outcomes and Risks of Treatments. *Ann Intern Med* 1997; 126(2): 97–106.

12

Oxygen in the palliation of breathlessness

Anna Spathis, Rosemary Wade
and Sara Booth

Introduction

Supplemental oxygen is commonly used for the palliation of breathlessness in advanced disease. It is by far the most frequently prescribed therapy for cancer patients with dyspnoea in the hospital setting.[1] Since a primary function of ventilation is transfer of oxygen from the environment to the blood, it is easy for healthcare professionals to assume that increasing the inspired oxygen concentration should inevitably lower the demand for ventilation, and therefore reduce dyspnoea. The widespread use of oxygen is, in part, a consequence of this intuitive assumption. In addition, patients anecdotally have high expectations of oxygen therapy, and often request it.[2]

Oxygen, however, is not a universal panacea for all breathless patients. Many patients do not experience relief with supplemental oxygen. Indeed, even some hypoxaemic patients will not experience palliation of dyspnoea, despite reversal of objective arterial hypoxaemia with oxygen. Equally surprisingly, some normoxic individuals do gain benefit from oxygen. Why does palliation of dyspnoea with oxygen not simply relate to correction of blood gas abnormalities?

Like any other pharmacological intervention, supplemental oxygen can have adverse effects. Furthermore, domiciliary oxygen is expensive to supply. Given that oxygen does not palliate breathlessness in all patients, it is clearly important to select patients for oxygen therapy carefully. As hypoxaemia does not predict benefit, how can appropriate patients be selected?

This chapter aims both to answer these questions by considering the mechanisms of action of oxygen, reviewing available research evidence, and describing methods to assess the effects of oxygen on individual patients. Negative aspects of oxygen therapy are then addressed. The chapter ends with a discussion of practical issues, such as the supply of oxygen, followed by pragmatic clinical guidelines.

Only the use of oxygen in chronic, stable disease will be considered. Oxygen is, of course, widely used in acute cardiopulmonary disease such as asthma and pneumonia, and in acute exacerbations of chronic disease such as heart failure. In the acute context, the primary aim of supplemental oxygen is usually to reverse acute hypoxaemia while the underlying disease is being treated. In chronic, stable disease, however, the underlying pathophysiology may not be reversible. Effective palliation of symptoms such as breathlessness then becomes of vital importance, in order to improve patients' quality of life.

Finally, it must be emphasized that oxygen therapy is only one of many approaches in the management of dyspnoea. As discussed in other chapters, many other strategies have important roles in the successful palliation of breathlessness. These include treatment of correctable underlying causes, judicious use of pharmacological agents such as opioids or benzodiazepines, and help with the psychological and social dimensions of breathlessness experienced by patients and their families.

Mechanism of action

How does oxygen reduce the sensation of breathlessness? Several mechanisms have been proposed which mostly relate to the underlying pathophysiological processes that lead to breathlessness itself. The pathophysiology of breathlessness has been described in detail in Chapter 1, and in relation to individual chronic diseases in Chapters 3–6. It is briefly summarized here, in order to provide a basis for the subsequent discussion of the mechanism of action of oxygen.

Pathophysiology of breathlessness

Dyspnoea is a complex symptom consisting of several qualitatively distinct sensations reflecting a variety of pathophysiological mechanisms.[3] Broadly speaking, dyspnoea occurs when the demand for ventilation is out of proportion to the patient's ability to respond to that demand.[4] The 'neuromechanical dissociation theory' suggests that dyspnoea is a consequence of mismatch between central respiratory motor activity (demand for ventilation), and incoming afferent information from receptors in the airways, lungs and chest wall structures (feedback on actual ventilation).[5] Dyspnoea can therefore be a consequence either of increased ventilatory demand, or impairment of the mechanical process of ventilation.

Most of the factors that increase ventilatory demand alter arterial blood gases or pH. Examples include:

◆ Hypoxaemia.
◆ Carbon dioxide (CO_2) retention e.g. due to increased physiologic dead space.

- Metabolic acidosis, such as lactic acidaemia.
- Deconditioning, causing increased oxygen consumption and CO_2 production.

Impairment of ventilation is generally caused by abnormal mechanics of the lung or chest wall. Examples include:

- Weakness of diaphragm and other respiratory muscles.
- Restrictive diseases of lung parenchyma, pleura and chest wall.
- Obstructive lung diseases.

It is important to remember that dyspnoea is a subjective sensation that is greatly influenced by higher cortical experience. Cognitive, emotional and behavioural factors all contribute to influence the central perception of dyspnoea.

Mechanisms of action of oxygen

Supplemental oxygen acts to reduce breathlessness by modifying several of the causes of breathlessness described above. Dyspnoea can be reduced by any action of oxygen that reduces ventilatory demand, improves the mechanical process of ventilation, or alters the central perception of dyspnoea. Some mechanisms of action are well established; others are unproven. The relative importance of each mechanism has not been well established.

Mechanisms that reduce ventilatory demand

Reversal of hypoxaemia Hypoxaemia is a potent stimulus of respiratory drive. A fall in the arterial partial pressure of oxygen (PO_2) is sensed by peripheral chemoreceptors in the carotid and aortic bodies. Signals from these chemoreceptors are transmitted to brainstem respiratory centres, increasing central respiratory motor activity (ventilatory demand). Supplemental oxygen increases PO_2 and prevents this process from occurring. This is postulated to be the primary mechanism by which oxygen reduces dyspnoea.[6]

It is worth noting that some investigators have found that the reversal of hypoxaemia with oxygen produces a relief in dyspnoea that is out of proportion to, or occurs earlier than the reduction in ventilation.[7,8,9,10] They have therefore proposed that hypoxia may have a direct 'dyspnogenic' effect, where stimulae from chemoreceptors act directly on the brainstem respiratory complex to cause a sensation of breathlessness that is independent of the increase in respiratory motor activity. Other researchers, who find good correlation between breathlessness and ventilation, refute this proposal.[6,11] Overall, it is unclear whether or not hypoxia has a separate, direct 'dyspnogenic' effect.

Reduced blood lactate levels This mechanism is important in exercise-induced dyspnoea. Lactic acid increases ventilatory demand, in an attempt to compensate for the metabolic acidosis. There is evidence that patients with chronic lung disease have impaired oxidative capacity of skeletal muscle, and generate significant lactic acidaemia compared with normals early in exercise.[12] Supplemental oxygen reduces anaerobic metabolism in peripheral muscles and therefore lowers lactic acid levels.[11]

Increased exercise training Many patients with chronic disease are significantly deconditioned. Exercise training lowers ventilatory demand and reduces dyspnoea by normalizing blood gases and pH. It improves the aerobic capacity of muscles (reducing lactic acidosis) and increases muscle efficiency (reducing oxygen consumption and CO_2 production). It is known that the physiological effects of training are greater in those patients who are able to train harder.[13] As, in many patients, ambulatory oxygen increases exercise capacity, oxygen should indirectly improve dyspnoea by allowing better exercise training. The evidence to support this assertion is conflicting.[14,15] Overall, endurance exercise training with oxygen appears to reduce dyspnoea only slightly. The limitation may be that anaerobic metabolism and lactic acid production appear to enhance the training effects on muscle. This may reduce some of the benefit otherwise received from training with oxygen.[13]

Reduced pulmonary artery pressure Oxygen is known to reduce pulmonary vascular resistance by reversing hypoxic pulmonary vasoconstriction. There is also evidence that supplemental oxygen delays and reduces exercise-induced increases in pulmonary artery pressure.[9] It has been hypothesised that a reduction in pulmonary arterial pressure may decrease afferent input to brainstem respiratory centres and may therefore reduce dyspnoea.[16]

Mechanisms that improve ventilation

Reduced dynamic hyperinflation Patients with chronic obstructive pulmonary disease (COPD) can develop dynamic hyperinflation (DH). During expiration in COPD, airways close prematurely at an abnormally high lung volume, which increases the residual volume (RV). The resulting resting hyperinflation exerts a restrictive mechanical disadvantage on respiratory muscles, and leads to a greater reliance on tachypnoea to increase ventilation. Tachypnoea further worsens hyperinflation by reducing the time for expiration. This increases the work of breathing, particularly during exercise, and leads to the sensation of dyspnoea. Oxygen delays the onset, and reduces the severity of DH during exercise.[17,18] It has been postulated that this occurs because oxygen reduces ventilation and lengthens expiratory time, and it may also have a bronchodilator effect which increases lung emptying (see below).[17]

Reduced ventilatory muscle and diaphragm fatigue There is evidence in patients with heart failure that respiratory muscle deoxygenation occurs during exercise.[19] Bye *et al.* have shown that some of the improvement in exercise capacity when exercising with oxygen is due to reduced respiratory muscle and diaphragm fatigue.[20] Although this study did not specifically measure dyspnoea, it is likely that oxygen can reduce breathlessness through the same mechanism.

Relief of bronchoconstriction Breathing supplemental oxygen has been shown to reduce hypoxia related bronchoconstriction and decrease pulmonary impedance.[21,22] This could be a mechanism by which it reduces breathlessness.

Mechanisms that alter the central perception of dyspnoea

Stimulation of facial, nasal or pharyngeal receptors There is evidence that the flow of cool air through the nose[23], mouth[24] or over the cheek[25] can reduce the perception of dyspnoea. This is not related to any fall in ventilation. Cool air is believed to stimulate nasal or pharyngeal mucosal receptors, or facial receptors in the region of the trigeminal nerve; afferent information is then projected to the sensory cortex, where it alters the perception of dyspnoea. It has been hypothesized that oxygen can reduce dyspnoea by this mechanism, simply by being a flow of cool gas. Evidence from Booth *et al.* appears to support this hypothesis; both cylinder oxygen and cylinder air were found to improve breathlessness, without there being a statistically significant difference between them.[26] If this indirect mechanism of action of oxygen does occur, it is probably not one of the more important ones, as several studies have found that cylinder oxygen is more effective at palliating dyspnoea than both cylinder air and room air.[27,28,29]

Exercise training In addition to reducing ventilatory demand as described above, exercise training is believed to alter the central perception of breathing discomfort. Exposure to greater than usual sensations of dyspnoea in a safe environment appears to lead to desensitization and a greater ability to cope with the symptom.[30] Oxygen may indirectly reduce dyspnoea by increasing the capacity to exercise train.

Placebo effect There is some evidence from clinical trials using cylinder air, that oxygen may have a placebo effect.[31] There is a widely held view that oxygen can help breathing; if a patient believes they are receiving oxygen, this in itself may reduce the severity of dyspnoea, by altering central processing.

Finally, knowledge of the mechanisms of action of oxygen can explain why, as mentioned in the introduction to this chapter, palliation of dyspnoea does not simply relate to correction of blood gas abnormalities. It is possible for normoxic patients to benefit from oxygen, and for hypoxaemic patients to fail to gain symptom relief. The existence of many other mechanisms of action of oxygen, in addition to reversal of hypoxaemia, explains relief of breathlessness in normoxic patients. For example, breathlessness in a normoxic patient may be due to dynamic hyperinflation, which can be improved by oxygen therapy. Although oxygen modulates many of the mechanisms of breathlessness, it does not influence them all. Breathlessness in any one patient is often multi-factorial. A patient may be hypoxaemic, but his breathlessness may be predominantly due to another cause not amenable to oxygen therapy, such as an increased physiological dead space. Although hypoxaemic, such a patient may therefore not benefit from oxygen.

Key points

◆ Supplemental oxygen has many mechanisms of action by which it can reduce dyspnoea.
◆ The primary mechanism is believed to be reversal of hypoxaemia, which reduces ventilation by depressing peripheral chemoreceptor mediated hypoxic drive.
◆ Other important mechanisms, particularly for exercise-induced dyspnoea, are a decrease in dynamic hyperinflation in COPD and a reduction of lactic acidaemia.
◆ An understanding of the mechanisms of action of oxygen helps explain why palliation of breathlessness with oxygen therapy does not necessarily relate to reversal of hypoxaemia.

Evidence for efficacy

The evidence base to support the use of supplemental oxygen in the palliation of dyspnoea is, at best, patchy. Most research has been done in patients with COPD and there is a small amount of evidence in cancer patients. There is, however, almost no research in patients with heart failure, interstitial lung disease, cystic fibrosis and other chronic diseases.

The interpretation of available evidence is hindered by the small numbers of trial participants, the short duration of oxygen supply during studies, and the considerable inter-study heterogeneity. Disease severity, degree of hypoxia, inspired oxygen tensions, nature and duration of exercise, oxygen delivery systems and study outcome measures all vary widely. Controlled studies with large patient numbers are being planned, but a degree of heterogeneity is hard to avoid.

Despite these issues, some conclusions can be drawn from the existing evidence, both in terms of the efficacy of oxygen in relieving dyspnoea, and to a lesser extent, criteria that can help guide patient selection.[32] The literature is reviewed according to both the underlying disease and the type of oxygen used. Only controlled studies are considered. The following definitions of oxygen therapy are relevant[33]:

- Short-burst oxygen therapy (SBOT) is the intermittent use of oxygen for relief of breathlessness at rest, before exercise or during recovery from exercise.
- Ambulatory oxygen refers to the delivery of oxygen during exercise or the activities of daily living.
- Long-term oxygen therapy (LTOT) is the provision of oxygen therapy at home on a continuous and long term basis, ideally for at least 15 hours daily, including time spent asleep.

Patients with COPD

Short-burst oxygen therapy

There have been five controlled studies in patients with COPD at rest, and eight controlled studies where oxygen was used before or after exercise (Table 12.1). All incorporate a crossover design.

At rest, only one study out of the five showed relief of breathlessness with oxygen.[35] This trial studied twelve significantly hypoxaemic inpatients who were 'severely disabled by respiratory distress' and had 'claimed subjective benefit of supplemental oxygen on the ward'. This may have influenced the results. All other controlled studies have shown no statistically significant benefit from oxygen.

Amongst studies using supplemental oxygen before or after exercise, three of the eight studies showed possible benefit with oxygen. Woodcock et al. showed that oxygen for 5 and 15 minutes before exercise reduced dyspnoea scores during an incremental treadmill test, but not after a 6 minute walk.[36] Evans et al. found a small but statistically significant reduction in recovery time when patients were given oxygen after exercise, but when retested under identical conditions the results of individual patients were not reproducible. They concluded that the number of patients with reproducible substantial benefit is likely to be very small.[27] Finally Killen and Corris reported a pragmatic

Table 12.1 Summary of studies using short-burst oxygen therapy in patients with COPD

Study first author	Design (number of patients)	Mean oxygenation on air at rest (exercise)	Intervention	Comparison	Effect of oxygen (outcome measure)
Liss (23)	SBRCT (8)	PaO$_2$ 7.05kPa	At rest, oxygen 2 l/min, 4 l/min for 5 min via nasal cannulae	At rest, CA zero flow, 2 l/min, or 4 l/min for 5 min via nasal cannulae	No reduction in SOB (VAS)
Kollef (34)	SBRCT (9)	PaO$_2$ 6.65kPa	At rest, oxygen 2 l/min, 4 l/min for 3–5 min via transtracheal catheter	At rest, CA zero flow, 2 l/min, or 4 l/min for 3–5 min via transtracheal catheter	No reduction in SOB (VAS)
Swinburn (35)	DBRCT (12)	PaO$_2$ 6.69kPa SaO$_2$ 86%	At rest, 28% oxygen for 10 min via mask	At rest, CA (same flow rate) for 10 min via mask	Reduction in SOB (VAS)
Booth (26)	SBRCT (13)	SaO$_2$ 80–99%	At rest, oxygen 4 l/min for 15 min via nasal cannula	At rest, CA 4 l/min for 15 min via nasal cannula	No reduction in SOB (VAS + Borg)
O'Donnell (17)	DBRCT (11)	PaO$_2$ 6.70kPa	At rest, 60% oxygen for 10 min via mouthpiece	At rest, RA for 10 min via mouthpiece	No reduction in SOB (Borg)
Woodcock (36)	DBRCT (10)	PaO$_2$ 9.65kPa (8.19kPa)	Before exercise, oxygen 4 l/min for 1, 5, 15 min via nasal cannula	Before exercise, CA 4 l/min for 1, 5, 15 min via nasal cannula	Reduction in SOB 5, 15 min oxygen (VAS)
Evans (27)	SBRCT (19)	PaO$_2$ 8.05kPa	After exercise, 67% oxygen during recovery via mask	After exercise, CA (same flow rate) or RA, during recovery via mask	Quicker recovery with oxygen (VAS)

Study	Trial (n)	Baseline	Intervention	Comparator	Outcome
McKeon (37)	DBRCT (20)	PaO_2 7.71kPa SaO_2 91% (83%)	Before exercise, oxygen 2.5 l/min for 10 min via nasal cannulae	Before exercise, CA 2.5 l/min for 10 min via nasal cannulae	No reduction in SOB (VAS)
Marques-Magallanes (38)	SBRCT (18)	PaO_2 6.8kPa	After exercise, 40% oxygen for 20 min via mask	After exercise, CA (same flow rate) or RA via mask	No reduction in SOB (VAS)
Killen (39)	SBRCT (18)	SaO_2 94% (86%)	Before + after exercise, oxygen 2 l/min for 5 min via mask	Before + after exercise, CA 2 l/min for 5 mins via mask	Reduction in SOB (VAS)
Nandi (40)	DBRCT (34 pre, 18 post)	PaO_2 7.7kPa SaO_2 92% (82%)	Before + after exercise, 28% oxygen for 10 min (before), 5 min (after) via mask	Before + after exercise, CA (same flow rate) for 10, 5 min via mask	No reduction in SOB (VAS)
Lewis (41)	SBRCT (22)	SaO_2 94% (83%)	Before + after exercise, oxygen 2 l/min for 5 min before/recovery via nasal cannulae	Before + after exercise, CA 2 l/min for 5 min before/recovery via nasal cannulae	No reduction in SOB (Borg)
Stevenson (42)	SBRCT (18)	SaO_2 96% (88–96%)	After exercise, 40% oxygen during recovery via mouthpiece or mask	After exercise, RA via mouthpiece, or CA (same flow rate) via mask during recovery	No reduction in SOB (Borg)

DB = double-blind; SB = single-blind; RCT = randomized controlled trial; PaO_2 = arterial partial pressure of oxygen; SaO_2 = oxygen saturation; CA = cylinder air; RA = room air; SOB = breathlessness.

study where either air or oxygen was given before and then after climbing stairs.[39] Three combinations were provided of 'air then air', 'air then oxygen' or 'oxygen then air'. There was no statistical difference in dyspnoea scores between these three groups, although a statistically significant improvement was seen when the 'air then oxygen' and the 'oxygen then air' subgroups were combined. Other than these three borderline positive results, all other studies report no benefit with SBOT before or after exercise.

No studies have been able to identify any factors that can predict which patients are most likely to benefit from SBOT.

Ambulatory oxygen

Nineteen controlled studies have examined the role of oxygen therapy during exercise, using severity of dyspnoea as an outcome measure (Table 12.2). Again, all incorporate a cross-over design.

Oxygen is known to significantly improve exercise capacity by 30–50 per cent (by increasing the endurance of submaximal exercise rather than by increasing the maximum workload achievable).[52] Assessment of the effect of oxygen on breathlessness is made more complicated by this effect on exercise capacity; oxygen allows patients to exercise harder, which in itself increases dyspnoea. Some studies correct for this. For example, in trials where patients on oxygen can exercise for a longer time than on air, dyspnoea scores can be compared at an equivalent time to the control ('isotime'), rather than at the end of exercise. Alternatively breathlessness scores can be compared at an equivalent work rate.

Out of the nineteen studies, fourteen revealed significant relief of dyspnoea when exercising with oxygen. Four studies appeared to show no improvement in dyspnoea score; however, all four studies demonstrated improved exercise capacity, but did not document breathlessness severity at 'isotime'.[6,45–47] Only one study showed no benefit at all, in terms of either exercise capacity or dypnoea score.[48]

Again, no studies have been able to find factors that can predict which patients are likely to experience symptom relief from supplemental oxygen. Response to oxygen does not correlate with the extent of dyspnoea at rest, level of hypoxaemia at rest, degree of desaturation on exercise, or any tests of lung function. The response to oxygen is extremely variable between individuals, although more reproducible on an individual level.[29] One study did find that most patients achieving an increase in exercise tolerance of more than 50 per cent were hypoxaemic at rest, or showed significant exercise desaturation. However, it cannot be inferred that these will be the same patients who benefit in terms of improved dyspnoea.

Table 12.2 Summary of studies using ambulatory oxygen in patients with COPD

Study first author	Design (number of patients)	Mean oxygenation on air at rest (exercise)	Intervention	Comparison	Effect of oxygen (outcome measure)
Woodcock (36)	DBRCT (10)	PaO_2 9.65kPa (8.19 kPa)	Portable oxygen 4 l/min via nasal cannulae	CA 4 l/min via nasal cannulae	Reduction in SOB (VAS)
Waterhouse (29)	SBRCT (20)	PaO_2 (8.9kPa)	Portable oxygen 2 l/min, 4 l/min via nasal cannulae	CA 3 l/min via nasal cannulae or RA	Reduction in SOB (VAS)
Swinburn (6)	DBRCT (5)	SaO_2 93% (86%)	60% oxygen via mouthpiece	RA via mouthpiece	No reduction in SOB at maximal work rate (VAS)
Lane (7)	SBCT (9)	PaO_2 8.9kPa	Oxygen at flow rate to just maintain resting SaO_2 via mouthpiece	RA via mouthpiece	Reduction in SOB (VAS)
Davidson (43)	DBRCT (17)	PaO_2 8.6kPa SaO_2 94% (88%)	Oxygen via mouthpiece 0, 2, 4, 6 l/min, and portable oxygen 4 l/min via mask or nasal cannulae	CA via mouthpiece 0, 2, 4, 6 l/min, and portable CA 4 l/min via mask or nasal cannula	Reduction in SOB, dose-response relationship (VAS)
McKeon (28)	DBRCT (21)	PaO_2 8.8kPa SaO_2 92% (83%)	Portable oxygen 4 l/min via nasal cannula	CA 4 l/min via nasal cannulae or RA	Reduction in SOB (VAS)
Leach (44)	SBRCT (20)	PaO_2 8.7kPa (7.8kPa)	Portable oxygen 2, 4, 6 l/min via mask	CA 4 l/min via mask	Reduction in SOB (VAS)
Dean (9)	DBRCT (12)	PaO_2 9.4kPa (8.4kPa)	40% oxygen via mouthpiece	CA via mouthpiece	Reduction in SOB at 'isotime' (Borg)
McDonald (45)	DBRCT (26)	PaO_2 9.2kPa SaO_2 94%	Portable oxygen 4 l/min via nasal cannula	CA 4 l/min via nasal cannulae	No reduction in SOB at end exercise (Borg)

(continued)

Table 12.2 (continued) Summary of studies using ambulatory oxygen in patients with COPD

Study first author	Design (number of patients)	Mean oxygenation on air at rest (exercise)	Intervention	Comparison	Effect of oxygen (outcome measure)
Roberts (46)	Unblinded RCT (15)	PaO_2 7.0kPa	Portable oxygen 2 l/min (continuous or demand delivery system)	RA	No reduction in SOB at end exercise (VAS)
O'Donnell (11)	DBRCT (11)	PaO_2 9.8kPa	60% oxygen via mouthpiece	RA via mouthpiece	Reduction in SOB at 'isotime' (Borg)
Garrod (14)	SBRCT (25)	PaO_2 8.5kPa SaO_2 92% (82%)	Portable oxygen 4 l/min via nasal cannulae	CA 4 l/min via nasal cannulae	Reduction in SOB (Borg)
Revill (47)	SBRCT (10)	SaO_2 91% (82%)	Portable oxygen 2 l/min via nasal cannulae	RA via nasal cannulae	No reduction in SOB at end exercise (Borg)
Knebel (48)	DBRCT (31)	SaO_2 97% (92%)	Portable oxygen 4 l/min via nasal cannulae	CA 4 l/min via nasal cannulae	No reduction in SOB (VAS)
Somfay (18)	SBRCT (10)	SaO_2 96% (92%)	30%, 50%, 75%, 100% oxygen via mouthpiece	CA via mouthpiece	Reduction in SOB, dose-response relationship (Borg)
Jolly (49)	DBRCT (20)	PaO_2 >7.8kPa	Oxygen at 3, 6, 9, 12 l/min (according to SaO_2) via nasal cannulae	CA at 3, 6, 9, 12 l/min (according to SaO_2) via nasal cannulae	Reduction in SOB (Borg)
Maltais (50)	DBRCT (14)	PaO_2 11.3kPa (9.3kPa)	75% oxygen via mouthpiece	RA via mouthpiece	Reduction in SOB (Borg)
O'Donnell (17)	DBRCT (11)	PaO_2 6.70kPa	60% oxygen via mouthpiece	RA via mouthpiece	Reduction in SOB at 'isotime' (Borg)
Eaton (51)	DBRCT (50)	PaO_2 9.2kPa SaO_2 94% (82%)	Portable oxygen 4 l/min via nasal cannulae	CA 4 l/min via nasal cannulae	Reduction in SOB (Borg)

DB = double-blind; SB = single-blind; RCT = randomized controlled trial; PaO_2 = arterial partial pressure of oxygen; SaO_2 = oxygen saturation; CA = cylinder air; RA = room air; SOB = breathlessness; 'isotime' = the time equivalent to the end of exercise on cylinder air.

There appears to be dose-response effect of supplemental oxygen. Studies that incorporate different inspired oxygen fractions have found that breathlessness reduces further as the inspired oxygen concentration increases up to approximately 50 per cent.[18,43,44] Above this point the relationship between dose and response appears to plateau. The mechanism for this has not been established, but it may relate to the onset of complete abolition of hypoxic drive.

Several studies have examined the use of portable ambulatory oxygen equipment.[36,43,44,47] The benefits of supplemental oxygen during exercise appear to outweigh the extra effort entailed in carrying the equipment. No studies have detected an increase in breathlessness caused by carrying a portable cylinder. One study did show a small reduction in exercise tolerance (breathlessness not measured).[44]

Long-term oxygen therapy

Long-term oxygen therapy (LTOT) conventionally refers to the long term and continuous use of oxygen for 15 or more hours each day. The use of LTOT is well established in severely hypoxic patients with COPD (PaO_2 less than 7.3 kPa), as landmark trials have shown that oxygen for 15 or more hours per day improves survival.[53,54] The benefit, in terms of survival, is not sustained in moderately hypoxic patients (PaO_2 7.4–8.7 kPa).[55] Breathlessness has never been used as an outcome measure in studies examining LTOT; there is no evidence on the effect on breathlessness of using oxygen continually over most hours of each day.

There have, however, been a small number of studies examining the effect of SBOT on breathlessness, when used over the longer term. Arguably, the effect on oxygen therapy on quality of life at home matters much more to patients than the acute effect of oxygen in a research setting. Almost all the evidence on the use SBOT has examined the acute response over a timescale of minutes, in artificial, often laboratory-like, conditions. Can it be assumed that acute responders will also gain benefit from oxygen when it is used over a longer time period at home? A retrospective survey in Denmark found that 75–80 per cent of patients using non-continuous oxygen therapy reported an improvement of quality of life and dyspnoea with oxygen.[56] There have, however, been only four controlled studies that have addressed this issue (Table 12.3).

In two studies, patients underwent pulmonary rehabilitation over 6 and 10 weeks and were randomised to use cylinder air or oxygen during the training.[14,15] Rooyackers et al. found that training using oxygen did not improve breathlessness any more than training using air. Garrod et al. did find a small benefit in terms of dyspnoea with oxygen-assisted training, but this did not translate into improved activities of daily living. In both studies, as has been

Table 12.3 Summary of studies using longer term oxygen in patients with COPD

Study first author	Design (number of patients)	Mean oxygenation on air at rest (exercise)	Intervention	Comparison	Effect of oxygen (outcome measure)
Rooyackers (15)	Unblinded RCT over 10 weeks (24)	PaO$_2$ 10.4kPa (7.3kPa)	Portable oxygen 4 l/min via nasal cannulae during pulmonary rehabilitation 5 times weekly	RA during pulmonary rehabilitation 5 times weekly	No reduction in SOB (Borg+CRQ)
Garrod (14)	SBRCT over 6 weeks (25)	PaO$_2$ 8.5kPa SaO$_2$ 92% (82%)	Portable oxygen 4 l/min via nasal cannulae during pulmonary rehabilitation 3 times weekly	CA 4 l/min via nasal cannulae during pulmonary rehabilitation 3 times weekly	Reduction in SOB (Borg)
McDonald (45)	DBRCT over 12 weeks (26)	PaO$_2$ 9.2kPa SaO$_2$ 94%	Portable oxygen 4 l/min via nasal cannulae during any activity normally causing SOB	CA 4 l/min via nasal cannulae during any activity normally causing SOB	No reduction in SOB (Borg)
Eaton (51)	DBRCT over 12 weeks (50)	PaO$_2$ 9.2kPa SaO$_2$ 94% (82%)	Portable oxygen 4 l/min via nasal cannulae during any activity normally causing SOB	CA 4 l/min via nasal cannulae during any activity normally causing SOB	Reduction in SOB (CRQ)

DB = double-blind; SB = single-blind; RCT = randomized controlled trial; PaO$_2$ = arterial partial pressure of oxygen; SaO$_2$ = oxygen saturation; CA = cylinder air; RA = room air; SOB = breathlessness; CRQ = chronic respiratory disease questionnaire.

well established, the pulmonary rehabilitation itself did lead to significant reductions in breathlessness.

Two other studies examined quality of life in patients randomised to receive either home oxygen or air over a 12 week period. Patients were instructed to use oxygen for any activity that would normally cause dyspnoea. Eaton *et al.*[51], using a study population with significant exercise desaturation and providing light oxygen cylinders, did find an improvement in quality of life in patients who had been receiving oxygen. An important finding was that an acute response to oxygen did not predict which patients would benefit when using longer term oxygen. McDonald *et al.*[45] recruited patients who desaturated less on exercise and they supplied heavier oxygen cylinders; they found no improvement in quality of life. Interestingly, Eaton *et al.* found that 41 per cent of patients who had had a response to oxygen declined to use it after the study, citing poor acceptability or tolerability.

Clearly, it cannot be extrapolated from studies revealing an acute benefit with oxygen, that patients will gain a longer term response in terms of quality of life or improvement in daily functioning. There is an urgent need for further research to investigate the effect of longer term oxygen in the home setting.

Patients with cancer

Short-burst oxygen therapy

Three controlled studies have examined the palliating effect of oxygen in cancer patients at rest[26,57,58] (Table 12.4). Both studies by Bruera *et al.* involved significantly hypoxaemic patients and revealed benefit with supplemental oxygen. Booth *et al.* also found relief of dyspnoea with oxygen, but this response was replicated with cylinder air.

Ambulatory oxygen

The effect of oxygen on dyspnoea during exercise has been investigated in two controlled trials.[59,60] Both studies involved non-hypoxaemic patients and failed to show any beneficial effect of oxygen on dyspnoea. Although Ahmedzai *et al.* found that 28 per cent oxygen was no more effective than medical air, they did find that a mixture of 72 per cent helium and 28 per cent oxygen caused a statistically significant decrease in breathlessness compared to air, perhaps due to the lower density and resultant reduced resistance to flow of the helium based gas mixture.

Patients with heart failure and other diseases

There have been just two controlled studies in patients with heart failure, both examining breathlessness on exertion[61,62] (Table 12.4). Although Moore *et al*

Table 12.4 Summary of studies using oxygen in patients with other advanced diseases

Study first author	Disease	Design (number of patients)	Mean oxygenation on air at rest (exercise)	Intervention	Comparison	Effect of oxygen (outcome measure)
Bruera (57)	Cancer	DBRCT (1)	SaO_2 84%	At rest, oxygen at 5 l/min for 5 min via mask	At rest, CA at 5 l/min for 5 min via mask	Reduction in SOB (VAS)
Bruera (58)	Cancer	DBRCT (14)	SaO_2 <90%	At rest, oxygen at 5 l/min for 5 min via mask	At rest, CA at 5 l/min for 5 min via mask	Reduction in SOB (VAS)
Booth (26)	Cancer	SBRCT (25)	Range SaO_2 80–99%	At rest, oxygen 4 l/min for 15 min via nasal cannula	At rest, CA 4 l/min for 15 min via nasal cannulae	No reduction in SOB (VAS + Borg)
Bruera (59)	Cancer	DBRCT (33)	SaO_2 98%	At rest, for 5 min, during exercise and recovery, oxygen 5 l/min via nasal cannula	At rest, for 5 min, during exercise and recovery, CA 5 l/min via nasal cannulae	No reduction in SOB (VAS)
Ahmedzai (60)	Cancer	DBRCT (12)	SaO_2 94% (median)	At rest, for 5 min, and during exercise, 28% oxygen via mask (also HeO)	At rest, for 5 min, and during exercise, CA (same flow rate) via mask	No reduction in SOB (HeO reduced SOB) (VAS + Borg)
Moore (61)	Heart failure	DBRCT (12)	(SaO_2 95%)	During exercise, 30%, 50% oxygen via mouthpiece	During exercise, RA via mouthpiece	Reduction in SOB, but statistical significance unclear (VAS)
Restrick (62)	Heart failure	DBRCT (12)	SaO_2 94% (90%)	During exercise, portable oxygen at 2 l/min, 4 l/min via nasal cannula	During exercise, CA 2 l/min via nasal cannula	No reduction in SOB (VAS + Borg)
Swinburn (35)	ILD	DBRCT (10)	PaO_2 6.38kPa SaO_2 86%	At rest, 28% oxygen for 10 min via mask	At rest, CA (same flow rate) for 10 min via mask	Reduction in SOB (VAS)
Leach (44)	ILD	SBRCT (10)	PaO_2 9.4kPa (8.1kPa)	During exercise, portable oxygen 2, 4, 6 l/min via mask	CA 4 l/min via mask	Reduction in SOB (VAS)

ILD = interstitial lung disease; DB = double-blind; SB = single-blind; RCT = randomized controlled trial; PaO_2 = arterial partial pressure of oxygen; SaO_2 = oxygen saturation; HeO = 72% helium 28% oxygen gas mixture; CA = cylinder air; RA = room air; SOB = breathlessness.

found consistently lower dyspnoea scores when patients exercised with oxygen, it was not stated whether these results were statistically significant. Restrick *et al.* found no benefit with supplemental oxygen despite the study population having significant arterial desaturation on exercise.

Two studies recruited patients with interstitial lung disease, as well as COPD[35,44] (Table 12.4). Oxygen appears to palliate breathlessness in both studies, but the evidence is very limited and involves few patients.

Key points:

- Interpretation of available evidence is limited by study heterogeneity, small patient numbers, and a lack of controlled studies in conditions other than COPD.
- In COPD, there is little evidence to support the use of SBOT for breathlessness at rest, before exercise or after exercise. Ambulatory oxygen does however appear to reduce breathlessness on exertion.
- Some patients with cancer and breathlessness at rest do appear to benefit from oxygen therapy.
- No predictive factors have been found in any disease that can help select the patients that are most likely to benefit from oxygen therapy.
- An acute benefit on breathlessness in an artificial research context, does not necessarily imply benefit when oxygen is used at home in the longer term.
- There is an urgent need for further more rigorous research, in particular to determine the effect of longer term oxygen at home, using outcome measures that assess quality of life as well as breathlessness.

Clinical assessment of the effects of oxygen

It is difficult to predict which patients may benefit from supplemental oxygen. Response to oxygen does not correlate with the extent of dyspnoea at rest, level of hypoxaemia at rest, degree of desaturation on exercise, or any tests of lung function. The only way to decide whether or not to prescribe oxygen for a particular patient is to perform an individual clinical assessment. This involves measuring breathlessness with and without oxygen, at rest or on exertion. Before discussing individual clinical assessments, this section describes assessment tools for breathlessness, use of exercise tests, and objective measurement of oxygenation. The focus is on assessment in the clinical context, rather than on tools used in research.

Assessment of breathlessness

Reliable quantification of breathlessness is made difficult by its complex, multidimensional and subjective nature. This topic is considered in detail in

Chapter 2. Only the two tools most widely used in determining the effects of oxygen therapy are described here.

Visual analogue scale (VAS)

A VAS is a vertical or horizontal line with anchors to indicate extremes of sensation. It is most commonly 100mm in length. Patients are asked to indicate their dyspnoea intensity by marking the line. The anchors used vary, and include 'no breathlessness' to 'worst imaginable breathlessness' and 'no difficulty breathing' to 'extreme difficulty breathing'. Patients must be given specific instructions about the exact sensation to be rated, such as effort of breathing, shortness of breath, etc. The VAS has been found to be valid and reproducible.[63]

Modified Borg Scale

The Borg Scale rating of perceived exertion has been modified to measure symptoms such as breathlessness.[64,65] This is a category ratio scale; descriptive terms are used to anchor responses, and the scale is non-linear. Extensive reports demonstrate its reliability, validity and sensitivity to treatment effects. It has a very strong correlation with the VAS in patients with COPD.[66] An advantage of the Borg Scale is that the adjectives used to anchor responses may help patients in selecting the symptom intensity, and also allow direct comparison between individuals.

Exercise tests

Exercise tests are used to standardise the degree of exertion, either for comparison of a patient's symptoms with or without oxygen, or to compare symptoms at different times. They are used widely in a research context to allow comparisons between patients, but do not necessarily reflect the experience of exercise in the home.

Maximal work rate tests

These tests involve externally paced, incremental exercise, until the point where patients are unable to continue. Examples include incremental treadmill or cycle ergometer exercise, or the incremental shuttle walk test (ISWT). The ISWT involves patients walking around two cones placed 10 metres apart, with pre-recorded audio signals providing an incrementally increasing walking speed.[67] It has been validated in several advanced diseases, including COPD, heart failure and cancer.[68]

Endurance tests

Patients are instructed to exercise at a fixed, externally paced work rate, usually set at a percentage of a previously calculated maximal work rate. They are asked to exercise for as long as possible, until limited by symptoms. The outcome of the test is measured in terms of time or distance exercised. Examples of endurance tests include fixed rate treadmill exercise and the endurance shuttle walk test (ESWT).[69]

Supplemental oxygen has been found to have a greater effect on endurance ability, than on maximal work rate. It appears to increase endurance by delaying the point at which the maximal work rate is reached. Endurance tests are more sensitive to change following an intervention such as oxygen therapy, as maximal work rate is likely to be limited mostly by the underlying chronic disease.

Self-paced tests

The two, six and twelve minute field walk tests are examples of self-paced exercise tests.[70] Patients are asked to walk as far as they can in the available time. Self-paced tests are less reliable than externally paced tests; patients may chose to reduce the work rate to limit the severity of symptoms. Such tests probably assess a combination of maximal performance and endurance capacity.

Measurement of oxygenation

Objective quantification of oxygenation is not an important part of the assessment of the effects of supplemental oxygen on breathlessness. The benefit from oxygen therapy does not relate to arterial oxygenation. Measurement of oxygenation simply allows one to determine whether, for an individual patient, palliation of breathlessness is related to reversal of hypoxaemia. Assessment of oxygenation can be determined by two techniques, arterial blood gas analysis and pulse oximetry.

Arterial blood gas analysis

Heparinized blood is taken from the radial, brachial or femoral artery, and the arterial partial pressures of oxygen (PO_2) and carbon dioxide (PCO_2) are measured using an automated analyser. The normal ranges of arterial PO_2 and arterial PCO_2 are 10.5–13.5 kPa and 4.7–6.0 kPa respectively. Hypoxaemia (arterial PO_2 less than 10.4 kPa) is caused by one or more of the following four reasons: ventilation-perfusion mismatch, hypoventilation, abnormal diffusion and shunts. Supplemental oxygen efficiently reverses hypoxaemia caused by the first three factors. A shunt, however, means that some blood reaches the arterial system without passing through ventilated areas of lung. Therefore an increased fraction of inhaled oxygen will not increase the arterial PO_2 as much as for other causes of hypoxaemia.

Pulse oximetry

This provides a convenient and continuous, non-invasive measure of peripheral haemoglobin oxygen saturation. Unfortunately there are many causes of inaccurate readings, which include poor peripheral perfusion, motion, excess light, nail varnish, skin pigmentation and dyshaemoglobinaemias. A further disadvantage is that pulse oximetry does not measure PCO_2; a rising PCO_2, such as in Type II respiratory failure, would not be detected.

Individual clinical assessments

All assessments should be tailored to the needs of each particular patient, using clinical judgement and consultation with the patient. A formal assessment, to determine the effect of supplemental oxygen for an individual patient, can be done using any of the tools described above. For example, a patient who is breathless only on exertion may be asked to perform the endurance shuttle walk test in an outpatient setting, on room air and on oxygen therapy, with Borg scores of breathlessness recorded before and during exercise. In view of the learning effects with walking tests, it is essential to perform practice walks before the test walks. For particularly rigorous assessment, the use of an 'N of 1 randomized controlled trial' has been described.[57] A single patient can undergo several brief randomized, double-blind, crossover trials between air and oxygen. Ideally, all assessments should be repeated after a rest period, to ensure reproducibility of results.

A more pragmatic approach is to assess breathlessness in the patient's own home. Patients can be instructed to keep a simple diary of the severity of breathlessness (using VAS or Borg scores) while performing selected usual daily activities such as climbing stairs. This can be done over a period of time, both with and without oxygen therapy. Since the aim of symptom palliation is to improve quality of life at home, it can be reasoned that the effect of oxygen on quality of life should be assessed in a patient's home, rather than in artificial hospital conditions. Formal exercise tests do not necessarily relate to the type of activities a patient would be attempting at home. Furthermore, there is evidence that the patients who gain acute benefit from oxygen are not necessarily the individuals who experience an increase in quality of life using oxygen therapy at home.[51]

The clinical condition of patients with advanced disease can change rapidly. After commencing supplemental oxygen, it is important to reassess patients regularly, to establish that the benefit from therapy is still outweighing any burden from the negative aspects of oxygen therapy.

Key points:

◆ Since no factors have been found that can help predict response of breathlessness to oxygen therapy, it is necessary to perform an individual clinical trial of oxygen, tailored to the needs of each patient.

- A formal assessment includes a measure of breathlessness severity using VAS or Borg scores, before and during oxygen therapy, at rest or on exertion.
- Endurance exercise tests, such as the endurance shuttle walk test, are more sensitive to the effects of supplemental oxygen than maximal work rate tests.
- Pragmatic home assessments are more likely to give an accurate reflection of the effect of oxygen on a patient's quality of life.
- Assessments should be regularly repeated after commencing oxygen therapy.

Negative aspects of oxygen therapy

Supplemental oxygen is often assumed to be safe; oxygen, after all, is a naturally atmospheric gas that is vital for the existence of life. However, it must not be forgotten that oxygen is a pharmacological agent, and like any other drug it can have adverse effects. Furthermore, it has a significant financial cost. This is why it is so important to give oxygen therapy only to those patients that will gain benefit from it.

Compliance with oxygen therapy is limited by its adverse effects. Eaton et al.[51] found that out of all study patients who responded to oxygen (in terms of less breathlessness, greater exercise capacity, or increased quality of life), 41 per cent chose not to continue oxygen after the end of the study, most citing poor acceptability or tolerability. However, there is evidence that patients who perceive that oxygen therapy relieves breathlessness are a particularly motivated group with higher compliance.[71]

Physical adverse effects

Carbon dioxide retention

It has been known for many decades that high-flow oxygen therapy is an important, although rare, cause of severe hypercapnia.[72] This is believed to be only a phenomenon of acute exacerbations of COPD, as there is no evidence that stable patients with COPD receiving continuous oxygen therapy develop further increases in arterial PCO_2.[53] It is routine practice in respiratory medicine to check arterial blood gas measurements before and after commencing oxygen therapy.

Controlled oxygen therapy, using a low concentration of 24–28 per cent, reduces the risk of carbon dioxide retention occurring.[73] It is worth noting that the consequences of severe hypoxia during acute exacerbations may be more dangerous for patients than the effects of hypercapnia. In such situations, higher concentrations of oxygen may need to be given to correct the hypoxaemia, and a degree of hypercapnia may need to be tolerated.

The two most important mechanisms for carbon dioxide retention are believed to be a reduction in ventilation due to removal of hypoxic respiratory drive, and release of hypoxic vasoconstriction causing an increased ventilation–perfusion mismatch and a larger alveolar dead space. The relative importance of these mechanisms remains controversial, as both have a considerable evidence base.[74] Recent work appears to support a reduction of ventilation as the predominant mechanism.[75]

Oxygen toxicity

High concentrations of oxygen over long periods are known to cause lung damage. In hyperoxia, cellular production of oxygen free radicals exceeds the capacity of antioxidant enzymes to detoxify them. These free radicals cause alveolar cell and microvascular injury. Early toxicity is almost completely reversible. Later, organization occurs, with interstitial fibrosis. Retrosternal pain, presumably from tracheal inflammation, appears to be an early indicator of oxygen toxicity.[76]

Significant oxygen toxicity appears to be a problem mainly in patients who are intubated and mechanically ventilated with high concentrations of oxygen. It has been suggested that oxygen concentrations of 50 per cent or higher for more than two days may produce toxic changes.[77] The clinical relevance of oxygen toxicity in non-ventilated patients with advanced disease is unclear. A long-term follow-up study of patients with COPD given continuous ambulatory oxygen did find histological changes suggestive of toxicity in 6 out of 12 patients, but importantly, survival was not shortened in these patients.[78]

Lung atelectasis

When an airway is obstructed, the trapped gas is gradually absorbed, causing absorption atelectasis. If a patient is breathing a high concentration of supplemental oxygen, the rate of absorption atelectasis is greatly increased. Nitrogen gas slows absorption because of its low solubility; replacement of nitrogen with a soluble gas such as oxygen increases the rate of atelectasis. The clinical importance of this adverse effect in oxygen users with stable chronic disease is not certain.

Drying of airways

Supplemental oxygen contains less water vapour than air. This can lead to discomfort from its drying effect, particularly on the nasal mucosa when using nasal cannulae. Humidifiers are noisy, bulky, ineffective and run the risk of bacterial contamination. In practice, humidification of oxygen is usually unnecessary, as the patient's upper respiratory tract can usually adequately humidify the inhaled gas. Drying of the nasal membranes and crusting of secretions can be improved by regular application of a water-based lubricant to the nose, or temporary use of a mask.

Combustibility

Oxygen promotes combustion, and is a significant fire hazard. Patients who continue to smoke while using oxygen therapy may suffer severe burns, and fatalities have been reported. Patients and their relatives must be warned not to smoke in the vicinity of oxygen, and patients must not use oxygen while close to sources of heat or open flame, such as gas stoves or lighted fireplaces.

Psychosocial adverse effects

Psychological dependence

Breathlessness is a frightening symptom, and it is easy for patients to become psychologically dependent on anything they perceive to be helping. Some patients become very frightened during even a short interruption of oxygen supply. This dependence can also make it difficult to withdraw oxygen therapy in patients where it is clear that it is no longer improving dyspnoea.

Social restriction

Cumbersome, heavy equipment may restrict movement and activities within the home, and may limit excursions outside. Use of an oxygen mask may impair communication between a patient and family. Some patients feel a sense of social stigma and embarrassment, which may further hinder inter-action and lead to isolation.

Misconceptions

Patients often have fears about oxygen therapy which, if known by health professionals, could easily be allayed. Some suspect that oxygen is in some way addictive, and the more it is used the more it is needed. Others fear, for example, that oxygen concentrators may reduce the amount of oxygen available for others in the vicinity.

Financial cost

Domiciliary oxygen therapy is expensive. Since the 1980s, when trials confirmed the survival benefit of LTOT in COPD, the costs of oxygen therapy have increased rapidly. Short-burst oxygen therapy is widely prescribed despite the lack of evidence for its efficacy, and it constitutes, for example, one of the most expensive therapies used in the NHS in the UK.[79] The process for funding oxygen therapy varies between countries, and depends on national healthcare reimbursement policy.

Key points:

◆ The cost of oxygen therapy can be measured not only in financial terms, but also in terms of physical and psychosocial adverse effects.

◆ Some patients with COPD are at risk of respiratory depression with supplemental oxygen. This risk is reduced by limiting the oxygen concentration to 24–28 per cent.

◆ Psychosocial adverse effects of oxygen therapy are the major cause of poor compliance with oxygen therapy.[70]

◆ The disadvantages of oxygen therapy make it particularly important to select patients carefully, in order to identify those who will gain significant benefit.

Practical issues

Once a decision has been made to commence a patient on oxygen therapy, several practical matters need to be considered by the health professionals involved. The best source of oxygen for an individual patient must be ascertained, the delivery device for the oxygen needs to be chosen, and the most appropriate flow rate must be prescribed

Oxygen source[33]

Oxygen concentrators

Oxygen concentrators are the most convenient and economical method of providing domiciliary long-term oxygen therapy. They are mains-powered machines, which concentrate oxygen from the atmosphere. A compressor filters atmospheric air and passes it under pressure through a chamber of zeolite, which removes nitrogen, in effect concentrating the oxygen. Each machine has two zeolite chambers, which it uses alternately to maintain a steady flow of oxygen; the chamber that is out of use recharges by releasing nitrogen back to the atmosphere. The oxygen flow rate is adjustable between 0 and 5 litres per minute. However, oxygen concentration falls with increasing flow rate. When a patient requires a higher flow rate, two concentrators can be linked using a Y connector. It is possible to attach long extension tubing to an oxygen concentrator, which allows patients to move within the house and sit in the garden. Oxygen concentrators are serviced by an engineer, usually three monthly, and have been found to be mechanically reliable.

Oxygen cylinders

These contain compressed oxygen, and deliver the gas through a regulator valve. The specification of the regulator determines whether the flow rate is variable or fixed. Cylinder capacity ranges from 170 to 6800 litres. A standard cylinder size of 1360 litres may only last 5–6 hours at a flow rate of 4 l/min. Thus, oxygen cylinders are more appropriate for SBOT than LTOT. Patients using LTOT from a concentrator need back up oxygen cylinders to be available in case electrical mains power is interrupted.

Several suppliers now produce lightweight portable cylinders for ambulatory use. These are refillable from a larger cylinder, and can be carried over the shoulder or in a backpack. In the UK, the British Lung Foundation produces a list of portable oxygen suppliers. A standard portable cylinder size is 220–240 litres, which can only provide oxygen at a rate of 2 l/min for two hours. However, oxygen-conserving devices have been developed, which supply a pulse of oxygen at the beginning of each inspiration. This means that during exercise, the increased respiratory rate triggers more frequent pulses of oxygen. Pulsed dose oxygen results in oxygen savings of 50 per cent or more, and has been found to be as effective as continuous oxygen.[80]

Liquid oxygen

This is provided in insulated tanks at a temperature of minus 240 degrees Fahrenheit. A vaporizer converts the liquid oxygen into gaseous oxygen when the system is used. Liquid oxygen systems contain a much larger volume than gaseous systems, and high oxygen flow-rates can be produced. The major disadvantage is that oxygen evaporates and cylinders have to be refilled, even if not used. Other problems include the cost of deliveries, the difficulty of regular delivery to isolated areas, and the risk of cold burns from the liquid oxygen.

Expensive liquid oxygen portable systems are available which supply oxygen for longer than compressed gas portable cylinders, particularly when used with oxygen conserving devices. They can supply approximately eight hours of oxygen at 2 l/min. Liquid portable units are refilled from the reservoir tank at the patient's home.

Oxygen delivery device

Nasal cannulae

These consist of two prongs that are positioned just inside the anterior nares of the nose, and supported with a light frame. These are usually comfortable, and allow patients to eat and communicate without difficulty. Only low oxygen concentrations, up to 30 per cent, can be supplied. The concentration received by the patient cannot be predicted as a higher inspiratory flow rate leads to a lower concentration of oxygen. Some patients develop nasal mucosal drying or dermatitis with nasal cannulae. An altered sense of taste and smell has also been reported.

Face mask

In general, masks are usually less well tolerated than nasal cannulae. Variable performance masks are simple masks that fit over the nose and mouth. They allow inspired oxygen concentrations of up to 60 per cent, but the oxygen concentration is not predictable. Some accumulation of carbon dioxide occurs within the mask, and some patients report a feeling of being smothered. Fixed performance masks are useful for delivering controlled oxygen concentrations. As oxygen enters the mask through a narrow jet, it sucks in a constant flow of air through surrounding holes, by the Venturi principle. With an oxygen flow of 4 l/min, a total flow of oxygen and air of approximately 40 l/min is delivered to the patient. This high flow rate enormously reduces rebreathing of expired gas, and carbon dioxide accumulation. Predictable fixed concentrations of oxygen of, for example, 24, 28 or 35 per cent can be supplied to patients.

Transtracheal oxygen (TTO)

A microcatheter can be inserted through the anterior tracheal wall with the tip lying just above the carina. TTO has been found to have several benefits. It decreases dead space, tidal volume and minute ventilation, and can reduce the necessary oxygen flow rates by up to 50 per cent. A study comparing TTO with oxygen via nasal cannulae found that COPD patients with TTO had improved exercise tolerance and less hospitalization. TTO does, however, have a number of disadvantages. Catheters require regular replacement and cleaning. They have been known to kink, and may be displaced or break off internally. There is some evidence that higher flow rates can cause a sensation of dyspnoea by stimulation of irritant tracheal receptors.[34] However, high flow rates by this route are rarely needed, and the clinical relevance of this finding is unclear. Overall, TTO may have a role in carefully selected patients at specialist centres.

Oxygen flow rate

Because of the adverse effects of oxygen described above, oxygen should be supplied at the lowest flow rate possible to produce benefit. When palliation of dyspnoea is the aim of therapy, the individual clinical assessment can measure breathlessness scores at different flow rates of oxygen. In practice, most patients use a flow rate of 2–4 litres/minute. These rates can provide symptom relief, but minimize the risk of adverse effects. In those patients that retain carbon dioxide when given supplemental oxygen it is vital to keep to a low flow rate. If necessary, a fixed performance mask providing a predictable oxygen concentration of 24 or 28 per cent may need to be used.

Prescribing issues

Every country has its own process by which home oxygen is prescribed. For example, in the UK responsibility for prescribing LTOT rests with specialists in hospital; General Practitioners can prescribe oxygen for short burst use. In some countries, prescription of supplemental oxygen is hindered by strict criteria for reimbursement of costs.

Key points:

◆ When prescribing oxygen therapy a decision must be made as to the most appropriate source, delivery device and flow rate for the oxygen.
◆ Oxygen concentrators are the most efficient source of oxygen for long-term oxygen therapy. Short-burst and ambulatory oxygen therapy is better provided by cylinders supplying compressed gas or liquid oxygen.
◆ Nasal cannulae are usually the most well tolerated form of oxygen delivery.
◆ Other practical aspects of prescription of oxygen are dependent on national regulations that vary between countries.

Clinical guidelines

The lack of good quality evidence makes it difficult to develop evidence-based guidelines. Several reports have published recommendations based on a combination of existing evidence and expert opinion.[32,33,78] Brief clinical guidelines are summarized below.

◆ Every patient in whom oxygen therapy is being considered should have an individual clinical assessment, to assess the efficacy of oxygen in palliating breathlessness.
◆ Short-burst oxygen therapy should be considered for any patient with advanced disease who is breathless at rest, if the breathlessness cannot be relieved by other treatments.
◆ The use of short-burst oxygen therapy immediately before and after exercise is not recommended.
◆ Ambulatory oxygen should be prescribed when there is a fall in SaO_2 of at least 4 per cent to a reading below 90 per cent during a baseline walking test whilst breathing air, and an improvement of at least 10 per cent in walking distance and/or breathlessness score when walking with supplemental oxygen compared with an air cylinder. A resting SaO_2 of 95 per cent or less may screen patients likely to desaturate below 90 per cent on exercise.[81]
◆ A decrease of 10 per cent or more in the score of a dyspnoea scale is considered a clinically significant change in breathlessness that warrants continued prescription of oxygen therapy.[31,57,82]

- Following a decision to provide domiciliary oxygen therapy, patients should be provided with education and written instructions, which include advice about the dangers of smoking near oxygen therapy.
- Longer term supplemental oxygen should only be instigated after assessment by a respiratory specialist.
- Arrangements should be made for an oxygen concentrator to be supplied, either if more than three oxygen cylinders a month are being used, or if more than one cylinder a month is being used and the duration of prescription is likely to be more than 12 months.[83]
- Ambulatory oxygen therapy should be supplied by a portable cylinder if duration of use is less than 90 minutes per day, by portable cylinder with oxygen conserving device if use is between 90 minutes and 4 hours per day, and by liquid oxygen if duration of use is more than 4 hours or if flow rates of more than 2 l/min are required.
- Individuals should be reassessed regularly after commencing therapy, to determine continuing efficacy of supplemental oxygen over the longer term.

Conclusion

Oxygen therapy does have a role in the palliation of dyspnoea in advanced disease. However, not all patients with advanced disease gain relief of dyspnoea with supplemental oxygen, and there is no way of predicting which patients will benefit. Furthermore, oxygen therapy is associated with significant adverse effects and financial cost. It is therefore of vital importance that patients who receive oxygen therapy are selected carefully, using an individual clinical assessment to determine the role of oxygen in that particular patient. Further research is urgently needed in order to define more clearly the role of oxygen in the palliation of breathlessness.

References

1. **Escalante C, Martin C, Elting L, et al.** Dyspnea in cancer patients. Etiology, resource utilization, and survival – implications in a managed care world. *Cancer* 1996; **78**: 1314–19.
2. **Roberts C.** Short burst oxygen therapy for relief of breathlessness in COPD. *Thorax* 2004; **59**: 638–40.
3. **Simon P, Schwartzstein R, Weiss J, et al.** Distinguishable types of dyspnea in patients with shortness of breath. *Am Rev Respir Dis* 1990; **142**: 1009–14.
4. **West J.** *Pulmonary Pathophysiology*, 7th edn, p. 45. Lippincott Williams &Wilkins; 2003.
5. **Schwartzstein R, Simon P, Weiss, J, Fencl V, Weinberger S.** Breathlessness induced by dissociation between ventilation and chemical drive. *Am Rev Respir Dis* 1989; **139**: 1231–7.

6. Swinburn C, Wakefield J, Jones P. Relationship between ventilation and breathlessness during exercise in chronic obstructive airways disease in not altered by prevention of hypoxaemia. *Clin Sci* 1984; **67**: 515–19.

7. Lane, Cockcroft A, Adams, L, Guz A. Arterial oxygen saturation and breathlessness in patients with chronic obstructive airways disease. *Clin Sci* 1987; **72**: 693–8.

8. Chronos N, Adams L, Guz A. Effect of hyperoxia and hypoxia on exercise-induced breathlessness in normal subjects. *Clin Sci* 1988; **74**: 531–7.

9. Dean N, Brown J, Hotelman, R *et al*. Oxygen may improve dyspnoea and endurance in patients with chronic obstructive pulmonary disease and only mild hypoxemia. *Am Rev Respir Dis* 1992; **146**: 941–5.

10. Kobayashi S, Nishimura M, Vasomotor M, *et al*. Relationship between breathlessness and hypoxic and hypersonic ventilatory response in patients with COPD. *Euro Respir J* 1996; **9**: 2340–5.

11. O'Donnell D, Bain D, Webb K. Factors contributing to relief of exertional breathlessness during hyperoxia in chronic airflow limitation *Am J Respir Crit Care Med* 1997; **155**: 530–5.

12. Malta's F, Samara A, Samara C, *et al*. Oxidative capacity of the skeletal muscle and lactic acid kinetics during exercise in normal subjects and in patients with COPD. *Am J Respir Crit Care Med* 1996; **153**(1): 288–93.

13. Casaburi R, Patessio A, Ioli F, *et al*. Reductions in exercise lactic acidosis and ventilation as a result of exercise training in patients with obstructive lung disease. *Am Rev Respir Dis* 1992; **143**: 9–18.

14. Garrod R, Paul E, Wedzicha J. Supplemental oxygen during pulmonary rehabilitation in patients with COPD and exercise hypoxaemia. *Thorax* 2000; **55**: 539–43.

15. Rooyackers J, Dekhuijzen P, Van Herwaarden C, Folgering H. Training with supplemental oxygen in patients with COPD and hypoxaemia at peak exercise. *Eur Respir J* 1997; **10**: 1278–84.

16. American Thoracic Society: Dyspnea: mechanisms, assessment, and management: a consensus statement. *Am J Respir Crit Care Med* 1999; **159**: 321–40.

17. O'Donnell D, D'Arsigny C, Webb K. Effects of hyperoxia on ventilatory limitation during exercise in advanced chronic obstructive pulmonary disease. *Am J Respir Crit Care Med* 2001; **165**: 892–8.

18. Somfay A, Porszasz J, Lee S, Casaburi R. Dose-response effect of oxygen on hyperinflation and exercise endurance in nonhypoxaemic COPD patients. *Eur Respir J* 2001; **18**: 77–84.

19. Mancini D, Ferraro N, Nazzaro D, Chance B, Wilson J. Respiratory muscle deoxygenation during exercise in patients with heart failure demonstrated with near infrared spectroscopy. *J Am Coll Cardiol* 1991; **18**(2): 492–8.

20. Bye P, Esau S, Levy R *et al*. Ventilatory muscle function during exercise in air and oxygen in patients with chronic air-flow limitation. *Am Rev Respir Dis* 1985; **132**: 236–40.

21. Libby D, Briscoe W, King T. Relief of hypoxia-related bronchoconstriction by breathing 30 percent oxygen. *Am Rev Respir Dis* 1981; **123**: 171–5.

22. Scano G, van Meerhaeghe A, Willeput R, Vachaudez J, Sergysels R. Effect of oxygen on breathing during exercise in patients with chronic obstructive lung disease. *Eur J Respir Dis* 1982; **63**(1): 23–30.

23. Liss H, Grant B. The effect of nasal flow on breathlessness in patients with chronic obstructive pulmonary disease. *Am Rev Respir Dis* 1988; **137**: 1285–8.

24. Simon P, Basner R, Weinberger S, *et al.* Oral mucosal stimulation modulates intensity of breathlessness induced in normal subjects. *Am Rev Respir Dis* 1991; **144**: 419–22.

25. Schwartzstein R, Lahive K, Pope A, Weinberger S, Weiss J. Cold facial stimulation reduces breathlessness induced in normal subjects. *Am Rev Respir Dis* 1987; **13**: 58–61.

26. Booth S, Kelly M, Cox N, Adams L, Guz A. Does oxygen help dyspnea in patients with cancer? *Am J Respir Crit Care Med* 1996; **153**: 1515–18.

27. Evans T, Waterhouse J, Carter A, Nicholl J, Howard P. Short burst oxygen treatment for breathlessness in chronic obstructive airways disease. *Thorax* 1986; **41**: 611–15.

28. McKeon J, Tomlinson J, Tarrant E, Mitchell C. Portable oxygen in patients with severe chronic obstructive pulmonary disease. *Aust NZ J Med* 1988; **18**: 125–9.

29. Waterhouse J, Howard P. Breathlessness and portable oxygen in chronic obstructive airways disease. *Thorax* 1983; **38**: 302–6.

30. Carrieri-Kohlman V, Douglas M, Gromley J, Stulbarg M. Desensitization and guided mastery: treatment approaches for the management of dyspnea. *Heart Lung* 1993; **22**: 226–34.

31. Lock S, Paul E, Rudd R, Wedzicha J. Portable oxygen therapy: assessment and usage. *Respir Med* 1991; **85**: 407–12.

32. Booth S, Wade R, Anderson H, *et al.* The use of oxygen in the palliation of breathlessness. A report of the expert working committee of the association of palliative medicine. *Respir Med* 2004; **98**: 66–77.

33. Wedzicha J. Domiciliary oxygen therapy services: clinical guidelines and advice for prescribers. Summary of a report of the Royal College of Physicians. *J R Coll Physicians Lond* 1999; **33**: 445–7.

34. Kollef M, Johnson R. Transtracheal gas administration and the perception of dyspnea. *Respir Care* 1990; **35**(8): 791–9.

35. Swinburn C, Mould H, Stone T, Corris P, Gibson G. Symptomatic benefit of supplemental oxygen in hypoxaemic patients with chronic lung disease. *Am Rev Respir Dis* 1991; **143**: 913–15.

36. Woodcock A, Gross E, Geddes D. Oxygen relieves breathlessness in 'pink puffers'. *Lancet* 1981; **1**: 707–9.

37. McKeon J, Murree-Allen K, Saunders N. Effects of breathing supplemental oxygen before progressive exercise in patients with chronic obstructive lung disease. *Thorax* 1988; **43**(1): 53–6.

38. Marques-Magallanes J, Storer T, Copper C. Treadmill exercise duration and dyspnea recovery time in chronic obstructive pulmonary disease: effects of oxygen breathing and repeated testing. *Respir Med* 1998; **92**(5): 735–8.

39. Killen J, Corris P. A pragmatic assessment of the placement of oxygen when given for exercise induced dyspnoea. *Thorax* 2000; **55**: 544–6.

40. Nandi K, Smith A, Crawford A, *et al.* Oxygen supplementation before or after submaximal exercise in patients with chronic obstructive pulmonary disease. *Thorax* 2003; **58**: 670–3.

41. Lewis C, Eaton T, Young P, Kolbe J. Short-burst oxygen immediately before and after exercise is ineffective in nonhypoxic COPD patients. *Eur Respir J* 2003; **22**: 584–8.

42. Stevenson N, Calverley P. Effect of oxygen on recovery form maximal exercise in patients with chronic obstructive pulmonary disease. *Thorax* 2004; **59**: 668–72.

43. Davidson C, Leach R, George R, Geddes D. Supplemental oxygen and exercise ability in chronic obstructive airways disease. *Thorax* 1988; **43**: 965–71.

44. Leach R, Davidson A, Chinn S, *et al.* Portable liquid oxygen and exercise ability in severe respiratory disability. *Thorax* 1992; 47: 781–9.
45. McDonald C, Blyth C, Lazarus M, Marschner I, Barter C. Exertional oxygen of limited benefit inpatients with chronic obstructive pulmonary disease and mild hypoxemia. *Am J Respir Crit Care Med* 1995; 152: 1616–19.
46. Roberts C, Bell J, Wedzicha J. Comparison of the efficacy of a demand oxygen delivery system with continuous low flow oxygen in subjects with stable COPD and severe oxygen desaturation on walking. *Thorax* 1996; 51(8): 831–4.
47. Revill S, Singh S, Morgan M. Randomised controlled trial of ambulatory oxygen and an ambulatory ventilator on endurance exercise in COPD. *Respir Med* 2000; 94(8): 778–83.
48. Knebel A, Bentz E, Barnes P. Dyspnea management in alpha-1 antitrypsin deficiency: effect of oxygen administration. *Nurs Res* 2000; 49(9): 333–8.
49. Jolly E, Di Boscio V, Aguirre L, *et al.* Effects of supplemental oxygen during activity in patients with advanced COPD without severe resting hypoxemia. *Chest* 2001; 120: 437–43.
50. Maltais F, Simon M, Jobin J, *et al.* Effects of oxygen on lower limb blood flow and O2 uptake during exercise in COPD. *Med Sci Sports Exercise* 2001; 33(6): 916–22.
51. Eaton T, Garrett J, Young P, *et al.* Ambulatory oxygen improves quality of life of COPD patients; a randomised controlled study. *Eur Respir J* 2002; 20(2): 306–12.
52. Rees P, Dudley D. Oxygen therapy in chronic lung disease. *BMJ* 1998; 317: 871–4.
53. Medical Research Council Working Party. Long-term domiciliary oxygen therapy in chronic hypoxic cor pulmonale complicating chronic bronchitis and emphysema. *Lancet* 1981; 1: 681–6.
54. Nocturnal Oxygen Therapy Trial Group. Continuous or nocturnal oxygen therapy in hypoxaemic chronic obstructive lung disease. *Ann Intern Med* 1980; 93: 391–8.
55. Borecka D, Gorzelak K, Slinwinski P, Tobiasz M, Zielinski J. Effect of long term oxygen therapy on survival in patients with chronic obstructive pulmonary disease with moderate hypoxaemia. *Thorax* 1997; 52: 674–9.
56. Ringbaek T, Viskum K, Lange P. Non-continuous home oxygen therapy: utilization, symptomatic effect and prognosis. Data from a national register on home oxygen therapy. *Respir Med* 2001; 95: 980–5.
57. Bruera E, Schoeller T, MacEachern T. Symptomatic benefit of supplemental oxygen in hypoxemic patients with terminal cancer: the use of the N of 1 randomised controlled trial. *J Pain Sy Manage* 1992; 7(6): 365–8.
58. Bruera E, de Stoutz N, Velasco-Leiva A, Schoeller T, Hanson J. Effect of oxygen on dyspnoea in hypoxaemic terminal cancer patients. *Lancet* 1993; 342: 13–14.
59. Bruera E, Sweeney C, Willey J, *et al.* A randomised controlled trial of supplemental oxygen versus air in cancer patients with dyspnea. *Pall Med* 2003; 17: 659–63.
60. Ahmedzai S, Laude E, Robertson A, Troy J, Vora V. A double-blind, randomised, controlled Phase 2 trial of Heliox28 gas mixture in lung cancer patients with dyspnoea on exertion. *Br J Cancer* 2004; 90: 366–71.
61. Moore D, Weston A, Hughes J. Effect of increased inspired oxygen concentrations on exercise performance in chronic heart failure. *Lancet* 1992; 339: 850–3.
62. Restrick L, Davies S, Noone L. Ambulatory oxygen in chronic heart failure. *Lancet* 1992; 340: 1192–3.
63. Mador M, Kufel T. Reproducibility of visual analog scale measurements of dyspnea in patients with chronic obstructive airways disease. *Am Rev Respir Dis* 1992; 146(1): 82–7.

64. **Borg G.** Psychophysical bases of perceived exertion. *Med Sci Sports Exerc* 1982; **14**(5): 377–81.
65. **Burdon J, Juniper E, Killian K, Hargreave F, Campbell E.** The perception of breathlessness in asthma. *Am Rev Respir Dis* 1982; **126**(5): 82–8.
66. **Muza S, Silverman M, Gilmore G, Hellerstein H, Kelsen S.** Comparison of scales used to quantitate the sense of effort to breathe in patients with chronic obstructive pulmonary disease. *Am Rev Respir Dis* 1990; **141**: 909–13.
67. **Singh S, Morgan M, Scott S, Walters D, Hardman A.** Development of a shuttle walking test of disability in patients with chronic airways obstruction. *Thorax* 1992; **47**: 1019–24.
68. **Booth S, Adams L.** The shuttle walking tests: a reproducible method for evaluating the impact of shortness of breath on functional capacity in patients with advanced cancer. *Thorax* 2001; **56**: 146–50.
69. **Revill S, Morgan M, Singh S, Williams J, Hardman A.** The endurance shuttle walk: a new field test for the assessment of endurance capacity in chronic obstructive pulmonary disease. *Thorax* 1999; **54**: 213–22.
70. **Butland R, Pang J, Gross E, et al.** Two-, six-, and 12-minute walking tests in respiratory disease. *BMJ* 1982; **284**: 1607–8.
71. **Earnest M.** Explaining adherence to supplemental oxygen therapy. The patient's perspective. *J Gen Intern Med* 2002; **17**: 749–55.
72. **McNicol M, Campbell E.** Severity of respiratory failure: arterial blood-gases in untreated patients. *Lancet* 1965; i: 336–8.
73. **Moloney E, Kiely J, McNicholas W.** Controlled oxygen therapy and carbon dioxide retention during exacerbations of chronic obstructive pulmonary disease. *Lancet* 2001; **357**: 526–8.
74. **Calverley P.** Oxygen-induced hypercapnia revisited. *Lancet* 2000; **356**: 1538–9.
75. **Robinson T, Freiberg D, Regnis J, Young I.** The role of hypoventilation and ventilation-perfusion redistribution in oxygen-induced hypercapnia during acute exacerbations of chronic obstructive pulmonary disease. *Am J Respir Crit Care Med* 2000; **11**: 1524–9.
76. **Montgomery A, Luce J, Murray J.** Retrosternal pain is an early indicator of oxygen toxicity. *Am Rev Respir Dis* 1989; **139**: 1548–50.
77. **West J.** *Pulmonary Pathophysiology,* 7th edn, p. 167. Lippincott Williams &Wilkins; 2003.
78. **Petty T, Stanford R, Neff T.** Continuous oxygen therapy in chronic airway obstruction. Observations on possible oxygen toxicity and survival. *Ann Int Med* 1971; **75**: 361–7.
79. **Chronic obstructive pulmonary disease:** national clinical guidelines on the management of chronic obstructive pulmonary disease in adults in primary and secondary care. *Thorax* 2004; **59**(Suppl 1): 1–232.
80. **Garrod R, Bestall J, Paul E, Wedzicha J.** Evaluation of pulsed dose oxygen delivery during exercise in patients with severe chronic obstructive pulmonary disease. *Thorax* 1999; **54**: 242–4.
81. **Knower M, Dunagan D, Adair N, Chin R.** Baseline oxygen saturation predicts exercise desaturation below prescription threshold in patients with chronic obstructive pulmonary disease. *Arch Intern Med* 2001; **161**: 732–6.
82. **Wilson R, Jones P.** Long term reproducibility of Borg scale estimates for breathlessness during exercise. *Clin Sci* 1991; **80**: 309–12.
83. **Heaney L, McAllister D, MacMahon J.** Cost minimisation analysis of provision of oxygen at home: are the drug tarrif guidelines cost effective? *BMJ* 1999; **319**: 19–23.

13

Pharmacological approaches to breathlessness

David C. Currow

Medications for the relief of dyspnoea at the end of life

There has been significant progress in the last decade in defining the benefits of treating refractory dyspnoea in people with life-limiting illnesses with agents including opioids. This continuing work around the world is ensuring that medications can be safely prescribed and adequately titrated to provide symptomatic relief.

In considering the evidence for use of pharmacotherapy for symptomatic breathlessness, it is important to consider the quality of the evidence (validity) and the population studied (generalizability). The palliative population is heterogeneous and each person has varying contributions to their breathlessness from the disease (primary life-limiting illness and comorbid causes), the interpretation of their situation (cortical input) and their response (what health professionals and caregivers/family see). None of this happens in isolation of the non-pharmacological approaches to people with dyspnoea in the face of advanced disease.

Many of the studies in the literature are single dose or short intervention studies of either healthy subjects or people with respiratory compromise who are in highly selected subpopulations. The number of participants in most studies is not adequate to answer the clinical question being asked. The ability to generalize these findings to many clinical situations is limited despite the advances that have occurred in better defining the mechanisms of breathlessness and its treatment. The concept of 'best evidence' is that we continue to adapt existing studies to current clinical practice while developing evidence through the conduct of more comprehensive clinical trials.

In trying to define an evidence base for practice, it is important to acknowledge the three distinct sources of information for the clinician:

1 data about interventions that will modify the course of the underlying disease
2 data from a broad range of studies in specialist areas other than palliative care that can inform practice and design of further studies
3 studies done specifically in palliative populations.

In clinical areas where there is a predominantly subjective experience like dyspnoea, there needs to be a distinction made between studies on healthy volunteers and those who are unwell and experiencing breathlessness. One cannot necessarily extrapolate from one to the other.

This chapter deals with breathlessness that is refractory – reversible causes have been addressed and despite this, breathlessness persists at rest or on minimal exertion.

The importance of addressing symptoms while at the same time defining and treating reversible components of breathlessness must be emphasized.[1]

A detailed overview of the characteristics of the palliative population with breathlessness is given in a prospective convenience sample study by Dudgeon and Lertzman.[2] As a referral-based specialty, this may not represent all breathlessness at the end of life. The heterogeneity of the palliative population with breathlessness is underlined when 100 consecutive cancer patients with shortness of breath in two inpatient units were examined. Seventy per cent of people with breathlessness at the end of life had more than a 20 pack-year history of smoking. Primary lung cancer accounted for half of the patients admitted to this study, but a reproducible denominator for the whole population (not just those referred to specialized palliative services) is difficult to determine. Almost one third had current cardiac problems that would be likely to add to breathlessness. Most patients had several identifiable contributing factors to their breathlessness on history, examination or from laboratory tests.

This was a group of unwell people. Median forced expiratory volume in one second (FEV_1) was 0.81 (range 0.16–2.35) and forced vital capacity (FVC) was 1.47 (range 0.15–4.29). Median maximum inspiratory pressure was $-16cmH_2O$ (normal $\leq -50cmH_2O$) suggesting that respiratory muscle weakness (any value $<25cmH_2O$) was a significant contributor to the sensation of dyspnoea as part of the cachexia/anorexia syndrome.

Reversible causes for breathlessness included bronchoconstriction, hypoxaemia and anaemia. No longitudinal intervention data were reported to reflect improvements obtained by addressing these deficits. Only one patient had anxiety as the sole cause of breathlessness. Anxiety, raised $PaCO_2$ and smoking were good predictors of breathlessness although the total variance contributed to breathlessness by these factors is relatively small. Median VAS scores were 53mm for breathlessness and 29 for anxiety. In modelling, anxiety accounted for only 10 per cent of changes in VAS scores of breathlessness. These findings need to be seen in tandem with the National Hospice Study where almost one quarter of people had no obvious cause for their dyspnoea (other than profound cachexia).[3]

There are no data currently to establish the nexus between the sensations caused by differing underlying pathologies causing dyspnoea and the best symptomatic intervention.[4,5] Despite the fact that the descriptors of dyspnoea in the English language differ depending on the underlying pathology, no work has been done to relate the type of sensation or its intensity with tailored pharmaceutical interventions. Breathlessness is still interpreted by most clinicians as a homogenous symptom. Any detailed clinical analysis is broadly of populations combining three clinical settings – cancer, chronic obstructive pulmonary disease and cardiac failure.

Given that there has been no 'gold standard' comparator, the best available evidence for pharmacological interventions for dyspnoea is drawn from placebo controlled randomized clinical trials. In the palliative management of dyspnoea, these vary in quality and power.

Opioids
Mechanisms of action of opioids
A clear distinction has to be made between the presence of opioid receptors and the dynamic process by which they may influence the perception of breathlessness. There are theoretical mechanisms by which opioids may exert an effect on the brainstem's respiratory centre, decrease discharge from the carotid body, reduce metabolic rate, decrease oxygen consumption and increase peripheral vasodilatation thereby reducing peripheral resistance.

To complicate the picture, studies generally confirm that there is, for the most part, a very poor relationship between the degree of functional impairment and the subjective sensation of dyspnoea.[6] Even the relationship between tachypnoea and the sensation of dyspnoea is not well established.[7]

Central mediation of breathing occurs in the brainstem respiratory centre, an area rich with opioid receptors. Central receptors in the brainstem are sensitive to CO_2 and pH. Blunting of a response to changes in partial pressure of these gases may be seen in response to opioids in healthy people.[8] The role of the right anterior insular cortex (part of the limbic system), cerebellar vermis and medial pons is still being defined although recent positron emission tomography (PET) scanning demonstrate dynamic changes not only when, but in proportion to induced dyspnoea.[9,10] Peripheral receptors include mechanoreceptors in the lungs and airways together with stretch receptors in the chest wall. The aortic arch and carotid body monitor oxygen tension. The lungs have opioid receptors that may be clinically relevant.[11]

Consensus documents

The WHO Global Initiative for the diagnosis, management, and prevention of chronic obstructive lung disease (GOLD) continues to recommend that opioids are contraindicated in chronic obstructive pulmonary disease (COPD) because of the risks of respiratory depression and the potential for increasing hypercapnia.[12] The American Thoracic Society, in its 1999 consensus document on the management of dyspnoea, did not state that opioids were contraindicated in chronic dyspnoea but recommended 'judicious use' for people 'in the terminal stages of cardiopulmonary disease'. They also stated 'because of safety concerns the use of (opioids and benzodiazepines) should be individualized to the patient'.[13] We need to be absolutely clear about the therapies we are using and by adopting a systematic approach (clear protocols that we share with our colleagues outside specialist palliative care) so a potentially important symptomatic treatment is not withheld from people who, despite best efforts, have refractory dyspnoea.[14]

By contrast, Therapeutic Guidelines in Palliative Care, a consensus document from palliative care clinicians and academics in Australia, recommends the use of low-dose opioids in people with intractable dyspnoea while closely monitoring them.[15]

Clinical data

There are several key studies that together help to define the use of opioids in the palliative population. The studies done to date are all efficacy studies and no effectiveness or safety studies have been performed. Efficacy studies – those in highly selected subpopulations to define a therapeutic benefit – need to be complemented with effectiveness studies – (large) studies that explore how the intervention works in real life practice for the whole population with dyspnoea at the end of life. Of note, there have been no safety studies in pharmacological treatment of dyspnoea. Such a study would be powered to ensure that there was no increase in adverse outcomes (e.g. death or respiratory depression) in people treated with, for example, opioids. These are large, complex studies that are still awaited.

Systematic reviews – opioids

There is only one systematic review published on the use of opioids in the palliative setting. A Cochrane review was published covering literature up until May 1999.[16] Although the primary outcome measure of the review was breathlessness, 10 of the 18 studies had as their primary outcome measure exercise or exercise endurance. One study was excluded because, although double-blind and randomized, it compared two doses of opioid rather than with placebo. Fourteen of the 18 included studies were for single doses of opioid only. Nine explored oral or parenteral opioids (eight studies for people with COPD) and nine studies examined opioids delivered by nebulizer (eight studies predominantly for people with COPD).

The target populations for the studies varied widely in diagnosis, comorbid condition and functional status. There was no evidence to support an improvement in exercise tolerance in opioids administered either orally or by nebulizer. Standardized mean differences (SMD) of the pooled data disclosed a reduction of 0.20 (CI: −0.42 to 0.03, p = 0.09). This result may be due to small numbers, but also suggests that any benefit is likely to be small and this may not be clinically significant, unless it is in a subpopulation yet to be defined. The relevance of breathlessness at maximal exertion to the palliative population if they have breathlessness at rest is open to question.

Oral opioids showed a consistent benefit in reducing dyspnoea across the populations studied. Dyspnoea was reduced in all studies when compared to placebo (SMD −0.31, CI: −0.50 to −0.13, p = 0.0008). This effect was greater if studies looking at nebulized administration of opioids were excluded from the studies (SMD −0.40, CI: −0.63 to −0.17, p = 0.006). How this translates to repeated doses or chronic administration is not clear. The systematic review would also support the need for further studies powered to detect the groups with either the underlying pathophysiology or subjective descriptors of dyspnoea that can generate a better focused approach to clinical practice.

Nebulized opioids delivered no benefit for either dyspnoea (SMD −0.11, CI: −0.32 to 0.10, p = 0.31) nor exercise (SMD −0.06, CI: −0.70 to 0.58, p = 0.86).

The magnitude of the change seen is approximately 8mm on a 100mm visual analogue scale. If all other avenues have been exhausted for modifying dyspnoea, a reduction of 8mm with a median starting point of between 50 and 55mm is a clinically significant reduction in dyspnoea if the treatment is well tolerated.

There was confirmation of transient nausea, vomiting and constipation in opioid-naive patients. Drowsiness caused withdrawal from studies for several people in the long term. One study highlights a rise in $PaCO_2$ but this was not above 40mmHg.[17]

Controlled clinical trials – morphine, cancer

Bruera and colleagues published a single-dose double-blind randomized controlled cross-over trial (RCT) in 1993 of people who were already on opioids for pain and had moderate dyspnoea at rest.[18] In this study, patients received a 50 per cent increment on their background opioid dose or placebo, switching to a single dose of the opposite arm the next day. The primary outcome was measured by 100mm visual analogue scale at 30, 45 and 60 minutes and compared to baseline. The maximum impact was seen by 45 minutes taking VAS readings from 30mm (+/– 23) to 14mm (+/–18). Background pain was comparable in both groups. There was no decrease in oxygen saturation or respiratory depression in the observation period.

The population from which the 10 patients in the study were drawn had progressive malignancy as the primary cause of their breathlessness. In one case, this was secondary to pleural effusion but in the other cases it was primary or metastatic lung cancer.

To take this study a step further, Allard and his team conducted a multi-site randomized continuous sequential clinical trial exploring paired preferences for supplementary opioids in dyspnoea.[7] Thirty-three patients with cancer, pain requiring stable doses of opioids and dyspnoea at rest despite oxygen were enrolled in the study. Details of comorbid lung conditions were not reported. A single additional dose of opioid at either a 25 or 50 per cent increment on their fourth hourly baseline dose by the route that they were already receiving was administered. Pairs at the two dose levels were assigned randomly using the same route of administration. Patients were followed for 4 hours with each subsequent measure of breathlessness anchored to the previous response, not generated *de novo*.

Both groups experienced a reduction in dyspnoea of 8.6mm (+/–1.1) and there was no statistical or clinical difference between the two groups for dyspnoea with maximum benefit seen at 60 minutes. In comparison to most other studies, it is of note that there was a statistically significant drop in the frequency of breathing in both groups compared to baseline. When stratified by the initial intensity of dyspnoea, it appears that people with mild to moderate dyspnoea may have had a greater response to the addition of opioids. Parameters for adverse effects were not systematically collected in this study.

Another efficacy study was a single-dose double-blind cross-over placebo controlled single-institution study in people with advanced cancer (primary cancer – 7 patients, metastatic disease – 2 patients) with significant comorbidities.[19] Seven opioid-naive patients (5mg subcutaneous morphine) and two people on established opioid analgesia (100 per cent increase on normal fourth hourly dose) with dyspnoea at rest were included in the study. Comorbid causes of dyspnoea were not outlined. Interventions were tested 24 hours apart and the primary outcome was a change in VAS. Outcomes showed a drop from 58mm (SD –16) to 33 (SD –15) at 45 minutes after administration. There were no clinically or statistically significant changes in physiological parameters and benefits were sustained for up to 180 minutes. Of note, three patients reported nausea on the active (blinded) arm and one reported somnolence at 60 minutes.

Controlled clinical trials – morphine, cardiac failure

In a double-blind, cross-over placebo controlled repeated dose RCT, Johnson and her team studied 10 male community patients with New York Heart Association grade 3 or 4 cardiac failure with an ejection fraction of less than 35 per cent.[20] In this study, 5mg of immediate release oral morphine solution was administered 4 times each day unless there was significant renal impairment (creatinine > 200micromol/l) when the dose was reduced to 2.5mg 4 times daily. Patients spent four days on either the active arm or the placebo arm before two days washout and the alternate arm. Blinded, 6 out 10 patients chose morphine as the intervention that best helped with their breathlessness. Median Visual Analogue Scale (VAS) fell by 23mm from 36 (15–51) to 13 (4–40) on morphine (p = 0.02) while breathlessness was unchanged at day four on the placebo arm. Sedation peaked on day three in the arm with people receiving morphine. There were no clinically or statistically significant changes in physiological parameters during the study and four patients continued on morphine at the same dose one year after completion of the study. One of the six patients who identified a benefit from morphine did not continue it because of continuing drowsiness.

Controlled clinical trials – morphine, varying aetiologies for breathlessness

There has been one adequately powered single site double-blind placebo-controlled cross-over study published in people with COPD, cancer and cardiac failure.[21] This study was in 48 opioid-naive patients with normal cognition, mean dyspnoea VAS scores 48mm, normal or mildly impaired renal function and stable respiratory disease. Thirty-eight patients completed both arms of the study. Eighty percent of patients had COPD as their primary life-limiting illness with three having cancer, two with restrictive lung disease and one with motor neuron disease. The study had four days on either 20mg of sustained release morphine each morning or placebo before changing to the other arm. The primary outcome was change in VAS from active to placebo interventions on day four morning and evening by which time steady state had been achieved for the active intervention.

In the evening, when the once-daily opioid was close to its maximum concentration, dyspnoea was 10mm (SD –19) better than placebo. In the morning, at the time of trough opioid levels, VAS scores were still 7mm

(SD −15) better than placebo. These findings are of the same order of magnitude as the only systematic review on this topic.[20]

Other than constipation, there was no excess of symptoms in the treatment group. Withdrawals from the study that were attributable to morphine included three people with nausea and one with sedation. Sedation as a side-effect peaked on the second day. Respiratory depression was not seen and the majority of patients continued on some form of opioid in the longer term.

A study to note is by Poole and her colleagues in which controlled release morphine (titrated over the first two weeks to a mean daily dose of 25mg) or placebo were administered for 6 weeks before a two-week washout and cross-over to the alternate arm. Sixteen participants (seven women) with COPD and relatively normal blood gases (PaO$_2$ of >65mmHg, PaCO$_2$ <40mmHg) were enrolled. The breathlessness of this cohort is difficult to judge. Two patients withdrew because of nausea and vomiting while on morphine. Most patients on morphine identified adverse events more frequently in the active arm. 'Mastery', fatigue and emotional subscales decreased on the active arm, and while the dyspnoea scale trended towards improvement with morphine this was not statistically significant. As power assumptions for power calculations were not given, this may be a Type II error.[21]

Controlled clinical trials – nebulized morphine, cancer

Although there are a relatively large number of reports in the literature[16] about the use of nebulized opioids, most focus on the ability to work before stopping due to breathlessness. This functional improvement may not be the best primary end-point to measure in people with dyspnoea due to advancing life-limiting illnesses such as cancer or end-stage organ failure.

One exception to this is the study by Davis and her group where 79 patients with lung pathology were enrolled in a double-blind, single dose, randomized placebo-controlled study exploring the effect on breathlessness at one hour after nebulized morphine.[22] The patients needed to have demonstrated lung pathology from cancer on chest x-ray and relatively normal renal function. On consecutive days, patients were administered nebulized saline or nebulized morphine (dose 5–50mg).

On an intention-to-treat basis, there were 66 paired sets of data for analysis. VAS scores were not significantly different, however, it is not clear whether the statistical comparison was for individual paired patient data or aggregate data for each arm. In this study there was no significant difference between nebulized normal saline and morphine sulphate. Of note, there was a trend towards benefit from morphine but also a trend towards a small (unquantified) drop in peak expiratory flow rate (PEFR) in the intervention arm. There was also a suggestion of a dose–response relationship. There was a cohort who derived significant benefit from the intervention arm but no clinical characteristics are given that help to identify this subgroup.

A challenge in this area of clinical exploration is that the droplet size delivered to the airways has a significant effect on the behaviour of the drug.[23] Recent work demonstrates that opioids can be predictably delivered systemically when a small enough droplet size is generated. This is in contrast to much of the research in palliative care that has sought to limit any systemic absorption of nebulized opioids and confine benefit (and side-effects) to the respiratory system.

Opioids in combination with other medications, people with COPD

Light and his group have explored very high dose morphine in a single dose single blinded study of a highly selected subgroup of patients with COPD.[24] In an attempt to minimize the significant drowsiness and confusion from an earlier study (that explored single dose 0.8mg/kg of immediate release morphine solution in opioid naïve patients with COPD), the group then explored combinations of morphine with prochlorperazine or promethazine.[25] Thirty mg of immediate release oral morphine solution was compared with placebo, morphine/promethazine or morphine/prochlorperazine in a randomized double-blind design. Maximum oxygen consumption, workload and maximum minute ventilation were better in all seven patients receiving morphine with prochlorperazine without apparent mental clouding. The Borg scale for breathlessness did not improve significantly in the active arms of the study again highlighting that the relationship between the sensation of dyspnoea and exertion is not highly correlated. This study was of a highly selected subgroup of patients in closely monitored laboratory conditions and, as such, its application to everyday clinical practice is not clear.

Likewise, the role of chlorpromazine is not fully defined clinically in this setting. Observations that there may be some benefit in reducing dyspnoea without affecting respiration have not been subsequently pursued.[26]

Other opioids

Dihydrocodeine – cardiac failure

Chua and his colleagues studied 12 men with severe impairment of their left ventricular ejection fraction in a double-blind RCT of a single dose of dihydrocodeine.[27] Importantly, a sub-study looked at chemosensitivity to hypoxaemia and hypercapnia one hour after administration during each arm. Both sensitivities fell in the active arm. Exercise duration and peak oxygen consumption increased significantly in the active arm. Most importantly, breathlessness as measured on a Borg scale at six minutes into a treadmill exercise test had fallen by 0.8cm (p = 0.003), the same magnitude as the systematic review concluded from pooled data.[16] An earlier properly blinded single dose study came to similar conclusions in 12 people with COPD. Of note, the addition of oxygen to dihydrocodeine helped to reduce breathlessness – 18 per cent reduction in breathlessness with dihydrocodeine, 22 per cent reduction with oxygen alone and 32 per cent reduction in both interventions given simultaneously.[17] A subsequent study by the same group used frequent 'as needed' dihydrocodeine or placebo in a double-blind algorithm. Exercise distance improved and breathlessness was reduced in this study.[28]

Diamorphine

A double-blind placebo-controlled RCT of diamorphine in 18 people (11 men, 7 women) explored two weeks of either 2.5 or 5mg of diamorphine 6-hourly orally. Daily diary cards reviewed a VAS score for dyspnoea, drowsiness, feeling of well-being, and how breathlessness disturbed sleep. The study failed to demonstrate any differences in dyspnoea, sleepiness nor well-being in the second week of the active arm. The study was not powered for the clinical benefit expected in the population.[29]

Morphine-6-glucuronide

An active metabolite of morphine is morphine-6-glucuronide. This has been studied prospectively in a single dose nebulized study at three dose strengths – 5, 10 and 20mg. There appears in the initial study to be an effect across 15, 30 and 60 minutes using both Borg and VAS.[30]

Fentanyl citrate

One unblinded single dose study of nebulized 25 micrograms of fentanyl in 2 mls of normal saline was carried out in 35 people with dyspnoea (20 women, 15 men) all but one of whom were on oxygen. Overall, people perceived an improvement in breathing in 26 of the 32 people reported, without adverse effect. This suggests that further studies are warranted.[31]

Other medications
Benzodiazepines

The use of benzodiazepines is poorly studied in palliative care despite their very widespread use for a number of 'indications'. In breathlessness (but not necessarily anxiety), a double-blind, placebo-controlled randomized trial on 24 people with COPD was carried out using 0.5 mg of alprazolam twice daily for one week and placebo for two weeks (including one week of washout).[32] Although exercise parameters were evaluated, the subjective sensation of dyspnoea at rest and with exercise was not significantly different on the final day of the active arm. This study was powered to detect only a major reduction in dyspnoea scores and, of concern, the trend for PaO_2 was downwards, and $PaCO_2$ upwards on the active arm.

A case study (that would have made a perfect n = 1 trial) suggests that in the presence of both breathlessness and anxiety, there may be a role for alprazolam without significant toxicity.[33] A single-blinded study in four patients with dyspnoea and COPD suggests that further investigation of diazepam may be warranted.[34]

Inhaled local anaesthetics

Given the complexity of the generation of the sensation of breathlessness, it is not surprising that there has been an attempt to use local anaethetics by nebulizer. The study by Stark highlights that it is imperative that the size of aerosol particle, or at least where it reaches in the respiratory tract is known.[35] (Perhaps much of the variation in reports on response to medications used palliatively by nebulizer relates to different aerosol particle size generated.) In a placebo-controlled trial, lignocaine was evaluated in six people four of whom had COPD and two diffuse alveolar pathology. The study was not powered to detect clinically relevant differences and although there was some broncho-constriction, some patients reported benefit. The only other studies are of well subjects to evalaute dyspnoea in response to exercise using much larger aerosol particles.[36,37]

Indomethacin

The use of indomethacin for dyspnoea illustrates the gulf between studies in patients with normal respiratory function and those with marked respiratory compromise. O'Neill and his group had demonstrated that in normal subjects, the perception of dyspnoea was blunted at submaximal exercise tolerance.[38] The purported mechanism was due to a reduction in prostaglandin production in the lungs given their local actions.

In both a single dose and repeated dose study, there was no evidence to support their use either on physiological (improved exercise tolerance) nor symptomatic grounds (measured by Borg scale) in populations of males with moderate to severe COPD.[39,40]

Azopirones – buspirone

As with most medications in the therapy of dyspnoea, there are limited data to inform the use of buspirone in clinical practice. Buspirone is a non-sedating anxiolytic with a gradual onset of action after it is commenced.

There are two double-blind, RCTs that explore the effect of buspirone in people with COPD. The first of these explored in a placebo-controlled study the use of 10–20mg of buspirone three times daily on dyspnoea measured on Borg scale and physiological parameters of exercise. The cohort of 11 males had moderate to severe COPD and anxiety. Neither dyspnoea scores nor anxiety scores (measured on the State Trait Anxiety Inventory) dropped by the end of the six-week study. There was no improvement in exercise workload including 12-minute walking distance.[41]

A study that was reported the same year explored the use of 20mg of buspirone per day in 16 people for 2 weeks. All had moderate to severe COPD with FEV1 of 1.15 +/– 0.42 and FEV1/FVC of 50.7 +/– 15.0 per cent. At the end of the study, although anxiety scores were reduced in the intervention group, there was no improvement in dyspnoea as measured by Borg scale or an incremental walk test on the treadmill.[42]

These findings may underline the observation by Dudgeon that anxiety accounts for a relatively small component of the total burden of breathlessness at the end of life.[2]

Methylxantines – theophylline

Theophylline is noted for its very narrow therapeutic index so that even with close monitoring and apparent therapeutic levels, people can experience significant toxicity. There are theoretical benefits for dyspnoea beyond any effect on airway constriction. These include the ability to improve the strength and efficiency of the muscles of respiration, especially the diaphragm, and to stimulate the respiratory centre.[43] There are studies that focus on symptomatic benefit in people with irreversible disease while other studies include people with significant reversibility in airway response to bronchodilators.[44]

A clinical trial of 12 patients with moderate to severe COPD without a reversible component crossed between placebo and active arms for four weeks each with a two-week washout in between. With therapeutic blood levels maintained on the active arm, overall dyspnoea was reduced by theophylline. Functional impairment was also reduced together with the threshold at which dyspnoea was perceived. The symptomatic improvement did not carry over to objective changes in lung function, gas exchange nor ability to exercise. The study suggests modest symptomatic benefit for dyspnoea in COPD where the mechanism is unrelated to bronchodilatation.[45] An Italian study of 236 patients taking oxtropium, theophylline or both in a double-blind, double-dummy RCT in people with moderate to severe COPD reported benefits for dyspnoea in all groups although this was most marked with the two groups who were taking oxitropium.[46] At two months, the combination of an anticholinergic agent and a methylxanthine gave both the most symptomatic and physiological benefit but also the most side-effects.

By contrast, the symptomatic benefits to patients who are on theophylline may not be sustained over time. Mahon and his research group compared continuation rates of theophylline for 31 people with stable non-reversible airways disease in terms of function but not the sensation of dyspnoea.[47] All patients had been on theophylline for 1–5 years yet almost half who participated in the 'n = 1' double-blind placebo RCTs to look at efficacy of theophylline discontinued treatment by 6 months.

Most importantly, this work builds on a rigorous blueprint of 'n = 1' studies for evaluating the clinical efficacy for many palliative interventions[48] where:

1 the evidence for the intervention is not established by rigorous, adequately powered trials
2 there may be some evidence of beneficial effect for subgroups of patients whose characteristics are ill-defined
3 the disease is stable enough to evaluate the intervention
4 the benefits may be marginal in the face of potentially significant toxicity.

In the studies done, there appears to be a dose–response relationship for theophylline and symptom control. This however means that serum theophylline levels are at the upper limit of normal with doses up to 10mg/kg/day to achieve significant reductions in dyspnoea over extended study periods.[49,44,50]

Other clinical causes of dyspnoea

The studies covered are predominantly in people with COPD or cancer. There are the cited studies of people with cardiac failure and a small number of participants who have restrictive lung disease or motor neurone disease. For people with cystic fibrosis, primary pulmonary hypertension, a range of restrictive lung diseases including systemic sclerosis, AIDS, valvular heart lesions and people with primary pleural malignancies there are no level I or II studies in this area.[51,52] There is an assumption that all breathlessness can be treated with a uniform approach. The literature to date really does not address this assumption well, but if we use pain as an analogy, it is an assumption unlikely to be sustained as studies focus on dyspnoea in people with varying underlying pathophysiology.

Gaps in the literature

The literature for such a devastating and frequently encountered symptom is sparse. Guidance for clinical practice is limited but improving. An assumption that adverse effects are mild or uncommon is not sufficient given the frailty of the population involved.

The fact that studies with relatively small numbers of patients can be adequately powered to answer key clinical questions suggests strongly:

- that the magnitude of benefit from appropriate interventions is quite large in the right patient population
- that we can develop much more responsive and sophisticated approaches to the symptomatic treatment of dyspnoea if we do well-designed studies to define subpopulations who will most benefit from intervention. These studies will also need to define populations in whom the burden of treatment may outweigh any symptomatic benefit.

For many years there has been recognition of the need for adequate efficacy and effectiveness studies that will only be achieved through research collaboration between highly motivated and well resourced units in true multi-centre studies.[53,54] Effectiveness studies that are longitudinal, of a wide cross-section of patients in the cohort being studied, that can document adverse events and withdrawal from treatment are now needed to complement studies in highly selected subpopulations.

Most of the studies reported in this chapter are under-powered, often single dose studies (and it was known 15 years ago that this leads to very inaccurate results in pain studies) with heterogeneous underlying causes for breathlessness. Although studies in healthy subjects can refine knowledge, their responses to interventions cannot be directly extrapolated to people with severe dyspnoea due to lung pathology.

Building this work to reflect both the underlying pathology and the descriptors with which the patient describes their breathing will add a level of sophistication that may well translate to better clinical outcomes for the patient and their caregivers. Making this match will improve the predictability of the response to a new treatment.

Comparisons between opioids for breathlessness will be an important area of study in the years ahead. As a better understanding of opioid receptor subtypes becomes available, such comparisons will be critical.

Medications in combination have hardly been explored. Many symptomatically burdensome respiratory diseases have not been studied and may respond differently to symptomatic interventions when compared with COPD, cancer or cardiac failure.

There are examples not only of improving knowledge but also of improving the care for this patient with 'n = 1' studies with an adequate therapeutic trial (dose and time) of a given intervention. Incorporating this into practice can further knowledge and remove much of the guesswork currently involved in the clinical care of someone with refractory breathlessness.[55,48]

Conclusions

Oral and parenteral opioids can be recommended to reduce breathlessness in the setting of a life-limiting illness where reversible causes for breathlessness have been adequately addressed. This includes both people who are opioid-naive and those on opioids for other indications. Their long-term use and the potential for tolerance have not been well defined. Their use in combination with other interventions is in its infancy. The use of nebulized opioids cannot be recommended at this time.

With the exception of theophylline, other interventions although widely used and widely recommended have few data to support them. Theophylline cannot be recommended for routine use in this setting as the studies that showed benefit were all using doses at the upper limit tolerated with significant side effects.

Rigorous high quality clinical research needs to continue to grow in this area.

Key points

1 Opioids have good Level 1 evidence to support efficacy in reducing refractory dyspnoea by approximately 20 per cent over baseline levels.
2 Underlying aetiologies that have been shown to benefit from opioid therapy include cardiac failure, chronic obstructive pulmonary disease and cancer.
3 Monitoring in the first few days of treatment with opioids for dyspnoea appears crucial to minimize side-effects and establish benefit.
4 There is no established link between underlying aetiology, intensity or descriptors of breathlessness and response to pharmacological interventions.
5 There are no consistent data to support any improvement in exercise tolerance with pharmacological interventions for refractory dyspnoea.

References

1. **Muers MF.** Opioids for dyspnoea. *Thorax* 2002; 57(11): 922–3.
2. **Dudgeon DJ, Lertzman M.** Dyspnea in the advanced cancer patient. *Journal of Pain and Symptom Management* 1998;16: 212–19.
3. **Reuben DB, Mor V.** Dyspnea in terminally ill cancer patients. *Chest* 1986; 89: 234–6.

4. Simon PM, Schwartzstein RM, Weiss JW, Lahive K, Fencl V, Teghtsoonian M, Weinberger SE. Distinguishable sensations of breathlessness induced in normal volunteers. *American Review of Respiratory Disease* 1989; **140**: 1021–7.

5. Simon PM, Schwartzstein RM, Weiss JW, Fencl V, Teghtsoonian M, Weinberger SE. Distinguishable types of dyspnea in patients with shortness of breath. *American Review of Respiratory Disease* 1990; **142**: 1009–14.

6. Burns BH, Howell JBL. Disproportionately severe breathlessness in chronic bronchitis. *Q J Med* 1969; **38**: 277–94.

7. Allard P, Lamontagne C, Bernard P, Tremblay C. How effective are supplementary doses of opioids for dyspnea in terminally ill cancer patients? A randomized continuous sequential clinical trial. *Journal of Pain and Symptom Management* 1999; **17**: 256–65.

8. Weil JV, McCullough RE, Kline JS, Sodal IE. Diminished ventilatory response to hypoxia and hypercapnia after morphine in normal man. *N Engl J Med* 1975; **292**: 1103–6.

9. Banzett RB, Mulnier HE, Murphy K, Rosen SD, Wise RJ, Adams L. Breathlessness in humans activates insular cortex. *Neuroreport* 2000; **11**: 2117–20.

10. Peiffer C, Poline JB, Thivard L, Aubier M, Samson Y. Neural substrates for the perception of acutely induced dyspnoea. *Am J Resp Crit Care Med* 2001; **163**: 951–7.

11. Zebraski SE, Kochenash SM, Raffa RB. Lung opioid receptors: pharmacology and possible target for nebulized morphine in dyspnea. *Life Sci* 2000; **66**: 2221–31.

12. Pauwels RA, Buist AS, Calverley PMA, Jenkins CR, Hurd SS. Global strategy for the diagnosis, management, and prevention of chronic obstructive pulmonary disease: National Heart, Lung, and Blood Institute and World Health Organization Global Initiative for Chronic Obstructive Lung Disease (GOLD): executive summary. *Respiratory Care* 2001; **46**: 798–825.

13. Anon. Dyspnea. Mechanisms, assessment, and management: a consensus statement. American Thoracic Society Position Statement. *Am J Respir Crit Care Med* 1999; **159**: 321–40.

14. Currow DC, Abernethy AP, Frith P. Morphine for management of refractory dyspnoea. *BMJ* 2003; **327**: 1288–9.

15. Mashford ML, Aranda S, Ashby M, Bowman J, Brooksbank M, Cairns W, *et al.* *Therapeutic Guidelines Palliative Care*, Version 1. North Melbourne, Victoria, Australia: Therapeutic Guidelines Limited, 2001.

16. Jennings AL, Davies AN, Higgins JP, Gibbs JS, Broadley KE. A systematic review of the use of opioids in the management of dyspnoea. *Thorax* 2002; **57**(11): 939–44.

17. Woodcock AA, Gross ER, Gellert A, Shahh S, Johnson M, Geddes DM. Effects of dihydrocodeine, alcohol, and caffeine on breathlessness and exercise tolerance in patients with chronic obstructive lung disease and normal blood gases. *N Engl J Med* 1981; **305**: 1611–16.

18. Bruera E, MacEachern T, Ripamonti C, Hanson J. Subcutaneous morphine for dyspnea in cancer patients. *Annals of Internal Medicine* 1993; **119**: 906–7.

19. Mazzocato C, Buclin T, Rapin CH. The effects of morphine on dyspnea and ventilatory function in elderly patients with advanced cancer: A randomized double-blind controlled trial. *Annals of Oncology* 1999; **10**: 1511–14.

20. Johnson MJ, McDonagh TA, Harkness A, McKay SE, Dargie HJ. Morphine for the relief of breathlessness in patients with chronic heart failure – a pilot study. *European Journal of Heart Failure* 2002; **4**: 753–6.

21. **Abernethy A, Currow D, Frith P, Fazekas B, McHugh A, Bui C.** Randomised double-blind placebo-controlled crossover trial of sustained-release morphine for the management of refractory dyspnoea. *BMJ* 2003; **327**: 523–8.

21. **Poole PJ, Veale AG, Black PN.** The effect of sustained-release morphine on breathlessness and quality of life in severe chronic obstructive pulmonary disease. *Am J Respir Crit Care Med* 1998; **157**: 1877–80.

22. **Davis C, Penn K, A'Hearn R, Daniels J, Slevin M.** Single dose randomised controlled trial of nebulised morphine in patients with cancer related breathlessness. *Pall Med* 1996; **10**: 64–5.

23. **Mather LE, Woodhouse A, Ward ME, Farr SJ, Rubsamen RA, Eltherington LG.** Pulmonary administration of aerosolised fentanyl: pharmacokinetic analysis of systemic delivery. *British Journal of Clinical Pharmacology* 1998; **46**(1): 37–43.

24. **Light RW, Muro JR, Sato RI, Stansbury DW, Fischer CE, Brown SE.** Effects of oral morphine on breathlessness and exercise tolerance in patients with chronic obstructive pulmonary disease. *American Review of Respiratory Disease* 1989; **139**: 126–33.

25. **Light RW, Stansbury DW, Webster JS.** Effect of 30 mg of morphine alone or with promethazine or prochlorperazine on the exercise capacity of patients with COPD. *Chest* 1996; **109**: 975–81.

26. **O'Neill PA, Morton PB, Strak RD.** Chlorpromazine – a specific effect on breathlessness? *Br J Clin Pharm* 1985; **19**: 793–7.

27. **Chua TP, Harrington D, Ponikowski P, Webb-Poploe K, Poole-Wilson PA, Coates AJS.** Effects of dihydrocodeine on chemosensitivity and exercise tolerance in patients with chronic heart failure. *JACC* 1997; **29**: 147–52.

28. **Johnson MA, Woodcock AA, Geddes DM.** Dihydrocodeine for breathlessness in "pink puffers". *Br Med J Clin Res* 1983; **286**: 675–7.

29. **Eiser N, Denman WT, West C, Luce P.** Oral diamorphine: lack of effect on dyspnoea and exercise tolerance in the "pink puffer" syndrome. *Eur Respir J* 1991; **4**: 926–31.

30. **Quigley C, Joel S, Patel N, Baksh A, Slevin M.** A phase I/II study of nebulized morphine-6-glucuronide in patients with cancer-related breathlessness. *Journal of Pain Symptom Management* 2002; **23**: 7–9.

31. **Coyne PJ, Viswanathan R, Smith TJ.** Nebulized fentanyl citrate improves patients' perception of breathing, respiratory rate, and oxygen saturation in dyspnea. *Journal of Pain and Symptom Management* 2002; **23**: 157–60.

32. **Man Cg, Hsu, K, Sproule BJ.** Effect of alprazolam on exercise and dyspnoea in patients with chronic obstructive pulmonary disease. *Chest* 1986; **90**: 832–6.

33. **Greene JG, Pucino F, Carlson JD, Storsved M, Strommen GL.** Effects of Alprazolam on respiratory drive, anxiety, and dyspnoea in chronic airflow obstruction: A case study. *Pharmacotherapy* 1989; 34–8.

34. **Mitchell-Heggs P, Murphy K, Minty Km Guz A, Patterson SC, Minty PS, Rosser RM.** Diazepam in the treatment of the 'Pink Puffer' Syndrome. *Q J Med* 1980; **49**: 9–20.

35. **Stark RD, O'Neill PA, Russell NJ, Heapy CG, Stretton TB.** Effects of small particle aerosols of local anaesthetic on dyspnoea in patients with respiratory disease. *Clin Sci* 1985; **69**: 29–36.

36. **Winning AJ, Hamilton RD, Shea SA, Knott C, Guz A.** The effect of airway anaesthesia on the control of breathing and the sensation of breathlessness in man. *Clin Sci* 1985; **68**: 215–25.

37. **Hamilton RD, Winning AJ, Perry A, Guz A.** Aerosol anesthsia increases hypercapnia ventilation and breathlessness in laryngectomized humans. *J Appl Physiol* 1987; **63**: 2286–92.

38. O'Neill PA, Stark RD, Morton PB. Do prostaglandins have a role in breathlessness. *American Review of Respiratory Disease* 1985; **132**: 22–4.
39. Schiffman GL, Stansbury DW, Fischer CE, Sato RI, Light RW, Brown SE. Indomethacin and perception of dyspnoea in chronic airflow obstruction. *American Review of Respiratory Disease* 1988; **137**: 1094–8.
40. O'Neill PA, Stretton TB, Stark RD, Ellis SH. The effect of indomethacin on breathlessness in patients with diffuse parenchymal disease of the lung. *Br J Dis Chest* 1986; **80**(1): 72–9.
41. Singh NP, Despars JA, Stansbury DW, Avalos K, Light RW. Effects of buspirone on anxiety levels and exercise tolerance in patients with chronic airflow obstruction and mild anxiety. *Chest* 1993; **103**: 800–4.
42. Argyropoulou P, Patakas D, Koukou A, *et al.* Buspirone effect on breathlessness and exercise performance in patients with chronic obstructive pulmonary disease. *Respiration* 1993; **60**: 216–20.
43. Murciano D, Auclair MH, Lecocguic Y, Pariente R. Effects of theophylline on diaphragmatic strength and fatigue in patients with chronic obstructive pulmonary disease. *N Engl J Med* 1984; **311**: 349–53.
44. Tsukino M, Nishimura K, Ikeda A, Hajiro T, Koyama H, Izumi T. Effects of theophylline and ipratropium bromide on exercise performance in patient with stable chronic obstructive pulmonary disease. *Thorax* 1998; **53**: 269–73.
45. Mahler DA, Matthay RA, Snyder PE, Wells CK, Loke J. Sustained release theophylline reduces dyspnoea in nonreversible obstructive airway disease. *American Review of Respiratory Disease* 1985; **131**: 22–5.
46. Bellia V, Foresi A, Bianco S, *et al.* Efficacy and safety of oxitropium bromide, thoephylline and their combination in COPD patients: a double-blind, randomized, multicentre study (BREATH trial). *Resp Med* 2002; **96**: 881–9.
47. Mahon J, Laupacis A, Donner A, Wood T. Randomised study of n of 1 trials versus standard practice. *BMJ* 1996; **312**: 1069–74.
48. Guyatt G, Sackett D, Taylor DW, Chong J, Roberts R, Pugsley S. Determining the optimal therapy – randomized trials in individual patients. *N Engl J Med* 1986; **314**: 889–92.
49. McKay SE, Howie CA, Thomson AH, Whiting B, Addis GJ. Value of theophylline treatment in patients handicapped by chronic obstructive lung disease. *Thorax* 1993; **48**: 227–32.
50. Murciano D, Auclair MH, Pariente R, Aubier M. A randomized, controlled trial of theophylline in patients with severe chronic obstructive pulmonary disease. *N Engl J Med* 1989; **320**: 1521–5.
51. Janahi IA, Maciejewski SR, Teran JM, Oermann CM. Inhaled morphine to relieve dyspnoea in advanced cystic fibrosis lung disease. *Pediatr Pulmon* 2000; **30**: 257–9.
52. Cohen SP, Dawson TC. Nebulized morphine as a treatment for dyspnea in a child with cystic fibrosis. *Pediatr* 2002; **110**: e38.
53. Davis CL. The therapeutics of dyspnoea. *Canc Surveys* 1994; **21**: 85–98.
54. Nicotra MB, Carter R. The use of opiates in chronic obstructive pulmonary disease. *Clin Pul Med* 1995; **2**: 143–51.
55. Robin ED, Burke CM. Single-patient randomized clinical trial. Opiates for intractable dyspnoea. *Chest* 1986; **90**: 888–92.

14

A palliative approach to the breathless patient

Sara Booth and Deborah Dudgeon

This book is concerned with the palliation of breathlessness associated with advanced disease – to finding the best way possible to help patients (and families) live as fully as possible with this distressing symptom and, when it is inevitable, to die as comfortably and peacefully as possible.

This chapter aims to give some pointers on managing the symptoms. Palliative care physicians (and other professionals) may see patients with intractable breathlessness who are many months or years from death or within hours of death, and in either case the first priority is to make an accurate assessment of the problem on which you are being asked to advise, so that the most appropriate and helpful treatment can be started. When a person with breathlessness presents it may be helpful to think of this series of questions.

What is causing the patient to be breathless? Is it his/her underlying disease or another process?

Prior to initiating treatment it is essential that a careful diagnosis is made. It has been emphasized throughout this book that breathlessness, particularly in patients with cancer, is multifactorial and that often there is no one, easily-reversible cause which can be treated to improve the symptom. As outlined in Chapter 2, a thorough assessment requires attention to not only the factors related to the underlying disease and other comorbid physical problems but also to the psychological, social and spiritual dimensions of the condition. Patients with intractable breathlessness will receive most benefit from the full range of therapeutic options available from a multiprofessional, multidisciplinary service who are considering not only the medical but also psychological, social and spiritual aspects of care. It is from this approach that the patient (and family) will gain most advantage and where specialist palliative care is distinctive from other specialities.

On occasion, patients referred to palliative care physicians may not have had a comprehensive work-up to exclude all reversible conditions as a sense of therapeutic nihilism may have guided the patient's management. This is more common in elderly patients who may themselves ascribe their symptoms to 'normal ageing' when further investigation with simple tests such as an electrocardiogram or chest X-ray may identify a condition that can be easily treated and this, in concert with other palliative interventions, will improve their symptoms. The choice of investigations should be appropriate to the stage of disease, prognosis, potential benefit and side effects of any treatment that would result from the knowledge gained from the investigation and the wishes of the patient and family.

What do the patient and family understand regarding the diagnosis and prognosis?

During the first assessment of the patient it is important to learn what the patient and family understand with regard to the person's diagnosis and prognosis. This will enable you to address any gaps in their knowledge or understanding, answer any questions they may have and set the stage for further communication.

If the patient needs further help from a another specialist (e.g. respiratory physician) to ensure that the medical treatment for their underlying condition is the best it can be, this does not preclude him or her receiving specialist palliative care as well. The key clinician from the specialist palliative care team may initially be the specialist nurse or physiotherapist working with the respiratory physician. Later the specialist palliative care team may take over care from the respiratory team. Another patient may need initial specialist treatment from a cardiology team but once stable, the best combination may be receiving most care from the primary care team and palliative care service with review at home from the cardiology specialist nurse.

It is worth explaining at the initial assessment, that the treatment plans set out initially will need regular review and altering as the patient's condition changes.

What are the priorities for the patient and family?

An essential part of the initial assessment is to discern what the patient and family expect, hope for or want the treatment to achieve as this may uncover unrealistic expectations of what is possible. Airing and discussing these expectations early on may help prevent later misunderstandings and frustration with the team, on the part of the patient and family, and enable the team to work with them towards achievable goals.

What is the plan of care?

After determining the aetiology of the person's breathlessness, possible treatment options, and priorities of the patient and family it is possible to establish a plan of care with them. When discussing it with them it is important to help them understand the possible benefits and side-effects of the proposed intervention(s). It is also helpful to discuss the goals of the treatment and establish a time limit to a trial of therapy after which the merits of continuing, changing or stopping will be assessed. This type of discussion helps to ensure that they understand what the potential benefits and limits of treatment are and allows you to more easily discontinue therapies when they are no longer providing meaningful benefit to the patient.

Improvement in the patient who is relatively fit may take some time as the treatment will usually be based around non-pharmacological care which needs some commitment and work from the patient and family and may involve a training effect or acquisition of some new coping skills by the patient and family.

In the dying patient or one with extreme breathlessness towards the end of life, treatment may be rapidly effective but may also make the patient sleepy – all this needs to be discussed with the individual (or family if the patient is very ill).

How often should treatment plans and priorities be reviewed?

Priorities for the patient will vary with their condition and the disease. Patients may live with a relatively stable level of breathlessness for months or years and the palliative care team may only be intermittently involved over that time – for example at the beginning of serious breathlessness when the patient needs more than usual advice or help with their symptom; perhaps again during an exacerbation when they are admitted to hospital and the family is distraught and needs help from specialist palliative care to come together and work together at a difficult time. These interventions may be months apart and triggered by the patient, family or other specialist team.

Patients with cancer or fibrosing alveolitis or end-stage cardiac failure may need review weekly and open access to the service. Some may be regular attendees at a day hospice or seen by a community team with inpatient stays in the hospice when necessary. As death approaches the symptom may escalate and treatment and the frequency of reassessment will need to reflect that escalation. Treatments may switch for a patient such as this from predominantly non-pharmacological to pharmacological management.

Who does the reassessing and reviewing?

It may not be the specialist palliative care team who takes the lead in reassessing patients with a chronic condition. The primary care physician, a community nurse, or the specialist who sees them in clinical regularly may be the best person. Patients with chronic conditions and comorbidities can find themselves overwhelmed with different clinic appointments and spend much of their time visiting clinicians. It is important, however, that patients know that they can self-refer back to a palliative care team if another team is carrying out the regular follow-up care.

With the increasing involvement of palliative care teams in the management of patients with non-malignant disease who have many years of ill-health, the development of new models of palliative care delivery may be necessary. This could include the introduction of drop-in palliative care rehabilitation centres or refresher courses for anxiety reduction techniques. The ups and downs of chronic non-malignant disease are different from the model of cancer care on which palliative care was founded and some types cancer now behave more like chronic disease with plateaus and exacerbations. This can make it difficult to identify when patients are at the end of their lives and when to change the emphasis of the therapies.

How to decide when a change of emphasis is needed?

It is important to know when to change tack and when to start having end of life discussions and start end of life planning. Patients and families expect the doctor, or other clinician, to initiate these discussions when the time is right and will not necessarily voice their fears unasked. Most patients do want to set their priorities for end of life care and it is important that palliative care teams recognize this and take on the responsibility of raising the issue in patients with non-malignant disease if nobody else has. Much research has shown that patients with a stable condition often want less intervention than their medical team would initiate and have views on whether they want to die in hospice, home or hospital. Leaving discussions about DNR orders and limitations of treatment until patients are very ill often excludes patients from the discussion and leaves the families with the burden and possible guilt. In a clinic or at home, when the decisions are not immediately needed, the emotion may be less heightened and the patient better able to make clear what they want and when. This also allows primary care and palliative care teams to make some plans for the patient's deterioration in line with their wishes, which although expected, could occur at any time.

It is generally much more difficult to prognosticate for patients with non-malignant disease and patients can seem near death one day and make a good recovery from an exacerbation, or conversely seem relatively stable and then die suddenly. This honest uncertainty may paradoxically make it easier to initiate the discussion about limitations of treatment and DNR orders as it will not be concerned with an imminent event.

What needs to be in place to help breathless patients die comfortably?

Expected deterioration, in a patient known to the service

If the palliative care service have been involved with a patient over a period of weeks or months, most of the questions outlined above should have been considered so that it is known, where the patient wants to die, the level of intervention that they consider appropriate at the end, their feelings about sedation, relatives that they would want to see, and who they want care from (i.e. mainly primary care team, or hospice inpatient care, or to be admitted to a familiar respiratory ward for example).

In the community good instructions should be left in the home (for example to prevent ambulance paramedics feeling obliged to initiate CPR if they are called out by someone unfamiliar with the plan). National laws vary, but it is sensible to have necessary drugs, including opioids, already in the home so that there is no need to contact unfamiliar out-of-hours services to prescribe drugs which relatives then have to travel to obtain leading to substantial delays and suffering for the patient.

Sometimes patients at home or in hospital may have non-invasive ventilation in place, for example in neurological disease or to help a patient over a respiratory infection. It is important to highlight again that when an intervention like this is used, preparation should be made at the time of its instigation (by discussion of its limitations and the treatment that will replace it) for removing it when the time is right. Sometimes the patient will initiate removal but often, the suggestion that drug therapy will now be more helpful in controlling symptoms, needs to come from the clinician. It would be usual to have a subcutaneous infusion established, or parenteral medication in regular use before removing another treatment that has helped contain dyspnoea.

Do not forget the relatives and carers: it has been highlighted at several points in the book, that they often feel neglected and alone and very frightened by their relative's dyspnoea. They need to understand fully the options for care available for their loved one and active support at home at the a time when the patient is deteriorating may prevent a panic-driven distressing admission in the last hours, to hospital. After years of urgent admissions to hospital for life-saving treatment it may be difficult to accept that the end of life has eventually come for their relative.

Unexpected or sudden deterioration

If the palliative care team is called to someone they have not met before and the patient is in extreme respiratory distress they are likely to walk in to a highly charged situation where history and examination of the patient will be minimal and treatment has to be speedily effective.

In this case the team needs to do their homework with the referring team and the clinical notes extensively before seeing the patient to satisfy themselves of the diagnosis and what needs to be done. They need to be confident when they walk into the patient's room (often surrounded by distressed and exhausted family) that they understand the diagnosis. The terminally breathless patient cannot give a detailed history and may only be able to signal or indicate their wishes –the clinician's needs to instil confidence and certainty that they can help and quickly offer choices about care. It is important to let the patient and family know that you have made a careful assessment of what is going on by talking to the referring senior clinician and being familiar with the patient's history (possibly checking the main details back with the patient after offering them the chance for relatives to answer if this would be helpful). Do not cut the patient out of the conversation (unless they are clearly comatose) but do give them the chance of either signalling answers or delegating answering to a relative.

At the very end of life, treatment with parenteral opioids and/or phenothiazines and/or benzodiazepines is likely to be the treatment of choice – often making the patient sleepy (see Chapters 5 and 13). Other interventions, such as oxygen, may well be stopped (although individual negotiation around initiating treatment is essential).

On a ward, or in a setting such as a nursing home where staff may not be familiar with the palliative treatment regimen started it is important to arrange early review e.g. give a dose of opioid/phenothiazines and then review after writing notes and talking to the relatives. Accurate handover to other community or hospital staff and keeping in touch by phone (if handing over care to another team) is very important. The relatives need to know how the treatment will be monitored and when they can expect to see a member of the palliative care service again routinely or if the patient's symptoms are not controlled. The relatives, and the patient, need to be confident that communication will be maintained to ensure that the patient's death is as peaceful as possible.

It is often helpful to explain to relatives (and perhaps to the patient, depending on the circumstances) what death is likely to be like and to help relatives to expect changes in breathing patterns and the pauses in breathing that can take place as death approaches.

Many people in the west have not seen a dead body or sat with someone who is dying – they may need help and support to do this (someone dropping by routinely just to see how they are etc.) and guidance or help about leaving the bedside, that reading a book or paper and ensuring regular meals and some sleep is important for them. They may need help to stay or see the body after death.

Deaths from breathlessness (and the time leading up to them) can be very distressing and the palliative care service may need to keep in touch, through bereavement services or with primary care team, with the relatives to help them with their grief, through explanation or answering questions about the medical circumstances of the death.

Key points

- Make the best diagnosis possible of the cause(s) of the patient's breathlessness
- Optimize the medical treatments for the underlying and any associated conditions
- Decide priorities for treatment and start treatment plan
- Review the patient and reassess the treatment plan regularly – priorities may change
- Remember all patients (and families) need non-pharmacological assessment and treatment
- Do not forget to use opioids, oxygen and other drugs to palliate breathlessness
- Do not forget to care for the family as actively as you care for the patient
- Always ensure the patient and family know who to contact, and how to do this, in case of query or emergency.

Index

Note: Page numbers in **bold** indicate tables, and page numbers in *italics* indicate figures.